OXFORD MEDICAL PUBLICATIONS

Oxford Handbook of
Palliative Care

Oxford Handbook list

Oxford Handbook of Clinical Medicine 6/e
Oxford Handbook of Clinical Specialties 6/e
Oxford Handbook of Accident and Emergency Medicine 2/e
Oxford Handbook of Acute Medicine 2/e
Oxford Handbook of Anaesthesia
Oxford Handbook of Applied Dental Sciences
Oxford Handbook of Clinical and Laboratory Investigation
Oxford Handbook of Clinical Dentistry 3/e
Oxford Handbook of Clinical Genetics
Oxford Handbook of Clinical Haematology 2/e
Oxford Handbook of Clinical Immunology
Oxford Handbook of Clinical Surgery 2/e
Oxford Handbook of Critical Care
Oxford Handbook of Dental Patient Care
Oxford Handbook of Dialysis 2/e
Oxford Handbook of Endocrinology and Diabetes
Oxford Handbook of General Practice
Oxford Handbook of Obstetrics and Gynaecology
Oxford Handbook of Oncology
Oxford Handbook of Operative Surgery
Oxford Handbook of Palliative Care
Oxford Handbook of Patients' Welfare
Oxford Handbook of Practical Drug Therapy
Oxford Handbook of Psychiatry
Oxford Handbook of Public Health Practice
Oxford Handbook of Rehabilitation Medicine
Oxford Handbook of Rheumatology
Oxford Handbook of Tropical Medicine 2/e

Oxford Handbook of
Palliative Care

Max S. Watson

Locum Consultant in Palliative Medicine,
Northern Ireland Hospice,
Research Fellow,
Belfast City Hospital,
Belfast, UK

Caroline F. Lucas

Deputy Medical Director,
Princess Alice Hospice, Esher, Surrey;
Clinical Director,
North Surrey Primary Care NHS Trust;
Honorary Consultant in Palliative Medicine,
St Peter's Hospital, Chertsey, Surrey, UK

Andrew M. Hoy

Medical Director,
Princess Alice Hospice, Esher, Surrey;
Consultant in Palliative Medicine, Epsom and
St Helier NHS Trust, UK

Ian N. Back

Consultant in Palliative Medicine,
Holme Tower Marie Curie Centre, Penarth;
Consultant in Palliative Medicine,
Pontypridd and Rhonda NHS Trust,
Mid Glamorgan, UK

OXFORD
UNIVERSITY PRESS

OXFORD

UNIVERSITY PRESS

Great Clarendon Street, Oxford OX2 6DP

Oxford University Press is a department of the University of Oxford.
It furthers the University's objective of excellence in research, scholarship,
and education by publishing worldwide in

Oxford New York

Auckland Cape Town Dar es Salaam Hong Kong Karachi
Kuala Lumpur Madrid Melbourne Mexico City Nairobi
New Delhi Shanghai Taipei Toronto

With offices in

Argentina Austria Brazil Chile Czech Republic France Greece
Guatemala Hungary Italy Japan Poland Portugal Singapore
South Korea Switzerland Thailand Turkey Ukraine Vietnam

Oxford is a registered trade mark of Oxford University Press
in the UK and in certain other countries

Published in the United States
by Oxford University Press Inc., New York

British Library Cataloguing in Publication Data

Data available

Library of Congress Cataloging in Publication Data

Data available

Typeset by Newgen Imaging Systems (P) Ltd., Chennai, India
Printed in Italy
on acid-free paper by Legoprint S.p.A

ISBN 0-19-850897-2 (flexicover)
ISBN 0-19-856989-0 (Pbk, Part 1)
ISBN 0-19-856990-4 (Pbk, Part 2)

10 9 8 7 6 5 4 3 2 1

This book is dedicated to computer-abandoned families in Dungannon, Esher, Epsom, and Cardiff. Without their patience and understanding support, this project could never have been completed.

MW, CL, AH, IB

You matter because you are you. You matter to the last moment of your life and we will do all we can not only to help you die peacefully but to live until you die.

(Dame Cicely Saunders)

Foreword

Derek Doyle
President Emeritus of the International Association for Hospice and Palliative Care,
Vice President of the National Council for Hospice and Specialist Palliative Care Services,
Medical Director/Consultant Physician St Columba's Hospice, Edinburgh, UK (retired)

Before his Cubist phase Picasso painted a moving scene, one that he had perhaps witnessed as a boy. He entitled it *Science and Charity* (words that will remind some readers of the motto of the Royal College of General Practitioners). An old doctor, in what is clearly a poor home, is sitting by the bedside of a dying patient. His expression is one of compassion and deep thought as he leans on the bed looking at the patient he has perhaps known for many years. It is impossible not to be moved by this image of a general practitioner in 'the old days' and tempting to compare him with us who care for the dying in a very different world.

Some will look at the painting and sigh with nostalgia for far-off days when, as young GPs, they too made time to sit by a bedside. Today, even if they wanted to, there is seldom sufficient time. They might smile to see so few pieces of equipment—no syringe drivers and drips, nebulisers or suction machines, or even catheter bags. Neither are there any nurses. Many might be surprised to see someone who looks so young dying at home—something that is getting less common in today's world in spite of the expressed wishes of so many patients and the personnel and resources being poured into community care.

Others will wonder if that old doctor ever felt as they often do today when caring for the dying; lonely, sometimes a little frightened, less confident and competent than at any other time in their work, and, in our secularized society, often at a loss to help with existential questions.

Junior hospital doctors (and, one would like to think, some consultants) will perhaps look at the painting and give a wry smile. The old man may have felt inadequate, poorly trained, and lonely but, they will ask themselves, is that any different from what they feel day in day out, caring for the dying in the wards of our hospitals? Yes, they have had a few lectures on palliative care and communication skills but their sense of inadequacy in the face of a spectrum of suffering is little assuaged. They have had tutorials on ethical decision-making but in today's real world most responses seem to be knee-jerk reactions made under pressure, not decisions talked through with colleagues in the luxury of a mutually supportive team.

It is tempting to wonder what Picasso's doctor would have thought about today's palliative care and this new book. We can be sure he would have smiled with disbelief at something so much a part and parcel of every doctor's life being glorified with a name like *palliative care*. After all, he might have asked, is that not what good care is all about; comforting, explaining, and listening, being there when needed and especially when the days of further tests and new therapies have long passed; sharing one's humanity with all its frailties with someone on the loneliest journey of life. He might be shocked to learn why 'the principles of all clinical care' as he knew them, had to be dignified with such a title in the last decades of the 20th century.

Given a copy of this new *Handbook* he would have been amazed and, hopefully, a little envious. Amazed at the cornucopia of drugs and formulations available to today's doctors to ease suffering. Amazed at how much scientific research has uncovered and made possible. Amazed at how many, other than doctors, now share in this ministry of caring and in doing so bring a richness of skills and compassion. Envious that, to his surprise, it is now possible to have so much information and guidance at one's finger tips, in a book small enough for his desk or his bag. Surprised and thrilled, one hopes, that underpinning this handbook is a yet more comprehensive *Oxford Textbook of Palliative Medicine*, the resource for the specialists in palliative medicine—the specialists across the country, eager to take away some of the loneliness and sense of inadequacy our old doctor felt at that bedside.

No, there is nothing new about the principles of palliative care. They are the age-old principles of all good care but, as this *Handbook* so beautifully illustrates, now enhanced by new knowledge, new drugs, new approaches, new insights—all available to every doctor, nurse, chaplain, professional allied to medicine privileged to share themselves with someone on their final journey. What a challenge but what a privilege, as Picasso's doctor would surely have reminded us. Picasso seems to have chosen the right words for us—palliative care is, before all else, science and charity in action.

Edinburgh, September 2004

Preface

Most clinical professionals have been affected by caring for patients with palliative care needs. Such patients may challenge us at both a professional and at a personal level in areas where we feel our confidence or competence are challenged.

'I wanted to help her, but I just didn't know what to do or say'

As in every other branch of medicine, knowledge and training can help us extend our comfort zone, so that we can better respond to such patients in a caring and professional manner. However, in picking up this handbook and reading thus far you have already demonstrated a motivation that is just as important as a thirst for knowledge, the central desire to improve the care of your patients.

It was out of just such a motivation that the modern hospice movement began 40 years ago, and it is that same motivation that has fuelled the spread of the principles of palliative care—in fact the principles of ALL good care—across the globe: respect for the person, attention to detail, scrupulous honesty and integrity, holistic care, team caring, and consummate communications (often more about listening than telling and talking).

'I knew we couldn't cure him, but didn't know when or how to start palliative care'

Increasingly it is being recognized that every person has the right to receive high quality palliative care whatever the illness, whatever its stage, regardless of whether potentially curable or not. The artificial distinction between curative and palliative treatments has rightly been recognized as an unnecessary divide, with a consequent loss of the border crossings that previously signified a complete change in clinical emphasis and tempo.

Medical knowledge is developing rapidly, with ever more opportunities for and emphasis on curative treatment, to the point when any talk of palliative care can sometimes be interpreted as 'defeatist'.

Today the principles of palliative care interventions may be employed from the first when a patient's illness is diagnosed. Conversely, a patient with predominantly palliative care needs, late in their disease journey, may benefit from energetic treatments more usually regarded as 'curative'.

'I just felt so helpless watching him die. Surely it could have been better?'

Governments and professional bodies now recognize that every nurse and doctor has a duty to provide palliative care and, increasingly, the public and the media have come to expect—as of right—high quality palliative care from their healthcare professionals irrespective of the clinical setting.

Many of these palliative care demands can best be met, as in the past, by the health care professionals who already know their patients and families well. This handbook is aimed at such hospital or community-based professionals, and recognizes that the great majority of patients with palliative needs are looked after by doctors and nurses who have not been trained in specialist palliative care but who are often specialist in the knowledge of their patients.

'Even though I knew she had had every treatment possible, still, when she died I really felt that we had failed her and let her family down.'

Junior healthcare staff throughout the world have used the Oxford Handbook series as their own specialist pocket companion through the lonely hours of on-call life. The format, concise (topic-a-page), complete and sensible, teaches not just clinical facts but a way of thinking. Yet for all the preoccupation with cure, no healthcare professional will ever experience greater satisfaction or confirmation of their choice of profession, than by bringing comfort and dignity to someone at the end-of-life.

'I had never seen anyone with that type of pain before and just wished I could get advice from someone who knew what to do.'

The demands on inexperienced and hard-pressed doctors or nurses in looking after patients with palliative care needs can be particularly stressful. It is our hope that this text, ideally complemented by the support and teaching of specialist palliative care teams, will reduce the often-expressed sense of helplessness, a sense of helplessness made all the more poignant by the disproportionate gratitude expressed by patients and families for any attempts at trying to listen, understand and care.

'It was strange, but I felt he was helping me much more than I was helping him'

While it is our hope that the handbook will help the reader to access important information quickly and succinctly, we hope it will not replace the main source of palliative care knowledge: the bedside contact with the patient.

It is easier to learn from books than patients, yet what our patients teach us is often of more abiding significance: empathy, listening, caring, existential questions of our own belief systems and the limitations of medicine. It is at the bedside that we learn to be of practical help to people who are struggling to come to terms with their own mortality and face our own mortality in the process.

Readers may notice some repetition of topics in the handbook. This is not due to weariness or oversight on the part of the editors, but is an attempt to keep relevant material grouped together—to make it easier for those needing to look up information quickly.

It is inevitable that in a text of this size some will be disappointed at the way we have left out, or skimped, on a favourite area of palliative care interest. To these readers we offer our apologies and two routes of redress: almost 200 blank pages to correct the imbalances, and the OUP website, http://www.oup.co.uk/isbn/0-19-850897-2, where your suggestions for how the next edition could be improved would be gratefully received.

Acknowledgements

This Handbook could not have been completed without the whole-hearted involvement of a team of healthcare professionals who freely shared of their time and expertise in advising, editing and contributing various chapters or sections.

That such writing was completed on top of existing heavy clinical work loads is a testimony to these advisors, their capacity for hard work and commitment to sharing knowledge and expertise.

The costs of such extracurricular activities as contributing to handbooks like this is ususally also paid for by the families and partners of those whom we have trapped in their studies—thank you.

We particularly thank Catherine Barnes and Georgia Pinteau at Oxford University Press for their patience through the long birthing process of the handbook, and their ready supply of encouragement.

We are indebted to Ian Back both for permission to use some of the material contained in his excellent *Palliative Medicine Handbook* and for his input into the project despite several other major commitments.

The South West London and The Surrey, West Sussex and Hampshire Cancer Networks gave permission to use material contained in their Adult and Paediatric palliative care guidelines.

Jan Brooman at the Princess Alice Hospice Library was an invaluable help in the painstaking task of checking through the references.

The management and colleagues at the Princess Alice Hospice and the Northern Ireland Palliative Medicine Training Scheme have been very supportive of this project.

Handbooks, by their very nature, are distillations of accumulated and shared clinical knowledge. There is no claim to originality in these pages. We must accredit the hundreds of palliative care professionals who have observed, researched, recorded and written in journals and textbooks, to create the palliative care knowledge base which has been our primary text—a text which, almost unbelievably, did not exist in medical literature only 40 years ago.

MW
CL
AH
IB

We are indebted for permission to reproduce material within the Handbook from the following sources.

I. Back (2001) *Palliative Medicine Handbook*, 3rd edition. Cardiff: BPM Books.

E. Bruera and I. Higginson (1996) *Cachexia-Anorexia in Cancer Patients.* Oxford: Oxford University Press.

D. Doyle, N. Hanks, and N. Cherny (eds.) (2004) *Oxford Textbook of Palliative Medicine*, 3rd edition. Oxford: Oxford University Press.

J-H. R. Ramsay (1994) A King, a doctor and a convenient death. *BMJ*, **308**: 1445.

The South West London and the Survey West Sussex and Hampshire Cancer Networks. M. Watson and C. Lucas (2003) *Adult Palliative Care Guidelines.*

K. Thomas (2003) *Caring for the Dying at Home: companions on the journey.* Oxford: Radcliffe Medical Press.

R. Twycross, A. Wilcock, S. Charlesworth, and A. Dickman (2002) *Palliative Care Formulary*, 2nd edition. Oxford: Radcliffe Medical Press.

Winston's Wish: supporting bereaved children and young people. *www.winstonswish.org.uk.*

www.rch.org.au/rch_palliative; www.rch.org.au.

Contents

Advisors and contributors

Jennifer Barraclough
Former Consultant in Psychological Medicine
Sobell House
Churchill Hospital
Oxford

Pauline Beldon
Nurse Consultant Tissue Viability
Epsom and St Helier NHS Trust
Surrey

Jo Bray
Former Occupational Therapist
Project Director
Royal Marsden Hospital
Chelsea

Jan Brooman
Librarian
Princess Alice Hospice
Esher

David Cameron
Associate Professor of Family Medicine
University of Pretoria
South Africa

Beverly Castleton
Medical Director for Specialist Services and Consultant Physician
Care of the Elderly and the Young Physically Disabled
Surrey Heath and Woking NHS PCT
Chertsey

Robin Cole
Consultant Urological Surgeon
St Peter's Hospital
Chertsey

David Conkey
Clinical Oncology Department
Belvoir Park Hospital
Belfast

Simon Coulter
Specialist Registrar
Palliative Medicine Training Scheme
Belfast

Jill Cooper
Head Occupational Therapist
Royal Marsden Hospital
Sutton

Elizabeth Cruickshank
Speech and Language Therapist
South Glasgow University Hospitals
NHS Trust
Glasgow

Dwipaj Datta
Specialist Registrar
Palliative Medicine Training Scheme
South Thames
London

Judith Delaney
Haematology/Oncology Senior Pharmacist
Great Ormond Street Hospital for Children NHS Trust
London

Julie Doyle
Consultant in Palliative Medicine
Northern Ireland Hospice and Mater Hospital
Belfast

Martin Eatock
Consultant Medical Oncologist
Belfast City Hospital
Belfast

Patricia Enes
Formerly Research Nurse
Princess Alice Hospice
Esher

Gill Eyers
Senior Principal Pharmacist
Princess Alice Hospice, Esher
Kingston Hospital NHS Trust
Surrey

Craig Gannon
Consultant in Palliative Medicine
Princess Alice Hospice
Ashford and St Peter's Hospitals NHS Trust
Surrey

Louise Gibbs
Consultant in Palliative Medicine
St Christopher's Hospice
Lawrie Park Road
Sydenham, London

J. Simon Gibbs
Senior Lecturer in Cardiology
National Heart and Lung Institute at
Imperial College London, and
Honorary Consultant Cardiologist
Hammersmith Hospital, London

David Head
Former Chaplain
Princess Alice Hospice
Esher

Irene Higginson
Professor of Palliative Care and Policy
King's College School of Medicine and Dentistry
London

Jenny Hynson
Consultant Paediatrician
Victorian Paediatric Palliative Care Program
Royal Children's Hospital
Melbourne
Australia

David Hill
Consultant in Anaesthesia and Pain Management
Ulster Hospital
Honorary Senior Lecturer
Queen's University
Belfast

Allan Irvine
Consultant Radiologist
Ashford and St Peter's Hospitals NHS Trust
Surrey

Aleen Jones
Consultant Physician
Care of the Elderly
South Tyrone and Craigavon Area Hospitals
Craigavon

Emma Jones
Consultant in Palliative Medicine
Phyllis Tuckwell Hospice
Farnham

Carol Katté
Stoma Care Specialist Nurse
Ashford and St Peter's Hospitals NHS Trust
Surrey

Sian Lewis
Senior Dietician
Velindre Hospital
Cardiff

Victoria Lidstone
Specialist Registrar
Palliative Medicine Training Schemes
South Thames/South Wales
Cardiff

Mari Lloyd-Williams
Professor, Honorary Consultant in Palliative Medicine
Director of Primary Care
University of Liverpool
Liverpool

Jayne Macauley
Consultant in Palliative Medicine
Antrim Area Hospital and Northern Health Board
Antrim

Sarah McKenna
Consultant Medical Oncologist
Belfast City Hospital Trust
Belfast

Pamela MacKinnon
Formerly at the Department of Human Anatomy and Genetics
University of Oxford
Oxford

Sarah MacLaran
Specialist Registrar
Palliative Medicine Training Scheme
Myton Hamlet Hospice, Warwick

Dorry McLaughlin
Lecturer in Palliative Care
Northern Ireland Hospice Care
Belfast

Penny McNamara
Consultant in Palliative Medicine
Sue Ryder Care—St John's
Bedford

Elaine McWilliams
Clinical Psychologist
Harrow Primary Care Trust
Harrow

Anne Miller
Consultant Haematologist
Ashford and St Peter's Hospitals NHS Trust
Surrey

Dan Munday
Consultant in Palliative Medicine
Honorary Senior Lecturer Warwick University
Coventry Primary Care Trust
Warwick

Simon Noble
Specialist Registrar Palliative Medicine
All Wales Higher Training Programme
Cardiff

Victor Pace
Consultant in Palliative Medicine
St Christopher's Hospice
Lawrie Park Road
Sydenham, London

Sheila Payne
Professor in Palliative Care
Sheffield Palliative Care Studies Group
University of Sheffield
Sheffield

Margaret Reith
Social Worker Team Manager
Princess Alice Hospice
Esher

Joan Regan
Specialist Registrar
Palliative Medicine Training Scheme
Belfast

Patti Stevely
Day Hospice Manager
Senior Physiotherapist
Princess Alice Hospice
Esher

Robert Sudderick
Consultant in Otolaryngology and Head
and Neck surgery
Royal Surrey County Hospital
Guildford

Keri Thomas
GP, National Clinical Lead Palliative Care
Cancer Services Collaborative of NHS Modernisation Agency
Macmillan Gold Standards Framework Programme
Associate Clinical Director Community Palliative Care, Birmingham
Senior Clinical Lecturer, Warwick University

Patrick Trend
Consultant Neurologist
Royal Surrey County Hospital
Guildford

Jo Wells
Nurse Consultant in Palliative Care
Princess Alice Hospice
Kingston Hospital NHS Trust
Surrey

Andrew Wilcock
Macmillan Clinical Leader in Palliative Medicine and Medical Oncology
Nottingham University
Consultant Physician, Hayward House Macmillan
Specialist Palliative Care Unit
Nottingham City Hospital
Nottingham

Abbreviations

AF	atrial fibrillation
AIDS	acquired immune deficiency syndrome
Amp.	ampoule
b.d.	twice daily
BNF	British National Formulary
BP	blood pressure
Caps.	capsules
CD	controlled drug
CHF	congestive heart failure
CMV	cytomegalovirus
CNS	central nervous system
CO_2	carbon dioxide
COPD	chronic obstructive pulmonary disease
COX	cyclo-oxygenase
CSCI	continuous subcutaneous infusion
C/T	chemotherapy
CT	computerized tomography
CTZ	chemoreceptor trigger zone
CVA	cerebrovascular accident
DIC	disseminated intravascular coagulation
DN	District Nurse
DVT	deep vein thrombosis
ECG	electrocardiogram
EDDM	Equivalent Daily Dose of Morphine
FBC	full blood count
FEV_1	forced expiratory volume in one second
FNA	fine needle aspiration
g	gram
GERD	gastro-oesophageal reflux disease
GI	gastrointestinal
GP	General Practitioner
Gy	Gray(s) a measure of radiation
h	hour or hourly
HAART	highly active anti-retroviral therapy
HIV	human immunodeficiency virus
HNSCC	head and neck squamous cell carcinoma

ICP	intracranial pressure
i/m	intramuscular
Inj.	injection
i/r	immediate release
i/t	intrathecal
i/v	intravenous
IVI	intravenous infusion
IVU	intravenous urogram
KS	Kaposi's sarcoma
kV	kilovolt
l	litre
L/A	local anaesthetic
LFT	liver function tests
LVF	left ventricular failure
MAI	Mycobacterium avium intracellulare
MAOI	monoamine oxidase inhibitor(s)
max.	maximum
MeV	mega electronvolt
mcg	microgram
MND	motor neurone disease
m/r	modified release
MRI	Magnetic Resonance Imaging
MUPS	multiple unit pellet system
MV	megavolt
m/w	mouthwash
NASSA	noradrenergic and specific serotoninergic antidepressant
neb	nebuliser
NG	naso-gastric
NMDA	N-methyl-D-aspartate
nocte	at night
NSAID	non-steroidal anti-inflammatory drug
NSCLC	non small cell lung carcinoma
NYHA	New York Heart Association
o.d.	daily
o.m.	in the morning
OTFC	oral transmucosal fentanyl citrate
PCA	Patient Controlled Analgesia
PCF	Palliative Care Formulary
PCT	Palliative care team
PE	pulmonary embolism
PEG	percutaneous endoscopic gastrostomy

PET	positron emission tomography
PHCT	primary healthcare team
p.o.	by mouth
PPI	proton pump inhibitor
PR	per rectum
p.r.n.	when required
PSA	prostate-specific antigen
PV	per vagina
q.d.s.	four times daily
QoL	quality of life
RBL	renal bone liver (investigations)
RCT	randomized controlled trial
RT	radiotherapy
SALT	speech and language therapy
SC	subcutaneous
SCLC	small cell lung carcinoma
S/D	syringe driver (CSCI)
SE	side-effects
SERMs	selective oestrogen receptor modulators
SL	sublingual
soln.	solution
SPC	specialist palliative care
SR	slow or modified release
SSRI	selective serotonin reuptake inhibitor
stat	immediately
Supps.	suppositories
Susp.	suspension
SVC	superior vena cava
SVCO	superior vena cava obstruction
Tabs.	tablets
TB	tuberculosis
TBM	tubercular meningitis
t.d.s.	three times daily
TENS	transcutaneous electrical nerve stimulation
TIA	transient ischaemic attack
TSD	therapeutic standard dose
U&E	urea and elecrolytes
URTI	upper respiratory tract infection
UTI	urinary tract infection
VTE	venous thromboembolism
WHO	World Health Organization

Introduction

Palliative care definitions

Palliative care is the active, holistic care of patients with advanced, progressive illness. Management of pain and other symptoms and provision of psychological, social and spiritual support is paramount. The goal of palliative care is achievement of the best quality of life for patients and their families. Many aspects of palliative care are also applicable earlier in the course of the illness in conjunction with other treatments.[1]

Palliative care:
- Affirms life and regards dying as a normal process
- Provides relief from pain and other symptoms
- Integrates the psychological and spiritual aspects of patient care
- Offers a support system to help patients live as actively as possible until death
- Offers a support system to help the family cope during the patient's illness and in their own environment.

Principles of palliative care

No single sphere of concern is adequate without considering the relationship with the other two. This usually requires genuine interdisciplinary collaboration.[2]

General palliative care is provided by the usual professional carers of the patient and family with low to moderate complexity of palliative care need. Palliative care is a vital and integral part of their routine clinical practice which is underpinned by the following principles:
- Focus on quality of life which includes good symptom control
- Whole person approach taking into account the person's past life experience and current situation

- Care which encompasses both the person with life-threatening illness and those that matter to the person
- Respect for patient autonomy and choice (e.g. over place of care, treatment options)
- Emphasis on open and sensitive communication, which extends to patients, informal carers and professional colleagues

Specialist palliative care

These services are provided for patients and their families with moderate to high complexity of palliative care need. The core service components are provided by a range of NHS, voluntary and independent providers staffed by a multidisciplinary team whose core work is palliative care.[2]

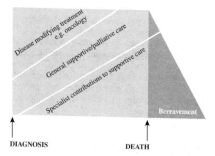

Disease modifying treatment e.g. oncology

General supportive/palliative care

Specialist contributions to supportive care

Bereavement

↑ DIAGNOSIS   ↑ DEATH

Supportive care is that which helps the patient and their family to cope with cancer and treatment of it—from pre-diagnosis, through the process of diagnosis and treatment, to cure, continuing illness or death and into bereavement. It helps the patient to maximize the benefits of treatment and to live as well as possible with the effects of the disease. It is given equal priority alongside diagnosis and treatment.

The principles that underpin supportive and palliative care are broadly the same.

Hospice and hospice care refer to a philosophy of care rather than a specific building or service and may encompass a programme of care and array of skills deliverable in a wide range of settings.

Terminal care is an important part of palliative care and usually refers to the management of patients during their last few days, weeks or months of life from a point at which it becomes clear that the patient is in a progressive state of decline.

1 World Health Organization (1990) *Cancer Pain Relief and Palliative Care*. Geneva: WHO: 11 (World Health Organization technical report series: 804)

2 National Council for Hospice and Specialist Palliative Care Services (2002) *Definitions of Supportive and Palliative Care*. London: NCHSPCS (Briefing Bulletin 11)

History of palliative medicine as a specialty

The specialty of palliative medicine as a specific entity dates from the mid 1980s. However, medical activity related to terminal care, care of the dying, hospice care and end-stage cancer is of course as old as medical practice itself.[1] Palliative medicine is the medical component of what has become known as palliative care.

The history of the hospice movement during the nineteenth and twentieth centuries demonstrates the innovations of several charismatic leaders. These practitioners were enthusiasts for their own particular contribution to care of the dying, and they were also the teachers of the next generation of palliative physicians. Although they were products of their original background and training, they all shared the vision of regarding patients who happened to be dying as 'whole people'. They naturally brought their own approaches from specific disciplines of pharmacology, oncology, surgery, anaesthetics or general practice. This whole person attitude has been labelled as 'holistic care'. Comfort and freedom from pain and distress were of equal importance to diagnostic acumen and cure. However, rather than being a completely new philosophy of care, palliative medicine can be regarded more as a codification of existing practices from past generations.

Histories of the development of palliative medicine illustrate the thread of ideas from figures such as Snow, who developed the Brompton Cocktail in the 1890s, to Barrett who developed the regular giving of oral morphine to the dying at St Luke's, West London, to Saunders who expanded these ideas at St Joseph's and St Christopher's Hospices. Worcester, in Boston, was promoting the multidisciplinary care of whole patients in lectures to medical students at a time when intense disease specialization was very much the fashion as it was yielding great therapeutic advances.[2] Winner and Amulree, in the UK in the 1960s, were promoting whole person care particularly for the elderly, first challenging and then re-establishing the ethical basis for palliative medicine.

The early hospice movement was primarily concerned with the care of patients with cancer who, in the surge of post-war medical innovation, had missed out on the windfall of the new confident and increasingly optimistic medical world.

That this movement was responding to a need perceived across the world, has been evidenced by the exponential growth in palliative care services throughout the UK and across the globe since the opening of St Christopher's hospice in south-east London in 1967.

The expansion is set to increase further, as the point has now been reached where patients, doctors and governments alike are calling for the same level of care to be made available to patients suffering from non-malignant conditions as for those with cancer.

If this new challenge is to be met, healthcare professionals from early in their training will need to be exposed to palliative care learning which can be applied across the range of medical specialities.

The essence of such palliative medicine learning both for generalists and specialists remains that of clinical apprenticeship. Alfred Worcester, in the preface to his lectures, notes that:

The younger members of the profession, although having enormously greater knowledge of the science of medicine, have less acquaintance than many of their elders with the art of medical practice. This like every other art can of course be learned only by imitation, that is, by practice under masters of the art. Primarily, it depends upon devotion to the patient rather than to his disease.[2]

1 Saunders C. (1993). Introduction—history and challenge. In C. Saunders, N. Sykes (eds) *The Management of Terminal Malignant Disease. 3rd edition*, pp. 1–14. London: Edward Arnold.

2 Worcester A. (1935) *The Care of the Aged the Dying and the Dead.* London: Bailliere & Co.

The death of Harold Shipman

> **Dr Harold Shipman died on 13 January in Wakefield Prison. He hanged himself on the day before his 58th birthday. He was convicted in January 2000 of the murder of 15 people. However, it is estimated that he killed at least 215 mainly elderly people. As well as being the UK's most prolific serial killer, what is most shocking is that his victims were his patients. They looked up to him as a trusted GP and friend. What significance does this have for those concerned with palliative care in both the UK and beyond?**

All medical practice, but particularly palliative care, relies on the establishment of a relationship of trust between patients and their healthcare professional advisors. This trust is threatened by dishonesty on the part of doctors or nurses. For this reason, the palliative care movement has embraced the philosophy of truthful disclosure of clinical information to patients if that is what is asked for. This philosophy is sometimes confused with total disclosure of every last documented outcome and complication of a proposed management plan, whether or not the recipient of the information is in an emotional or intellectual state to process it. This offloading of detail may be advocated as part of the process of obtaining informed consent, or it may be the result of defensive practice to protect against future litigation. Neither is in the patient's best interest. Furthermore, frank disclosure does not imply brutal use of stark prognostic details, without first listening carefully to the patient's informational requests. So honesty and truthfulness are prerequisites for trust. Trust in turn is essential to prevent advice from becoming paternalism.

Harold Shipman used opioids to kill his victims. We will never know the details of dose and methods, but it is safe to assume that he gave very large doses to opioid-naïve patients. This fact has not always been reported to the public, with the unfortunate consequence that there is now increasing suspicion of strong opioids even when such drugs would relieve severe pain. This makes palliative care more difficult and results in increased suffering especially for the vulnerable.

Although Shipman showed no remorse or inclination to collaborate in establishing his motives, while he was still alive there was still the chance that we might eventually have gained some insight into his psychopathology. Now he has killed himself, we are simply left to speculate that in death as in life his motive was the need to exert control over all those around him.

The popular press has named his activity as 'euthanasia without consent'. This term is unfortunate for several reasons. We do not have evidence that all his victims died peacefully and without anguish. They were certainly not given any opportunity to complete unfinished business with family and friends. In the immediate aftermath of Shipman's death, anger and resentment among relatives has increased not diminished. There would seem to be no sense of closure which either understanding or remorse might have brought. The use of the word euthanasia only muddies the water in a debate which is difficult in any event. Finally, although death can be viewed as the inevitable relinquishment of autonomy, at least in a physical sense, choices can be exercised before such relinquishment. Shipman removed consent, choices and therefore all autonomy and self-determination. His activity was murder with or without an understandable motive.

Since the conviction four years ago, there has been an exhaustive judicial inquiry of current law and regulations relating to death registration, monitoring of single-handed general practice, prescription, availability and supply of controlled drugs. The Prime Minister has already said that the recommendations of this review will be implemented in full. There is, however, considerable anxiety that this may result in a straitjacket for sensible community palliative care. It would be doubly tragic if Shipman's legacy of murder resulted in the frustration of good palliative care. An exceptional case makes for bad law.

Reproduced with kind permission from the *European Journal of Palliative Care*.

Communication

Effective symptom control is impossible without effective communication

Buckman 2000

Communication is fundamental to good palliative care, but difficulties can arise that need to be understood and addressed.

Society's attitudes towards death and dying can hinder open communication. Health professionals may be uneasy with issues of death and dying: they may wish to protect themselves and others, and feel a sense of discomfort with strong emotions.

It is easy for the busy health professional to use a variety of blocking tactics which inhibit communication, such as hiding behind task-focused practice. An additional hazard may arise if the setting is not conducive to privacy with space and time to listen.

Information-giving can take the place of hearing the underlying feelings and emotions. The essence of good communication is not what we say, but how we listen. The quality of listening empathically to patients should not be underestimated if patients are to feel understood and cared for.

Communication in palliative care is necessary to achieve accurate assessment of patients' physical, emotional and psychosocial needs. If we are to be able to find ways of supporting patients and families facing change and uncertainty, we as health professional needs to find out about the patient's expectations and goals.

Enabling people to make informed choices and to make future plans involves careful listening and sensitive responses. Attending to cultural and language issues, and helping people face some of the strong emotions aroused by their situation such as anger, denial, depression and fear, are essential in providing holistic PALLIATIVE CARE.

Buckman, R. (2000) Communication in palliative care: a practical guide.
In D. Dickenson, M. Johnson and J. S. Katz (eds.) *Death, Dying and Bereavement*, 2nd edn.
pp 146–73. London: Sage.

Prognostication in end-of-life care

The natural history of disease has been documented over many years. This has become increasingly less relevant as successful therapies have developed. In present day palliative medicine, prognosis frequently relates to chronic progressive disease in patients with multiple co-morbidities, and not to the recovery prediction of a young adult with an acute illness, as was more common in the nineteenth century.

The reasons for making an attempt at predicting how long a patient with incurable disease might live include:

- Providing information about the future to patients and families so that they can set goals, priorities and expectations of care
- Helping patients develop insight into their dying
- Assisting clinicians in decision-making
- Comparing like patients with regard to outcomes
- Establishing the patient's eligibility for care programmes (e.g. hospice) and for recruitment to research trials
- Policy-making regarding appropriate use and allocation of resources and support services
- Providing a common language for healthcare professionals involved in end-of-life care.

Prognostic factors in cancer

There is a good literature on the probability of cure for the different cancers.

- Although individual cancers behave differently, as a generalization, predictions relate to tumour size, grade and stage
- Other factors include hormonal status (for hormone-dependent tumours such as cancer of the breast and prostate)
- Age
- Biochemical or other markers
- The length of time taken for the disease to recur.

In palliative care such prognostic indices may not be so relevant.

Factors such as physical dependency (due to e.g. weakness, low blood pressure), cognitive dysfunction, paraneoplastic phenomena (e.g. anorexia–cachexia, cytokine production), certain symptoms (weight loss, anorexia, dysphagia, breathlessness), lymphopaenia, poor quality of life and existential factors (either 'giving up' or 'hanging on' for symbolically important times) may be more important.

Some patients may survive for a long time (months and years) with a seemingly high tumour load, while others succumb within a short time (days) for no obviously identifiable reasons.

Several scores have been developed to aid prediction of survival. The Palliative Prognostic (PaP) score is predictive of short term survival and summarizes scores for dyspnoea, anorexia, Karnovsky performance status, the clinician's estimate of survival (in weeks), total white count, and percentage of lymphocytes.

Oncologists rely on prognosis assessments in order to predict which patients are likely to benefit from oncological interventions. Many of their decisions are based on the patient's functional status.

Patients with an ECOG score greater than two are usually deemed unsuitable for most chemotherapy interventions.

Eastern Co-operative Oncology Group (ECOG)

Fully active; able to carry on all activities without restriction	0
Restricted in physically strenuous activity but ambulatory and able to carry out work of a light or sedentary nature	1
Ambulatory and capable of all self care; confined to bed or chair 50% of waking hours	2
Capable of only limited self-care; confined to bed or chair 50% or more of waking hours	3
Completely disabled; cannot carry on any self care; totally confined to bed or chair	4

Prognostic factors in non-malignant disease

Predicting prognosis in patients with a non-cancer diagnosis is very difficult. These patients often remain relatively stable, albeit at a low level, only to deteriorate acutely and unpredictably. They are usually then treated acutely in hospital, and the disease course may consist of acute exacerbations from which recovery may take place.

One study showed that even in the last 2–3 days of life patients with congestive heart failure (CHF) or COPD were given a 80 per cent and 50 per cent chance respectively of living six months.

There are, however, general and specific indicators of the terminal stage approaching.

General predictors

Those predicting poorer prognosis include reduced performance status, impaired nutritional status and a low albumin (greater than 10 per cent weight loss over six months).

Specific predictors

Congestive heart failure (CHF)
- More than 64 years old
- Left ventricular ejection fraction less than 20 per cent
- Dilated cardiomyopathy
- Uncontrolled arrhythmias
- Systolic hypotension
- CXR signs of left heart failure
- A prognosis of less than six months is associated with NYHA Class IV (chest pain and/or breathless at rest/minmal exertion) and already optimally treated with diuretics and vasodilators

Chronic obstructive pulmonary disease (COPD)
- Advanced age
- FEV_1 less than 30 per cent
- Pulmonary hypertension with cor pulmonale/right heart failure
- Other factors NHO sob at rest
- On 24 hour home O_2 with pO_2 less than 50 mm Hg and/or pCO_2 more than 55 mm Hg and documented evidence of cor pulmonale

Cortical dementias (Alzheimer's disease)
- Functional status—the onset of being unable to walk unaided
- Unable to swallow
- Unable to hold a meaningful conversation
- Increasing frequency of medical complications, e.g. aspiration pneumonia, urinary tract infections, decubitus ulcers

Stroke
- Impaired consciousness
- Lack of improvement within three months of onset
- Age
- Incontinence
- Cognitive impairment
- Dense paralysis

Communicating prognosis

Prognostication is a notoriously difficult task to perform accurately. The world abounds with stories of patients who have been told by their physicians that they have only a matter of months to live who twenty years later can recount in vivid detail the day they were given the news.

One of the reasons that prognostication is so difficult is that it is fraught with uncertainty and also with opportunities for misunderstandings between doctors and patients, who often have very different agendas as to what they want to get out of the interview.

> Mr. Jones listened carefully as the consultant went into great detail about the nature and the extensive spread of his metastatic prostate tumour. The explanations were detailed and scientific and long. Eventually the consultant stopped. 'Now Mr. Jones, do you have any more questions'
>
> 'Well, I didn't like to interrupt you but I was only asking how long I had before I needed to go down to get my X-Ray.'

Over the past 20 years there has been a huge shift in attitudes regarding disclosure of information to patents, and a culture of complete disclosure has now become the norm. Yet prognostication does not just involve passing on clinical details and predictions of disease progression; it also involves assessing:
- What does the patient actually want to know? (Giving too much information to a patient who does not want to have the exact details spelt out is as unprofessional as the patronising attitudes of 'best not to trouble the patient'
- How is the patient dealing with the information that is being given?

- How can the patient be helped to deal with the implications of the news?

To pass on facts without regard for the implications of those facts is to increase the risk of dysfunctional communication taking place. (📖 See Chapter 2)

Risk and chance

While doctors are used to describing risk in terms of percentages, when such percentages are measuring out your own longevity it is hard to translate the mathematical chances into personal experience.

A doctor may feel that he has provided the patient with the clear facts when he states that in 100 patients with the particular malignancy, 36 will be alive after five years following treatment. Such sentences can be easily misunderstood, and the patient may hear something very different from what the doctor is saying.

Professional discomfort

Doctors are also particularly vulnerable to miscommunication at the time of passing on prognostic information.

- Society in the west is now death-denying, and if the prognosis is poor it can be uncomfortable for the doctor to pass on the information and confront the patent with their imminent death
- There is increasing fear of litigation, particularly if disease is not responsive to treatment, and any admission of failure may come across as an admission of guilt
- Doctors may feel uncomfortable in dealing with the emotional impact that their news may have on the patient, and develop techniques to protect themselves from this discomfort

Prognostic information can be extremely important to patients as it allows them to focus on tasks and goals which they want to achieve before their disease takes over: communicating such information effectively is a skill which all healthcare professionals should covet.

Ethical issues

An ethical framework
- Respect for autonomy (self-determination)
- Beneficence (do good)
- Non-maleficence (do no harm)
- Justice (fairness)

The concept of exploring end-of-life issues is inherent to palliative care. With good communication and trust in the patient/professional relationship, patients' attitudes and concerns can be discussed sensitively, confusion unravelled and fears dispelled. Some patients like to consider writing a formal Advance Directive or 'living will', which should give a more formative clearly defined record of patients' wishes in order to facilitate more informed decision-making. In practice, when patients ask for euthanasia there may be areas of 'unfinished business', fear, guilt or other issues that need to be explored. After sensitive and open communication, most patients feel a sense of relief and their need to press for a deliberate ending of their life diminishes.

We live in a world which has become increasingly complex. Ethical issues that arise towards the end-of-life are often fraught with difficulty in an increasingly technological age in which the process of dying may be prolonged. In healthcare, there is often no right or wrong decision, but only a consensus view of a clear aim, considered on the basis of ethical principles. The most widely used ethical framework in health issues in the West comprises:
- **Autonomy** (the patient should be informed and involved in decision-making)
- **Beneficence** (do good)
- **Non-maleficence** (do no harm)
- **Justice** (balancing the needs of individuals with those of society)

In the abstract, these principles can seem straightforward; in the heat of a clinical situation their application can be anything but clear. It is, however, very useful to have a framework with which to deal with ethical crises.

The following clinical scenarios are examples which occur commonly. Applying the principles of ethics in order to reach a balanced compromise can help provide a path through uncertainty.

Example 1: 'My father is not drinking adequately. Why are you not giving him extra fluids?'

Ethical issues
- **Beneficence**: Will artificial fluids help the patient?
- **Non-maleficence**: Will giving or not giving artificial fluids cause the patient harm?
- **Autonomy**: Does the patient want a drip?

It is instilled in all of us, from childhood years onwards, that food and drink are essential for life. There are clinical situations in palliative care when extra systemic fluids might be useful, for instance in hypercalcaemia or profuse diarrhoea and vomiting. These may be salvageable clinical situations where we are expecting the patient to return to his 'normal', albeit generally deteriorating, state of health.

Artificial hydration
- A blanket policy of artificial hydration, or of no artificial hydration, is ethically indefensible
- If dehydration is thought to be due to a potentially correctable cause, the option of artificial hydration should be considered
- The appropriateness of artificial hydration should be weighed up in terms of harm and benefit on a day-to-day basis

When someone is considered to be dying irreversibly, however, the routine of giving systemic fluids may not be in the patient's best interests.

Background information
There are a few studies addressing this issue, but there is no proof that either the giving or withholding of fluids interferes with the length of remaining life or affects comfort.
- Biochemical parameters show that only 50 per cent of patients have any evidence of dehydration within the final 48 h of life and, even then, only in mild to moderate degree
- There is no evidence that thirst or dry mouth (particularly) improve with artificial hydration
- The extensive experience of nurses working in hospices suggest that systemic fluids at best make no difference and, at worst, may actually contribute to suffering at the end-of-life
- The more fluid available, the more likely it is that it will gather in lungs and dependent parts of the body particularly in the presence of hypoalbuminaemia, which is common in advanced malignancy
- Artificially increasing fluids at the end-of-life, when the body physiology is winding down, may lead to worsening respiratory secretions, increased vomiting, raised intracranial pressure in the presence of intracerebral disease, and an uncomfortable urinary output

- Families can spend precious time worrying about intravenous infusions running out or plastic cannulae being displaced and causing discomfort, instead of concentrating on quality time with the patient

Discussion

Withholding systemic fluids is inevitably a very emotive issue signifying finally and clearly, perhaps for the first time to the family, that their loved one is now entering the final stages of their life. In practice, patients are often able to take small amounts of fluids until shortly before death. It should be explained to families that the body is gradually shutting down and is unable to handle an extra fluid load. They need to be aware that the patient will not be allowed to suffer from pain or other discomfort and they will need explanations of the measures that will be taken to avoid discomfort. These will include medication where necessary and most importantly meticulous mouthcare to prevent the common symptom of a dry mouth.

Palliative care is neither about shortening life nor prolonging the dying period.

Occasionally, families cannot bring themselves to accept the inevitability of death and insist on artificial hydration. Although healthcare professionals must act only in the best interests of the patient, it would be unwise to ignore the views of the family, who have to go on surviving with vivid memories of the dying phase. On occasion, if it is felt that extra fluids will not adversely affect comfort, it is sometimes helpful to have a contract with the family for a relatively small volume of fluid to be used subcutaneously or intravenously for a defined short period, on the understanding that it would be discontinued at any time if it was thought to be causing the patient distress.

As in most ethical crises, a balance has to be made—in this situation, between the harm caused by withholding or giving artificial hydration.

- Acknowledge family distress
- Explore concerns
- Discuss the above points
- Reassure the family that the patient will be looked after and kept comfortable whether fluids are given artificially or not

Example 2: 'How long have I got left?'

Ethical issue
- **Autonomy**: Is every attempt beng made to inform the patient adequately?

This type of question usually relates to prognosis. As ever, however, it is always important to make sure that the question has been entirely understood, since to enter into a conversation about how long a patient has to live when all they want to know is when they are going to leave hospital can cause unnecessary distress.

> Centuries of systematic insensitive deception cannot be instantly remedied by a new routine of systematic insensitive truth telling.
>
> Buckman

When it is certain that the patient is talking about prognosis, first find out what they already know, how they see the situation, why they are asking the question and how much they really want to know.

The following questions can be useful:
- 'What have the doctors told you so far?'
- 'What has prompted you to ask this question now?'
- 'How do *you* see the situation?'
- 'Are there other specific issues, related to how long there is left, on your mind that you would like to talk about?'
- 'Are you the kind of person who likes to know everything?'

In practice, patients often say that they have not been told anything by the doctors: this may be true, or they may have inadvertently used denial mechanisms to 'forget' the bad news. The patient may also deny knowledge in an attempt to find out more information. It is important to explore what they understand accurately thus far. Patients often want to achieve goals such as writing a will, attending a family wedding, reaching a wedding anniversary, being reunited with old friends and family who they have not seen for a long time or seeing their religious adviser. Patients may not find it easy to discuss these issues, with even close family members, and may need help to facilitate discussions. They may need help in setting realistic and achievable goals while planning their limited future.

Before addressing prognosis directly, it is important to be aware of the full medical history and to build up a picture of the pace of clinical deterioration. Questions such as 'I believe you have not been feeling so well recently' or 'the doctors/your medical notes tell me that you feel that life has become more difficult over the past few weeks' open up these issues, giving you and the patient a chance to estimate prognosis. Remember that studies show that health professionals tend to overestimate prognosis.

Background
Literature on determining prognosis is available, especially for patients with cancer. For a population presenting with a defined stage, grade, cancer type and histology, five year survival rates are available and often

quoted to families. Many other factors have been studied singly and in combination in an attempt to categorize patients into prognostic groups, and this can be helpful in broad terms. In practice, however, it is not possible to predict prognosis for an individual accurately, because there are so many different influencing factors—including psychosocial, emotional and existential issues—all of which defy measurement of any kind.

- Make sure that you are answering what the patient wants to know
- Stress that you are not evading the question but that is is difficult to answer
- Find out specific issues that should be addressed e.g. weddings, wills etc.
- Do not be specific but use weeks/months, etc.

Despite all these pitfalls, it is still important to answer the patient's question. It is still relatively common for a precise prognosis, for example 'six months', to be given and this is invariably inaccurate. If the patient dies before the due date, the family feel cheated of time that they would otherwise have spent differently had they known that time was so short. If the patient survives longer than the due date, both patient and family may feel proud that they have defeated the odds and take comfort from this; on the other hand, if the family have altered their lifestyles including giving up work (and salary) to look after a patient who has not significantly deteriorated by the due date, family tensions inevitably build up alongside all the normal feelings of guilt and anger.

It is not helpful to give a precise date, which patients and families often take literally, but to talk in terms of days/weeks, weeks/months and months/years. It is also important to say that even within these broad terms we may still be innacurate.

It is also useful to talk about the pace of deterioration and to say that the pace may continue at the same rate but it may also either stabilize for a while or speed up.

Example 3: 'Don't tell my mother the diagnosis. I know her better than you.'

Ethical issues

- **Autonomy**: Does Granny not need to be told regardless of what the family think?
- **Benificence**: Would it help Granny to know her diagnosis?
- **Non-malevolence**: Would it harm Granny to know her diagnosis?

It is common to be caught in the hospital or health practice corridor by anxious relatives who (possibly wrongly) have been told that their relative has cancer, before this information has been given to the patient. There is increasing evidence that patients want to know what is wrong with them and to be involved in decisions. Generally speaking, we have moved away from a paternalistic approach in truth-telling whereby doctors often avoided telling patients they had cancer, to a more open approach, respecting the principle of autonomy.

However, the family have known the patient over many years and are aware of how she has responded to bad news in the past. They may feel that there is no point in discussing the diagnosis, particularly if the patient is very elderly and there is no available treatment.

- For understandable reasons the family want to protect the patient from bad news, but very often they want to protect themselves from further hurt and the reality that the patient may now be entering the last stages of life
- It needs to be acknowledged with the family that this is a difficult area but that the patient may have important things to say or do (financial, wills, gifts etc.) or opinions to voice (regarding both medical and after-death decisions)
- The family also need to know that patients pick up non-verbal clues from professionals and relatives; they are often aware of the diagnosis and are not unduly surprised if it is confirmed
- Patients often want to protect the family, denying that they know anything
- The family need to be aware that patients are often comforted by a 'label' to their illness, even if it is cancer, because it explains why they have been feeling so unwell. This gives them a genuine reason for feeling so wretched
- Families need to know that it becomes more difficult to conceal the truth from the patient as time goes on and as more professionals, family members and friends share the secret. There are increasing opportunities for the truth to slip out and for the patient to lose trust in and be angry with the family for not having been more honest in the first place
- Families also need to know that patients are not always frightened of death but of the process of leading up to it, over which they may want some control
- It is very important not to lie to the patient as this breaks all communication and confidence

- Acknowledge family anxiety
- Inform family of the issues as above
- Stress that it is important for neither professionals nor family to lie if the patient starts asking direct questions

If there are no particular decisions to be made, the patient has dealt with his or her affairs and is living with the family, there may be no pressing need to try to discuss the issue and invite family disquiet. However, if the patient begins to ask direct questions, the family should be advised not to lie. The family also needs to be aware that family tensions reduce considerably when there are open discussions about diagnosis.

The professional is able to override family views if it is clearly in the interests of the patient to do so, but it is also always advisable and prudent to listen to and take account of the views of the family. If it is felt important to discuss the diagnosis, it is usually acceptable to families to say that we will try to find out what the patient understands by their illness and whether or not they would like more information.

Example 4: 'I want full resuscitation if my heart or lungs fail.'[1]

Ethical issues
- **Autonomy**: Does the patient have the right to demand treatments from nursing and medical staff?
- **Beneficence**: Would it be in the patient's best interests to initiate resuscitation?
- **Non-malevolence**: Would it do the patient any harm to initiate resuscitation?
- **Justice**: Would it be an appropriate use of resources to initiate resuscitation measures and appropriate a bed in ITU?

Background
Patients and families are increasingly aware of the many ethical issues surrounding cardiopulmonary resuscitation. These have been highlighted recently with 'DNR' (Do Not Resuscitate) notices being recorded in patients' notes without the patients being aware that they had been thus assigned. This has caused much concern, particularly among the weakest and most vulnerable sections of the community.

The issues have caused marked unease within hospices where, until very recently, resuscitation was regarded as an unacceptable practice. Patients with non-malignant disease and patients with cancer in the early stages, however, are increasingly requiring specialist palliative care. Such patients may feel very strongly that, in the event of a sudden cardiac or respiratory collapse, they want full resuscitation.

Litigation anxiety can cause a dilemma and increase the strain on staff to make the right decision. The need to document the resuscitation status of patients, following full discussion, can of itself lead to increased stress for all involved in handling what can be a very distressing issue.
- **Autonomy**: Patients have the right to ask for whatever treatment they choose. Medical and nursing staff are not obliged to comply with such expressed wishes if:
  - they feel it would not be in the patient's best interests
  - the intervention is deemed to be futile

Good practice would dictate that such matters are addressed by the whole multiprofessional team, though the senior doctor has ultimate responsibility for the decision.[2]

Achievement of success from CPR in any setting:

In hospital	15%
In community	1–5%
In hospices	1%

1 Willard C. (2000) Cardiopulmonary resuscitation for palliative care patients: a discussion of ethical issues. *Palliat Med* **14**: 308–12.

2 National Council for Hospice and Specialist Palliative Care Services. *Ethical decision-making in palliative care. Cardiopulmonary Resuscitation (CPR) for people who are terminally ill.* London: NCHSPCS.

A king, a doctor, and a convenient death

Lord Dawson of Penn was the most admired and respected doctor of his generation. The skill with which he managed King George V's respiratory illness in 1928 undoubtedly saved the king's life and made Dawson a national celebrity. He was also respected within the medical profession. He was president of the Royal College of Physicians, elected twice president of the BMA, and honoured with a viscountcy.

His reputation would have been considerably diminished, however, had it been known that when the king was suffering from cardiorespiratory failure in January 1936 he administered a lethal combination of morphine and cocaine at a time when the king was already comatose and close to death. His action remained a well kept secret and the truth came to light only 50 years later when his private diary was opened, Dawson having died in 1945.

The king had been in failing health for several weeks when Queen Mary summoned Dawson to Sandringham on 17 January. Contemporary accounts of the king's last days given by the Archbishop of Canterbury and others tell of days that were tranquil and pain free with the king sitting in an armchair before a log fire for much of the time but becoming steadily weaker and with consciousness gradually slipping away.

At 9:25 pm on 20 January Dawson issued the memorable bulletin stating that the king's life was moving peacefully towards its close. The action which he took one and a half hour later is described in his diary thus:

'At about 11 o'clock it was evident that the last stage might endure for many hours, unknown to the patient but little comporting with the dignity and serenity which he so richly merited and which demanded a brief final scene. Hours of waiting just for the mechanical end when all that is really life has departed only exhausts the onlookers and keeps them so strained that they cannot avail themselves of the solace of thought, communion or prayer. I therefore decided to determine the end and injected (myself) morphia gr.3/4 and shortly afterwards cocaine gr. 1 into the distended jugular vein.'

Dawson did not consult the other two doctors in the case, and his diary indicated that he was acting entirely on his own. To her credit, Sister Catherine Black of the London Hospital, who was present and who had nursed the king since the 1928 illness, refused to give the lethal injection, which is why Dawson had to give it himself. Nevertheless, faced with conflicting loyalties, she kept quiet about what had been done and her autobiography published in 1939 made no mention of what must have been the most poignant and unforgettable episode in her long and distinguished career.

The reason for his action, which Dawson frankly admits in his diary, was to ensure that the announcement of the king's death should appear first in the morning edition of the Times and not in some lesser publication later in the day. To make doubly sure that this would happen Dawson telephoned his wife in London asking her to let the Times know when the announcement was imminent.

Nevertheless, it was surely special pleading to claim that he also acted to reduce the strain on the royal family. Apart from the Prince of Wales, who was unhappy at being separated from his mistress Mrs Wallis Simpson, there was no evidence of such strain and in particular, as Dawson noted in his diary, Queen Mary remained calm and kindly throughout. The earlier death suited Dawson. Having issued his famous bulletin he had a vested interest in ensuring that death occurred sooner rather than later. At the same time it allowed him to get back to his busy private practice in London.

1 grain≡65mg

Although Dawson spoke against euthanasia when it was debated in the House of Lords in December 1936, he clearly felt that it or something similar might sometimes be appropriate for his own patients and there is no reason to think that King George V was the only patient he treated in this way. He described his management of the king's final illness as 'a facet of euthanasia or so called mercy killing.' But even the most ardent supporter of euthanasia would hesitate to describe the killing of an unconscious patient, without the patient's prior knowledge or consent, as mercy killing. Indeed, when examined closely this and almost all similar cases turn out in the end to be examples, not of mercy killing but of convenience killing. This was so in this case and the person most convenienced was Dawson.

The ethical line which separates acceptable from unacceptable conduct is sometimes a narrow one. What caused Dawson to stray across the line is a matter of speculation but the likely answer is that he was guilty of the besetting sin of doctors and that is of arrogance. Although in daily contact with the great and good of the land, including the Archbishop of Canterbury who was living at Sandringham at the time, he arrogantly assumed that he, and he alone, had the special insight to appreciate the importance of the timing of the king's death. It was also unfeeling of Dawson to involve Sister Black in his plan and arrogant to assume that her conscience was as elastic as his own.

This whole episode seems a piece of pointless folly which Dawson was wise to conceal at the time. The emergence of the truth 50 years later did nothing to enhance his reputation nor did his half hearted espousal of euthanasia do anything to diminish the opprobrium which rightly attaches to doctors who break the sixth commandment.

J H R Ramsay

BMJ (1994); **308**: 1445, with permission from the BMJ Publishing Group.

Consent and competence

> A patient is able to give *valid consent* to a procedure if he is *informed*, *uncoerced*, and *competent*.

'Informed' means that a patient has all the relevant information, given in an appropriate form, with which to make a decision.

'Uncoerced' means that the person is free to make decisions without any undue influence or pressure from any other person.

'Competence' (the medical term) or 'capacity' (the legal term) may conveniently be considered in five sections:

1 The patient must be able to understand the issue in question
2 The patient needs to be able to retain the information in memory for long enough to use it in making a decision
3 The patient needs to be able to *believe* the information given
4 The patient needs to be able to weigh the information in the balance and aggregate arguments for and against in order to reach a decision
5 The patient must be able to express the decision in some form

If a patient is not competent to be involved in discussions regarding medical care, in England a medical decision should be taken in the 'best interests' of the patient. It is best practice for the multidisciplinary team and the family to be involved in these discussions. The family cannot make decisions for incompetent patients but, where possible, they should be consulted to find out what the patient would have wanted. It often focuses the minds of a distressed family to ask questions such as 'What do you think your mother would want, given this situation?'

Points to :
- It is perfectly in order to provide all measures to enhance competence by managing the environment e.g. optimize the senses (glasses/ hearing aids), comfortable familiar environment with good lighting and heating, and bringing an advocate to the meeting, writing materials, interpreter etc.
- Patients are entitled to make seemingly illogical decisions provided they are made with competence
- Patients may be competent even if they are mentally ill
- Patients may have lucid intervals

Specific situations

In palliative medicine we may be asked to assess competence in order that a patient can, for instance, make a will, change a codicil to a will, execute an Enduring Power of Attorney or write an Advance Directive. All the above points apply.

Making a will

Clinical staff are generally advised not to witness the signing of a will for fear of legal complications. In palliative care, however, we are endeavouring to support patients and their families through a very difficult time and it may be helpful for us to assist. In this situation, a senior doctor, if witnessing a signature, would be advised to do this only if they have assessed competency. The competency then needs to be documented.

Enduring Power of Attorney

As above, doctors witnessing the signing of these documents should ensure and document that the patient is fully competent. (📖 See also Chapter 16.)

Advance Directives (Living Wills)

Again, doctors need to assess and document competency. (📖 See also Chapter 16.)

Euthanasia

He jests at scars, that never felt a wound.

Shakespeare, *Romeo and Juliet*

Etymologically, the term euthanasia derives from the ancient Greek, '*Eu*', meaning good and '*thanatos*', meaning death, thus a 'good death'. Today, the term euthanasia refers to the administration of death, the active intentional ending of life. It is a final and irreversible step and the subject of great debate, engendering on one hand strong feelings about the right to demand death and, on the other, strong feelings that life is so precious that we have a duty to preserve it at all costs. It must not be forgotten that patients are often making decisions regarding euthanasia on the basis of inadequate prognostic information, since medical advances will never be able to identify accurately when an individual patient will die naturally.

Proponents of euthanasia feel that
Euthanasia is the only alternative to avoiding a painful death
Comment: Although the control of pain is not perfect, patients can usually achieve a degree of relief acceptable to them. Public education has started to erode the myth that all patients with cancer inevitably die in considerable pain, although this fear is still held strongly by some.

In practice, even patients with distressing symptoms and an apparent high level of suffering rarely request euthanasia consistently.

Euthanasia is the only answer to the fear of being kept alive at all costs
Comment: Extraordinary advances in medicine over the last few centuries have pushed forward the frontiers, extending the quantity of life and potentially, therefore, the extension of an 'unacceptable' poor quality of life. Medical ethics, however, has also advanced, allowing competent patients to refuse treatment and supporting the concept that burdensome, futile treatment is bad medicine. Assuming that healthcare professionals act with multidisciplinary support within an ethical framework, the fear of being kept alive at all costs should be minimized.

Euthanasia is the only way to die with dignity
Comment: Families are torn between not wanting to see their loved ones deteriorate and wanting them to survive as long as possible to nurture precious time. A natural death and all the potential healing and strengthening of family unity that so often occurs during the final days is often worthwhile and dignified, a sentiment supported by most healthcare professionals experienced in the care of the dying. Furthermore, the efficacy of drugs used to carry out euthanasia is unpredictable. There are literature reports of failure to achieve coma and patients reawakening in considerable discomfort, which can hardly be described as dignified.

Euthanasia should be legalized to uphold the principle of autonomy
Comment: In the West, individual rights have been elevated to a central tenet of society, implying that the individual has the right to control their own destiny. In society, however, others also have rights and the concept of a healthcare professional delivering euthanasia as a technical act may not be in the best interests of individuals or society.

Euthanasia, if carried out, should rightly occur only when the patient is fully competent and consistently requests it. However, patients who are ill, often bed-bound, unable to care for themselves and wholly reliant on others for care may feel a burden and under pressure to acquiesce.

A diagnosis of a reversible clinical depression may be missed if families and healthcare professionals are slow to recognize it. The concept of the 'slippery slope' argument, in which patients may be subjected to euthanasia without their expressed consent and within a short time of having had the discussions, has already been reported in the literature.

Whatever the arguments, the fundamental principles are that life is infinitely precious and that the vulnerable deserve protection. We should always consider the views of our competent patients and act in the best interests of those who are not able to give consent.

It is also fundamentally important to recognize what is *not* euthanasia, which includes the following, where the primary intention is to prevent suffering.

Euthanasia is not

- Witholding or withdrawing futile, burdensome treatment including nutrition and hydration if the patient is dying and is unable to swallow
- Giving opioids, or any other medications, to control symptoms including pain, fear, and overwhelming distress
- Sedating a patient in the terminal stages if all other practical methods of controlling symptoms have failed
- Issuing a *Do Not Resuscitate* order

The Royal Dutch Medical Association has formulated five requirements that must be fulfilled for euthanasia to be acceptable or legally excusable. These are:

1 There is voluntary, competent and durable request on the part of the patient
2 The request is based on full information
3 The patient is in a situation of intolerable and hopeless suffering (physical or mental)
4 There are no acceptable alternatives
5 The physician has consulted another physician before performing euthanasia

The physician has to notify the local medical examiner and complete an extensive questionnaire. It is then reported to the public prosecutor who decides if prosecution is necessary. This notification procedure has formal legal status and also covers cases involving euthanasia without the patient's explicit request.

In some States in the USA, physicians are allowed to prescribe medication to hasten death in terminally ill adults.

A Time to Go

Doctor you must help me,
And there's something you must know,
My mind's made up I'm certain,
It's time for me to go.

I'm old and tired and weary,
I've lived a life first rate,
But there's just no denying,
I'm well past my sell-by date.
Just give me the tablet,
Just send me off to sleep
For I don't want to go on living
And I want to 'shut-eye' for keeps.

Now Doctor I've been thinking,
How I'd like it all to be.
Vivaldi in the background
Test Match special on TV.
With the smell of cut grass wafting
And a cup of Earl Grey tea,
Doctor you've got to help,
You've got to help poor me.

Now Doctor please, please listen.
I know you think euthanasia's wrong,
But just between ourselves
How d'you expect me to carry on?
My bridge partners just left me.
My son's off in Ceylon,
English cricket's just appalling
And my get up and go has gone.
To crown it all last Thursday,
A lady from meals on wheels,
Came offering gammon and pineapple,
I mean Doc, how would *you* feel?

So pronto I called my GP
Something must be done no doubt
And I was sent to Hospice,
As he said 'To get sorted out'.

So Doctor I am waiting
I don't want this to drag on and on
I've made up my will, killed the cat,
And my mind is set upon,
A peaceful departure from this long dark vale of tears
And just in case you'll ask me,
I've no doubts, no bills, no fears.

Doctor you've got to help me.
Last night I couldn't sleep.
There was such an infernal racket
And I thought I heard someone weep.

And then again this morning,
That nice woman in number nine?
She wasn't there to talk to
About her illness which was a bit like mine.
I glimpsed a hearse pass by the window
Please tell me it's not true
Are people here really dying?
O what am I to do?

Doctor you've got to help me
I've got to get out of here.
Though you're all most pleasant
This is just not for me I fear.
My pains have eased
My mind is clear
Doctor,
Why on earth are you keeping me here?

Doctor you must help me,
And there's something you must know
My mind's made up I'm certain
It's time for me to go.

M. Watson
2002

Breaking bad news

> I have received two wonderful graces. First, I have been given time to prepare for a new future. Secondly, I find myself—uncharacteristically—calm and at peace.
>
> Cardinal Basil Hume, breaking the news of his imminent death from cancer to the priests of Westminster diocese, 16 April 1999

Patients and relatives need time to absorb information and to adapt to bad news. Health professionals need good communication skills, including sensitivity and empathic active listening.

Breaking bad news takes time, and issues often need to be discussed further and clarified as more information is imparted.

There is increasing evidence that most patients want to know about their illness. Many patients who have been denied this knowledge have difficulty in understanding why they are becoming weaker and are then relieved and grateful to be told the truth. They may be angry with the family who have known about the illness all along and have not thought it right to tell them.

Professionals often become involved unwittingly in a potential conspiracy of silence when the family demand information before the patient has been appraised of the situation. The family might say, 'Do not tell him the diagnosis/prognosis because he will not be able to cope with it. We know him better than you do.' The family needs to know that their concerns, of not wanting to cause any more hurt to the patient, have been heard. They also need to be aware that the bad news may be more painful for themselves than for the patient. The family also need to know that it would be unwise for clinical staff to be untruthful if the patient appeared to want to know the truth and was asking direct questions, because of the inevitable breakdown in trust that this could cause.

Advising patients and families with regard to prognosis is important since they may want (and often need) to organize their affairs and plan for the time that is left. However, it is *not possible to be accurate with prognosis*. Overestimating or underestimating the time that someone has to live can cause untold anguish. It is therefore more sensible to talk in terms of days/weeks, weeks/months, and months/years as appropriate.

There is a balance to be made between fully informing the patient about their disease and prognosis, completely overwhelming them with facts and figures, or providing only minimal and inadequate information.

While it is important to avoid being patronizing, it is also important not to cause distress by 'information overload'.

It is important to be aware that people have divergent attitudes to receiving bad news and that this needs sensitive handling. Patients and families respond badly to being told bad news in a hurried, brusque and unsympathetic manner with no time to collect their thoughts and ask questions. However sensitively bad news is imparted, patients and families are naturally devastated and the impact of the news can obliterate a great deal of the communication that took place. Patients may either not remember or misinterpret what has been said, particularly if they use denial as a coping technique.

A strategy for breaking bad news

Nothing in all the world is more dangerous than sincere ignorance and conscientious stupidity.

Martin Luther King 1929–68: *Strength to love (1963)*

Outlining a strategy for breaking bad news is difficult because it turns a process which should be natural and unforced into something which seems constrained and awkward. The following advice encompasses the techniques that health professionals have found, through trial and error, to be helpful. It can be used as a guide to develop an individual's personal confidence and skills in breaking bad news.

The goals of breaking bad news

The process of breaking bad news needs to be specifically tailored to the needs of the individual concerned, for every human being will have a different history and collection of fears and concerns. The goal of breaking bad news is to do so in a way that facilitates acceptance and understanding and reduces the risk of destructive responses.

The ability to break bad news well involves skills which need to be coveted and trained for, audited and kept up to date with as much objective determination as that shown by a surgeon in acquiring and maintaining surgical skills. The consequences of performing the process badly may have immediate and long term damaging effects for all involved, every bit as catastrophic as surgery going wrong. For example, patients and families may lose trust. Having awareness of strategies to complete the process well is vital, but breaking bad news must never become so routinized that patients, or their families, detect little individual caring compassion.

Break bad news well and you will always be remembered, break bad news badly and you will never be forgotten.

Preparing to tell bad news

Acquire all the information possible about the patient and their family. (A genogram is particularly useful in quickly assimilating the important people in the patient's life, and the web of relationships within the family.)

Read the patient's notes for

- Diagnostic information
- Test results
- Understanding of the patient's clinical history
- The support system for the individual
- Background knowledge of the patient's life—making basic mistakes will undermine the patient's confidence)
- Understanding of spoken language, e.g. English. If not, arrange for an interpreter to be present

Discuss with other members of the team, and then select the most appropriate team member to break the bad news. Decide which other member of the team should be present during the interview. Ensure there is an interpreter or advocate present for those with special needs or language difficulties.

Check that you have

- A place of privacy where there will be no interruptions. Unplug the telephone and switch off the mobile phone etc.
- Tissues, a jug of water, and drinking glasses
- Time to carry out the process
- Your own emotional energy to do so—this job is better done earlier in the day than late
- Pressing tasks are completed so that there will be minimal interruptions

Plan

Prepare a rough plan in your mind of what you want to achieve in the communication, and what you want to avoid communicating. Having a rough goal will bring structure to the communication, though it is important to avoid imposing your agenda on the patient's agenda.

Setting the context

- Invite the patient to the place of privacy
- Introduce yourself clearly
- Let the patient know that they have your attention and how long you have got
- Ensure that the patient is comfortable and not distracted by pain or a full bladder etc.
- Give a 'warning shot' indication that this is not a social or routine encounter
- Sit at the same eye level as each other within easy reach

A *warning shot* is concerned with preparing a patient that bad news is coming. This allows them to be more receptive than if it comes 'out of the blue'. An example would be, 'I'm sorry to say that the results were not as good as we had hoped.'

Assess

- How much the patient knows already
- How much the patient wants to know
- How the patient expresses him/herself and what words and ways he/she uses to understand the situation

'Are you the sort of person that likes to know everything?'

Acquire empathy with the patient

- What would it be like to be the patient?
- How is the patient feeling?
- Is there anything that is concerning the patient which he or she is not verbalizing?
- What mechanisms has the patient used in the past to deal with bad news?
- Does the patient have a particular outlook on life or cultural understanding which underpins his or her approach to dealing with the situation?

- Who are the important people in the patient's life?
  Respond to *non-verbal* as well as *verbal* clues

Encourage the patient to speak by listening carefully and responding appropriately.

Sharing information

- Having spent time listening, use the patient's words to recap the story of the journey so far, checking regularly with the patient that you have heard the story correctly

'Would you mind if I repeated back to you what I have heard you tell me to make sure I have understood things correctly?'

- Slowly and gradually draw out the information from the patient while regularly checking that they are not misunderstanding what you are saying
- Use the 'warning shot' technique to preface bad news to help the patient prepare themself
- Use diagrams to help understanding and retention of information if appropriate and acceptable to the patient
- Avoid jargon and acronyms which are easily misunderstood
- Do not bluff. It is acceptable to say 'I do not know, and I will try to get an answer for you for our next meeting'

Remember to ensure that

- The patient understands the implications of what you are saying
- The patient is in control of the speed at which information is being imparted
- The patient can see that you are being empathic to their emotional response. It can be very appropriate to say something like 'Being told something like this can seem overwhelming'
- You address the patient's real concerns, which may be very different from what you expect them to be
- You offer a record of the consultation, for example a tape recording or short written notes if appropriate

Response

- You should respond to the patient's feelings and response to the news
- You should acknowledge the patient's feelings
- You should be prepared to work through the patient's emotional response to the bad news with them

'It can be very distressing to get such news, and it is not unusual to feel very angry, or lonely or sad on hearing such news.'

Let the patient speak first

Use open questions, such as:-
'How are you feeling today?'
'Can you tell me how this all came about?'
'How do you see things going from here?'

Make concrete plans for the next step

'Your appointment to see Dr. Brown the oncologist is provisionally booked for next Thursday at 2 o'clock. How would that fit in with your other arrangements?'

Immediate plans

'What are you doing now?' 'How are you getting home?' 'Who will you tell?' 'How will you tell them?' 'What will you say?' 'How will they cope?'
Such questions can help the patient to start formulating the answers that they will need for their family or friends.

Summarize

For the patient
- Try to get the patient to repeat the key points to ensure they have understood

For other healthcare professionals
- Record details of the conversation in the patient's notes clearly
- Convey information quickly to those who need to know, most importantly the GP

Deception is not as creative as truth. We do best in life if we look at it with clear eyes, and I think that applies to coming up to death as well.

Cicely Saunders, in *Time* 5 September 1988

Deal with questions
- 'Are there any questions which you would like me to deal with at this point?'

Contract for the future

'I know the news today was not what you were hoping for but you are not going to go through this on your own. We are there for you, your family is there for you and we are going to go through this together. Dr. Brown will be seeing you next Thursday and I'll see you back here on Monday morning.'

- Closing remarks should identify support networks, including contact telephone numbers and times of easy access. Be fairly concrete about the next meeting but also allow the patient the option to postpone if they do not feel able to attend

10 Steps to breaking bad news (Adapted from Peter Kaye, 1996)

1 Preparation
Know all the facts before the meeting. READ THE MEDICAL RECORDS. Find out who the patient wants to be present. Ensure comfort and privacy. Minimize the risk of interruptions.

2 What does the patient know?
Ask the patient for a brief narrative of events (e.g. 'how did it all start?').

3 Give a warning shot
e.g. 'I am afraid it looks rather serious'—then allow a pause for the patient to respond.

4 Allow denial
Allow the patient to control the amount of information and to proceed at his/her own pace.

5 Explain (if requested) and check understanding
Narrow the information gap step-by-step. Use diagrams if the patient thinks it would be helpful. Use simple language.

6 Is more information wanted?
It can be very frightening to ask for more information and the patient may not want to know any more. Inquire gently, by asking if they would like further information.

7 Listen to concerns
Ask, 'what are the things that bother you most at the moment?'. This could be to do with their physical or emotional health or relate to social or spiritual issues.

8 Encourage ventilation of feelings
This conveys empathy and may be the key phase in terms of patient satisfaction with the interview. Check that there is nothing else that the patient wants to talk about.

9 Summary and plan
Summarize concerns, plan treatment, and foster hope. Check with the patient that he/she would have no objection to your talking with the family either alone or together.

10 Offer availability
Most patients need further explanation (the details will not have been remembered) and support (adjustment takes weeks or months), and benefit greatly from a family meeting.

Further reading

Books

Bacon F. (1912) *Of Death*. In *Essays*, London: Black.

Heaven C. and Maguire P. (2003) Communication issues. In M. Lloyd Williams (ed.) *Psychosocial Issues in Palliative Care*. pp. 13–34. Oxford: Oxford University Press.

Kaye P. (1996) *Breaking bad news. A 10 step approach*. Northampton: EPL Publications.

Wilkes E. (1982) *The Dying Patient: The medical management of incurable and terminal illness*. Lancaster: MTP Press.

Worden J. W. (2002) *Grief Counseling and Grief Therapy*, 3rd edn. London: Routledge.

Reviews

Saunderson E. M., Ridsdale L. (1999) General Practitioners' beliefs and attitudes about how to respond to death and bereavement: qualitative study. *BMJ*, **319**: 293–6.

Articles

Charlton R. and Dolamn E. (1995) Bereavement: a protocol for primary care. *British Journal of General Practice*, **45**: 427–30.

Jewell D. (1999) Commentary: Use of personal experience should be legitimized. *BMJ*, **319**: 296.

Raphael B. (1977) Preventive intervention with the recently bereaved. *Archives of General Psychiatry*, **34**: 1450–4.

Research in palliative care

In the culture I grew up in you did your work and you did not put your arm around it to stop people from looking—you took the earliest opportunity to make knowledge available.

James Black, On modern medical research, *Daily Telegraph*, 11 December 1995

Good medical practice requires evidence of effectiveness to address deficits in care, strive for further improvements, and justly apportion finite resources.

The Declaration of Helsinki was drawn up by the World Medical Association in 1964 in response to the need for a code of ethics on human experimentation. This is particularly pertinent in the field of palliative care, where the core practice is looking after the dying. It acknowledges the need for guidance for the physician caught in the conflict between patients' own best interests and the necessity to advance knowledge for society as a whole. Research must conform to strict ethical principles and be scrutinized by independent assessors.

The origins of palliative care research in the modern UK Hospice movement date from the founding of St Christopher's Hospice in 1967. Dame Cicely Saunders advocated scientific observation and systematic research as an essential component of the specialty. The burgeoning interest in the provision of palliative care services and the national agenda for practising evidence-based care has stimulated the development of collaborative, often multidisciplinary, research committees between clinical units and academic institutions.

The Palliative Care Research Forum of Britain and Ireland developed in 1991; the science committee for the Association for Palliative Medicine and the Palliative Care Forum of the Royal Society of Medicine were created in 1996 and 1997 respectively. On a local palliative care network level, there are numerous research committees which are either self standing or have grouped in response to the initiatives of the Supportive and Palliative care remit of the National Cancer Plan. The importance and principle of research is now inherent in specialist training.

Palliative care research largely encompasses: the control of symptoms, ethical issues, clinical decision making, communication, family and carer issues, interdisciplinary team issues, health systems and services and existential and spiritual concerns both before and after death.

Evidence-based medicine

Evidence-based practice is the conscious, explicit and judicious use of current best evidence in making decisions about the care of individual patients.

The gold standard of evidence for the harm or efficiency of an intervention is the randomized controlled trial (RCT), though RCTs are not the only method of such assessment. There are many factors apart from the results of RCTs which must be accorded due weight in decisions affecting the care of patients. The key element of evidence-based medicine is to integrate the best available evidence with patient preference. The nature of palliative care lends itself more readily to investigation by those methods which are considered by some to hold less weight such as the descriptive study. An overview of quantitative and qualitative research methodology and the difficulties encountered in palliative care research will be outlined.

Table 3.1 The five strengths of research evidence

Type	Strength of evidence
I	Strong evidence from at least one systematic review of multiple well-designed randomized controlled trials
II	Strong evidence from at least one properly designed randomized controlled trial of appropriate size
III	Evidence for well designed trials without randomization, single group pre-post, cohort, time series or matched case-control studies
IV	Evidence from well-designed non-experimental studies from more than one centre or research group
V	Opinions of respected authorities, based on clinical evidence, descriptive studies or reports of expert committees

The Agency for Health Care Policy and Research (AHCPR) 1997

Quantitative methodology

The biomedical model of scientific research aims to define objective reality which can be discovered, measured and understood through scientific method. Rigorous, systematic examination allows the identification and assessment of the probability of causal relationships between variables through statistical analysis. Quantitative researchers are rigid in adhering to the original focus of the research question and maintain an objective distance from the research itself. Quantitative research is *deductive* and based on questions/hypotheses of existing theory and knowledge. Examples of quantitative designed research include RCTs, experiments and surveys on representative samples.

Arguments against over reliance on quantitative trials in palliative care include the following:

1 Quantitative trials should not be considered as the only method of assessing scientific validity.
2 Quantitative trials do not lend themselves to issues such as quality of life, emotional distress, and other domains of the patient's experience.
3 It would be impractical and unethical to engender doubt on the efficacy of almost all already widely-used treatments in palliative care solely on the basis that they had not been submitted to quantitative trials.
4 It is almost impossible to isolate a single variable and watch the effect of it changing, particularly in the frail, elderly, clinically deteriorating and dying. A variety of methods is needed to assess the usefulness of interventions.
5 It is frequently not possible to recruit the number of patients that are required for statistical significance to a quantitative trial.
6 Quantitative research, while extremely important, is not suited to answering all types of research question, particularly those relating to patient experience.
7 It could be considered as unethical to subject patients to a trial with a placebo arm—i.e. a trial arm with no active treatment—especially in dying patients.

In order to encompass these difficulties in palliative care, research methods other than purely quantitative must be used.

Systematic reviews

These aim to locate and appraise research evidence to provide informative empirical answers to scientific research questions. They adhere to strict scientific design to make them more comprehensive, to minimize bias and to ensure reliability. The protocol defines a clear question and the methodology is explicit. Research from all sources is obtained and this may involve the use of electronic databases as well as personal searches according to a pre-defined protocol. Systematic reviews can be regarded as reliable summaries of research evidence.

Qualitative research

He uses statistics as a drunken man uses lampposts—for support rather than for illumination

Andrew Lang, 1844–1912, attributed

'Quantitative' research uses often uncritically respected, 'tried and tested' techniques of measurement, data collection and analysis. 'Qualitative' research techniques, which are often more suited to palliative care, incorporate the subjective experience, which cannot be measured so easily within a mathematical framework. Evidence from qualitative research studies has not been bestowed with the weight of evidence attributed to quantitative research, although the techniques are rigorous and are gradually becoming more accepted. Qualitative research can be extremely demanding if carried out well, with major time and cost implications, especially for the process of analysis. Specific aims (generic goals) and objectives (specific ends or outcomes) and precision and clarity are important whether or not the methodology, data collection and analysis is qualitative or quantitative.

Qualitative research takes account of ways in which the research subject makes sense of their individual experience. There is interaction between the researcher and the subject. Ideas and concepts develop as the research progresses and these may then be redirected back to further inform the research findings. Words are used as opposed to numerical data. The method is *inductive*, to discover new knowledge and to ground it in the subjective experience. Qualitative research has the power to disrupt existing assumptions and to challenge what has been considered as reliable, factual material. It also lends itself to the imaginative expression of language, making research findings more widely interesting and relevant to those accustomed to the more precise biomedical model of research reporting.

Qualitative and quantitative research methods can be combined to offer a different perspective and to enhance knowledge in a more holistic way.

A range of techniques, guided by set principles, exist. Examples of such techniques include:

1 Observation—Researchers are involved in a field work setting within, for instance a ward, recording conversations, encounters, non-verbal communication, spatial arrangements and physical environment. Aspects such as the quality of care of patients can be explored in this way.

2 Participant observation—Researchers become an active subject within the study group. For instance, they may join in with practical tasks in a ward or day hospice setting with the sole purpose of observing and not influencing.

3 Interviews—This is the most widely adopted method within qualitative research. Interviews may be interactive, with opportunities to develop or deepen the discussion according to the subject in question. Bereavement issues may usefully be conducted in this way.

4 Focus groups—Group interviews have the capacity to generate large amounts of data. Tape-recorded transcripts may be analysed. A number of computer packages exist to sort and code items for analysis, which facilitates the handling of large volumes of data. The researcher acts as the facilitator, usually for a group of about eight people. Ideas and experiences can be explored. For instance, a multidisciplinary group of healthcare professionals might explore issues surrounding the attitudes to such issues as organ donation at the end-of-life.

5 Documentary analysis.

6 Case studies—Case studies serve to structure research problems and can involve observation, interviewing and the analysis of documentary sources. Detailed explanation of a single case can accrue data from a variety of perspectives, using different qualitative methods to focus on a common issue or research question. The particular case can then be understood in its wider context. For instance, a case study of a single hospice might look at defined aspects of care and how they interrelate across different care settings to provide consistent, holistic care for patients.

Quantitative and Qualitative Research Differences

QUANTITATIVE RESEARCH	QUALITATIVE RESEARCH
Tests theories	Develops theories
Rigid methods	Flexible methods
Experiments	In depth interviews
Surveys	Observation
Large samples	Small samples
Numbers	Words
Statistics	Meaning

Argument for palliative care research

Basic research is what I am doing when I don't know what I am doing.

Wernher von Braun, A Random Walk in Silence, 1973

Research is an unavoidable imperative if progress is to be made.
- The terminally ill should not be considered as 'special' and shielded from studies (although there should be stringent criteria for the research design and ethical scrutiny)
- Patients receive considerable attention which they may appreciate
- A new treatment might benefit the patient
- Autonomy—patients should be given the chance to be involved in studies
- Patients and families often genuinely want to 'give' in order that others can get better care

Difficulties in palliative care research

Practical considerations

- Attrition of patients from studies leading to difficulties in recruiting adequate numbers of patients, particularly to quantitative studies
- Eligibility criteria for inclusion into studies, particularly if the patient is deteriorating, restricts the inclusion of adequate numbers
- Measures of end points and outcomes are often complicated in an already complex clinical scenario
- Funding has been limited
- Compliance of deteriorating patients may be difficult to sustain

Ethical and emotional considerations

- Patients are often considered too unwell, with distressing symptoms, to be asked to partake in research
- Some professionals feel that patients with a short prognosis should not have extra burdens placed on them
- Patients are vulnerable and may be exploited
- The research may be of no benefit to the patient taking part
- Questionnaires if used may be painful and intrusive either for patients, families or in bereavement
- Fully informed consent may be difficult to obtain; patients may try to please researchers by agreeing to take part without really wanting to; some patients feel that they may be punished or ignored if they do not take part; acute symptoms do not allow for adequate time for patients to decide whether or not they want to be involved; patients are not infrequently cognitively impaired
- Trying a new treatment may engender false hope
- Research may encourage the patient to focus on their illness instead of enjoying precious time
- Information given by the patient's proxy may be misleading

There is limited evidence based in the delivery of palliative care, thus potentially exposing patients to toxic treatment of unknown benefit. We have an ethical imperative to provide the best care for our patients. Although research in palliative care is fraught with practical, ethical and emotional issues, we can only improve care by carrying out studies; these must be carefully designed to be of minimal burden and to provide maximum use of precious research opportunities.

Despite the difficulties, an evidence base is forming in such areas as ethical issues, control of symptoms, palliative rehabilitation, clinical decision-making, communication, family and caregiving issues, interdisciplinary team working, health systems and existential and spiritual issues.

Provided that palliative care investigators compassionately apply ethical principles to their research, there is no justification for not endeavouring to improve the standards of palliation.

Further reading

Dollery C. T. (1979) A bleak outlook for placebos (and for science). *European Journal of Clinical Pharmacology*, **15**: 219–21.

Greenhalgh T. and Donald A. (2000) Evidence based healthcare workbook: understanding research: for individual and group learning. London: BMJ Books.

Jones B., Jarvis P. Trials to assess equivalence: the importance of rigorous methods. *BMJ*, **313**: 36–9.

Rothman K. J. and Michels K. B. (1994) Sounding board: the continuing unethical use of placebo controls. *NEJM*, **331**: 394–8.

Principles of drug use in palliative medicine[1]

We can no more hope to end drug abuse by eliminating heroin and cocaine than we could alter the suicide rate by outlawing high buildings or the sale of rope.

Ben Whittaker, *The global fix*, 1987

Drugs are not the total answer for the relief of pain and other symptoms. For many symptoms, the concurrent use of non-drug measures is equally important, and sometimes more so. Further, drugs must always be used within the context of a systematic approach to symptom management, namely:

- evaluation
- explanation
- individualized treatment
- attention to detail

In palliative care, the axiom 'diagnosis before treatment' still holds true. Even when the cancer is responsible, a particular symptom may have different causes, e.g. in lung cancer vomiting may be caused by hypercalcaemia or by raised intracranial pressure—to name but two of many possible causes. Clearly, treatment will vary according to the cause.

Attention to detail includes *precision in taking a drug history*. It is important to ascertain, as precisely as possible, the drug being taken, the dose and the frequency and to confirm that the drug alleviates the symptom throughout the day and night. It is very common for patients to be non-compliant with medication for many different reasons. In palliative care, patients may not have understood the reason for taking medication regularly to prevent symptoms. The medication consequently may not help adequately, leaving him/her either to suffer in pain, thinking that the drug does not work, or to take inappropriately large extra doses which cause side-effects. Patients may also stop taking the drugs because of the side-effects. Vicious circles may develop, adding to patient and family despair. As the patient becomes weaker and less well they may become less able to swallow large numbers of tablets, leading again to less than optimal symptom control.

Attention to detail also means *providing clear instructions for drug regimens*. 'Take as much as you like, as often as you like', is a recipe for anxiety and poor symptom relief. The drug regimen should be written out in full for the patient and his family to work from (Figure 4.1). This should be in an ordered and logical way, e.g. analgesics, antiemetics, laxatives, followed by other drugs. The drug name, times to be taken, reason for use ('for pain', 'for bowels' etc.) and dose (x ml, y tablets) should all be stated. The patient should also be advised how to obtain further supplies e.g. from the General Practitioner.

[1] General guidance about the use of drugs in palliative care (www.palliativedrugs.com).

When prescribing an additional drug, it is important to ask:
- What is the treatment goal?
- How can it be monitored?
- What is the risk of adverse effects?
- What is the risk of drug interactions?
- Is it possible to stop any of the current medications?

Good prescribing is a skill, and makes the difference between poor and excellent symptom control. It extends to considering size, shape and taste of tablets and solutions; and avoiding awkward doses which force:
- patients to take more tablets than would be the case if doses were 'rounded up' to a more convenient tablet size. For example, it is better to prescribe m/r morphine 60mg (a single tablet) rather than 50mg (3 tablets: 30mg + 10mg + 10mg)
- nurses to spend more time refilling syringes for 24h infusions. For example, in the UK, it might be appropriate to prescribe diamorphine 100mg (a single ampoule) instead of 95mg (60mg ampoule + 30mg ampoule + 5mg ampoule)

It is necessary to be equally thorough when re-evaluating a patient and supervising treatment, because it is often difficult to predict the optimum dose of a symptom relief drug, particularly opioids, laxatives and psychotropic drugs. Some drugs, e.g. steroids, may be given as a trial only and continued or stopped as appropriate after a certain time. Arrangements must be made, therefore, for continuing supervision and adjustment of medication.

Finally, it may be necessary to compromise on complete symptom relief in order to avoid unacceptable adverse effects. For example, the sedative side-effects of levomepromazine or the dry mouth caused by octreotide may limit dose escalation in inoperable bowel obstruction. The patient may prefer to reduce the frequency of nausea or vomiting to an acceptable level (i.e. vomit once a day) rather than to tolerate side-effects of higher doses of effective medication.

The drugs mentioned in this text are listed alphabetically in the formulary and are based on as robust evidence as is currently available. Many of these drugs are used outside their current product licences.

Medication
Information
Chart

Patient details/Identification label

Mr Albert Brown

1 Park Road

Anytown AB1 2CD

General Advice

- Keep this chart with you so that you can show your doctor or nurse a list of your medications.
- If you need a further supply, give your GP at least 48 h notice.
- If your chemist has difficulty in obtaining your medicines, please ask him to contact the palliative care pharmacist, on tel: .... or in the evening/at weekends contact the on-call pharmacist at .... Hospital via the switchboard on tel: ....
- Occasionally your medication may be supplied in different strengths or presentations. If you have any concerns about this, check with your local pharmacist or district nurse.
- If you need to see a doctor, telephone your GP first unless advised otherwise.
- If you, or your family doctor, need any advice, please ring tel: .... and ask to speak to the Hospice Community **Team nurse.**

Regular Medication

Description (Trade Name)	STRENGTH	REASON	ON WAKING	LUNCH 2pm	TEA 6pm	BED TIME
Morphine Sulphate MR (MST) Purple tablet	30mg	Pain Relief *take 12 h apart*	1			1
Diclofenac Round brown tablet	50mg	Bone Pain	1		1	1
Sodium Valproate (Epilim) Lilac tablet	200mg	Nerve Pain				2
Codanthramer Orange liquid	Strong	For Bowels			TWO 5ml spoons	
Domperidone (Motilium) Small white tablet	10mg	Stop Sickness	2	2	2	2

As Needed

Morphine Solution (Oramorph) Clear liquid	10mg in 5ml	Breakthrough Pain	Take ONE 5ml spoon every 2–4 h if needed			
Avilone suspension White liquid		Indigestion	Take TWO 5ml spoonfuls FOUR times a day			

Completed by: _S Thorp_   Nurse/Pharmacist   Checked by _M Smith_   On: _24.2.05_

Fig. 4.1 Sample Medication Information Chart. Adapted with permission from HAYWARD HOUSE Macmillan Specialist Palliative Care Unit, City Hospital NHS Trust Nottingham.

The use of drugs beyond licence

If a lot of cures are suggested for a disease, it means that the disease is incurable.
Anton Chekov, *The cherry orchard*, 1904

The Medicines and Healthcare Products regulatory Agency in the UK grants a product licence for a medical drug. The purpose of the drug licence is to regulate the activity of the pharmaceutical company when marketing the drug. The licence does not restrict the prescription of the drug by properly qualified medical practitioners. Licenced drugs can be used legally in clinical situations that fall outside the remit of the licence (referred to as 'off-label'), for example a different age group, a different indication, a different dose or route or method of administration. Use of unlicenced drugs refers to those products that have no licence for any clinical situation or may be in the process of evaluation leading to such a licence.

A recent audit in palliative care found that 'off-label' use is common (around 25 per cent of prescriptions affecting 66 per cent of patients in one specialist palliative care unit), but the use of unlicenced drugs is rare. Recommendations from bodies such as the General Medical Council and the medical defence organizations place a duty on doctors to act responsibly and to provide information to patients on the nature and associated risks of any treatment, including 'off-label' and unlicenced drugs.

Guidance also recommends that such drugs are prescribed by a consultant or GP, following informed consent by the patient, and that this decision is recorded in the patient's notes. This may not be practical in palliative care where the use of 'off-label' medication is routine.

Prescribing outside the licence

In the UK, a doctor may legally:
* prescribe unlicenced medicines
* in a named patient, use unlicenced products specially prepared, imported, or supplied
* supply another doctor with an unlicenced medicine
* with appropriate safeguards, use unlicenced drugs in clinical trials
* use or advise the use of licenced medicines for indications or in doses or by routes of administration outside the licenced recommendations
* override the warnings and precautions given in the licence

The responsibility for the consequences of these actions lies with the prescribing doctor.[2,3]

It has been recommended that when prescribing a drug outside its licence, a doctor should:[4,5]
* record in the patient's notes the reasons for the decision to prescribe outside the licenced indications
* where possible explain the position to the patient (and family as appropriate) in sufficient detail to allow them to give informed consent (the Patient Information Leaflet obviously does not contain information about unlicenced indications)

- inform other professionals, e.g. pharmacist, nurses, general practitioner, involved in the care of the patient to avoid misunderstandings

In addition to clinical trials, prescriptions beyond licence may be justified:

- when prescribing generic formulations (for which indications are not described)
- with established drugs for proven but unlicenced indications
- with drugs for conditions for which there are no other treatments (even in the absence of strong evidence)
- when using drugs in individuals not covered by licenced indications, e.g. children

2 Anonymous (1992) Prescribing unlicensed drugs or using drugs for unlicensed applications. *Drug and Therapeutics Bulletin* **30**: 97–9.

3 Cohen P. J. (1997) Off-label use of prescription drugs: legal, clinical and policy considerations. *European Journal of Anaesthesiology* **14**: 231–50.

4 Atkinson C. V. and Kirkham S. R. (1999) Unlicensed uses for medication in a palliative care unit. *Palliative Medicine* **13**: 145–52.

5 Association of Palliative Medicine, Pain Society (2002) *The use of drugs beyond licence in palliaitive care and pain management.* Southampton and London: APM and Pain Society.

Drug interactions in palliative care

It may seem a strange principle to enunciate as the very first requirement in a hospital that it should do the sick no harm.

Florence Nightingale, *Notes on Hospitals*, 1863

The potential for drug interactions is high in palliative care due to polypharmacy. The following are some selected drug interactions which are pertinent to palliative care prescribing:

Warfarin

The anticoagulation effect of warfarin can be affected by many drugs. Anticoagulation may increase with:

- amiodarone
- erythromycin, clarithromycin
- cranberry juice
- dextropropoxyphene (co-proxamol)
- fluconazole, itraconazole, miconazole, ketoconazole
- metronidazole
- NSAIDs
- paracetamol
- quinolone antibiotics (e.g. ciprofloxacin)
- St. John's Wort
- testosterone

Amiodarone

A number of drugs used concomitantly with amiodarone increase the risk of ventricular arrhythmias and the advice is to avoid them:

- tricyclic antidepressants (amitriptyline etc.)
- phenothiazines, haloperidol
- flecainide
- quinine
- erythromycin (parenteral)

The low doses of haloperidol as an antiemetic, and tricyclic antidepressants for neuropathic pain, used in palliative care, probably carry a reduced risk, but one that cannot be completely dismissed.

MAOIs (antidepressants) and selegiline

There is a serious and potentially fatal interaction (serotonin syndrome) between pethidine and MAOIs. A similar reaction is seen with selegiline, an MAO-B inhibitor.

No adverse interaction normally occurs in patients on MAOIs given morphine, but there are isolated and unexplained reports of patients who became hypotensive and subsequently unconsciousness and who rapidly improved with naloxone. Some very limited evidence also suggests that no interaction occurs with methadone.

The concurrent use of MAOIs and phenothiazines is usually safe and effective. The exception appears to be levomepromazine (methotrimeprazine) which has been implicated in two fatal reactions with pargyline and tranylcypromine.

Anticonvulsants

Carbamazepine levels are increased (risk of toxicity) with:

- clarithromycin
- dextropropoxyphene (co-proxamol)
- erythromycin
- fluoxetine
- fluvoxamine

Phenytoin levels are increased (toxicity) by:

- amiodarone
- aspirin
- clarithromycin
- diltiazem
- fluconazole
- fluoxetine
- fluvoxamine
- metronidazole
- miconazole
- nifedipine
- omeprazole
- trimethoprim

Carbamazepine and phenytoin levels are decreased (risk of fits) by corticosteroids.

Carbamazepine, phenytoin and phenobarbital can reduce the efficacy of corticosteroids. This two-way interaction is common when managing patients with cerebral tumours.

Antifungal drugs

- fluconazole, miconazole increase phenytoin levels
- fluconazole and miconazole increase the effect of sulphonylureas e.g. gliclazide, glibenclamide (risk of hypoglycaemia)
- fluconazole increases celecoxib levels—halve celecoxib dose
- itraconazole, ketoconazole and possibly fluconazole increase sedation with midazolam
- fluconazole, miconazole, itraconazole, and ketoconazole all enhance warfarin anticoagulation

Proton pump inhibitors (PPIs)

- omeprazole increases blood diazepam levels (increase in sedation)
- omeprazole enhances anticoagulation effect of warfarin

Metronidazole

- disulfiram-like reaction with alcohol
- enhances anticoagulation with warfarin
- increases phenytoin blood levels (toxicity)
- increases blood levels of fluorouracil increasing toxicity

SSRI antidepressants

- fluoxetine and fluvoxamine increase carbamazepine and phenytoin blood levels (toxicity)
- fluoxetine increases plasma levels of flecainide
- serious reaction with MAOIs, selegiline (serotonin syndrome)
- increased serotonergic effects with St. John's Wort (avoid)

St. John's Wort

- increased serotonergic effects with SSRIs (avoid)
- reduced anticoagulant effect of warfarin
- reduced plasma levels of carbamazepine, phenytoin, phenobarbital (risk of fits)
- reduced plasma levels of digoxin

Dextropropoxyphene (in co-proxamol)

- increases blood levels of carbamazepine up to sixfold (toxicity)
- enhanced anticoagulation effect of warfarin

Regular paracetamol may also affect warfarin anticoagulation.

Torsades de pointes

An increasing number of drugs have been recognized to prolong the QT interval and potentially cause torsades de pointes, a serious cardiac arrhythmia. A register of drugs that cause QT prolongation is available on the internet at http://www.torsades.org

Corticosteroids

The use of corticosteroids in palliative care varies considerably from unit to unit and physician to physician. Traditionally they have been used to reduce oedema, to promote appetite and well-being; and for their specific use in disease processes such as asthma, or chronic lymphatic leukaemia or in emergency situations where their use can buy time until a more definitive treatment can be instituted.

Corticosteroids are produced by the adrenal gland and have a number of physiological rôles including catabolic effects on protein, carbohydrate and fat metabolism, and anti-inflammatory effects. They influence water and electrolyte balance and suppress immunity.

Dexamethascne is the corticosteroid of choice in palliative care.

Indication for use	Daily dose of dexamethasone
Anorexia	2–4mg
Weakness	
Pain (where caused by tumoral oedema)	
Improvement in well being/mood	
Nerve compression pain	4–8mg
Liver capsule pain	
Nausea	
Bowel obstruction	
Post-radiation inflammation	
Raised intracranial pressure	12–16mg
Superior vena caval obstruction	
Carcinomatosa lymphangitis	
Malignant spinal cord compression	

Side-effects of corticosteroids include a rise in blood glucose, increased susceptibility to infection (especially oral thrush) fluid retention and additive insult to the gastrointestinal mucosa with NSAIDs. Insomnia and agitation sometimes lead to a disturbed mental state.

Steroids may also give rise to proximal myopathy often manifesting as difficulty in standing from a sitting position. Classical Cushingoid effects may develop including a very frail skin which bleeds easily on contact. If patients are expected to be on long term steroids (longer than 6 months or so) such as patients with cerebral tumours, consideration may need to be given to prophylaxis for osteoporosis.

Equivalent anti-inflammatory effects of steroids
- Prednisolone   5mg
- Hydrocortisone   20mg
- Methylprednisolone   4mg
- Dexamethasone   750mcg
- Cortisone acetate   25mg
- Betamethasone   750mcg
- Triamcinolone   4mg

Reducing steroids

Dexamethasone above 2mg daily—reduce by 2mg every 5–7 days (and check for symptoms before the next dose reduction), until reaching 2mg

Dexamethasone doses of 2mg or less—reduce by 0.5mg every 5–7 days or on alternative days for a more conservative approach.

Consider:
- Doubling the dose for patients on phenytoin, carbamazepine or phenobarbital
- Giving steroids before midday since they may disturb sleep
- Prophylactic gastric mucosal protection if also taking NSAIDs
- Switching from dexamethasone to prednisolone if myopathy develops
- The possibility that steroids may be masking the clinical signs of perforation of an abdominal viscus or sepsis
- Carefully weigh up the burden/benefit of continuing steroids subcutaneously should the patient become unable to swallow
- Checking blood glucose if any relevant symptoms occur

Always:
- Reduce dose of steroids to the minimum possible
- Review treatment every week, stopping after one week if no benefit
- Reduce dose slowly every few days if the patient has taken steroids for longer than two weeks or has been taking a relatively large dose

In the terminal care situation the patient's inability to swallow oral medication is often the provoking factor which leads to stopping steroids. The continuing of steroids by injection should be considered on an individual basis.

Side-effect risks of steroids

Doses of dexamethasone >4mg o.d. are likely to lead to significant side-effects after several weeks

Doses <4mg o.d. are often tolerated in patients with a prognosis of months

Doses <4mg can be stopped abruptly IF used for less than three weeks

Further reading

Book

Back I (2001) *Palliative Medicine Handbook*. 3rd edn. Cardiff: BPM Books pp. 126–9.

Formulary

Drugs in **bold** can be given in a syringe driver

Drug	Route	Dose	Frequency	Indications/Side-effects/Remarks
Alfentanil	**CSCI**	Titrate	24h	Synthetic opioid working on similar opioid receptors to fentanyl. Alternative CSCI-delivered opioid for patients unable to tolerate diamorphine. e.g. in renal failure
				Alfentanil 1mg = diamorphine 10mg
Aminophylline				Theophylline
i/r	p.o.	100–300mg	t.d.s.	Reversible airways obstruction
m/r	p.o.	225–450mg	b.d.	Theophylline concentration for optimal response is 55–110micromol/l
				Narrow therapeutic/toxicity margin
				Half life increased in heart failure, the elderly, and with drugs such as erythromycin and ciprofloxacin.
				SE: Tachycardia, palpitations, nausea, CNS stimulation.
Amitriptyline	p.o.	10–50mg	nocte	Neuropathic pain. Start at 10–25mg. Faster effect at lower doses than for depression. Salivary dribbling in MND.
				SE: Blurred vision, dry mouth, hypotension. Caution if cardiac disease, or history of urinary retention
Artificial saliva	Spray, gel, pastilles		As required	Contains mucin, an animal product not suitable for some religions
Arthrotec (see also diclofenac)	p.o. p.o. (m/r)	50mg 75mg	t.d.s. b.d.	Contains diclofenac + misoprostol (for prophylaxis against NSAID gastro-duodenal ulceration).
				SE: Diarrhoea. May enhance the anticoagulation effect of warfarin

Baclofen	p.o.	5–10mg max. 100mg/day	t.d.s.	Spasticity i.e. in MND Increase dose slowly SE: sedation and weakness
Benzydamine	0.15% oral rinse spray	15ml 4–8 puffs	1.5–3h p.r.n.	Local analgesic spray Dilute with water if stings
Bethanecol	p.o.	25mg	t.d.s.	Dry mouth
Bicalutamide (Casodex)	p.o. p.o.	50mg 150mg	o.d. o.d.	Anti-androgen With orchidectomy or gonadorelin therapy start three days beforehand Prostate cancer SE: GI upsets, nausea, vomiting, depression, loss of libido
Bisacodyl	p.o. PR	5–20mg 10mg	nocte— b.d. o.d.	Stimulant laxative. 5mg Tabs—action 10–12h. 10mg Supps—action 20–60 mins. Avoid in bowel obstruction
Bupivacaine	neb.	5ml 0.25%	6 h	Useful for persistent dry cough, not breathlessness. Beware reflex bronchospasm. (Pretreat with nebulised salbutamol.) No food for one hour after treatment because of pharyngeal anaesthesia
Buprenorphine	SL	0.2–0.4mg	t.d.s.	0.4mg t.d.s. Equivalent to 10–15mg morphine 4 h **Beware use in palliative care as it is a partial agonist, i.e. it can displace more effective opioids from their receptor sites**
Buprenorphine	Transdermal matrix patch	35, 52.5, 70 mcg/h	Every three days	Maximum dose = 140mcg/h For breakthrough buprenorphine SL, or other opioids can be used
Buscopan see Hyoscine butylbromide				

Drug	Route	Dose	Frequency	Indications/Side-effects/Remarks
Capsaicin	topical	0.075% cream	q.d.s.	Neuropathic pain/post herpetic neuralgia. May cause stinging. Wear gloves to administer. Avoid contact to sensitive areas
Carbamazepine	p.o.	100–200mg (max. 1.2g)	b.d.	Tonic-clonic/partial seizures; neuropathic pain. Build up dose slowly. Check serum levels. Watch drug interactions. Tabs./chewtab/Supps. SE: Ataxia and blood, hepatic and skin disorders
Carbenoxolone	m/w	1% sachet	q.d.s.	Mild oral and perioral ulcers
Carbocisteine	p.o.	750–1500mg	t.d.s.	Reduces sputum viscosity and increases expectoration. SE: Gastric irritant. Avoid if peptic ulceration
Celecoxib	p.o.	100–200mg	o.d.–b.d.	Cyclo-oxygenase-2 inhibitor. Pain and inflammation with reduced gastric side-effects
Chlorphenamine	p.o.	4mg	4–6h	Sedating antihistamine. Allergic reactions SE: Sedation
Chlorpromazine	p.o. PR	25–50mg 100mg	o.d.–t.d.s.	Severe agitation. Tenesmus (low dose). Hiccup (low dose). SE: sedative/hypotensive. Half dose in elderly. Supps. available by special order

Drug	Route	Dose	Frequency	Notes
Clonazepam	p.o.	0.5–2mg	nocte or b.d.	Neuropathic pain, anticonvulsant, sedative.
	CSCI	**1–4mg**	**24h**	May stick to plastic of syringe making titration difficult
Co-codamol Weak 8/500 (Not recommended for palliative care patients)	p.o.	1–2 Tabs.	4–6 h Max 8 in 24h	Codeine phosphate 8mg + paracetamol 500mg. Soluble preparations available. There is no evidence that 'weak co-codamol' is any more efficacious in pain control than paracetamol alone.[6]
Co-codamol **Strong 30/500**	p.o.	1–2 Tabs.	4–6 h Max 8 in 24h	Codeine phosphate 30mg + paracetamol 500mg e.g. Tylex, Solpadol. Soluble preparations available
Co-danthramer	p.o.	5–10ml 1–2 Caps.	nocte nocte	Stimulant (dantron) 25mg + softener (poloxamer) 200mg per Caps. or 5ml. Useful for drug induced constipation. 'Strong' capsules and Susp. also available. SE: May colour urine red. Do not use if incontinent as is associated with burning of perineal skin and excoriation Not licenced for patients with non-malignant disease as danthron is a potential carcinogen.
Co-danthrusate	p.o.	1–3 Caps. 5–15ml	nocte nocte	Stimulant (dantron) + softener (docusate) See co-danthramer
Co-dydramol	p.o.	1–2	4–6h max 8 in 24h	Dihydrocodeine 10mg + paracetamol 500mg. There are also combined preparations containing dihydrocodeine 20mg and 30mg

Drug	Route	Dose	Frequency	Indications/Side-effects/Remarks
Colestyramine	p.o.	4–8g	o.d.	Anion-exchange resin Pruritus associated with biliary obstruction, diarrhoea associated with ileal resection, radiation SE: Constipation and nausea
Cyproterone acetate	p.o. p.o.	300mg/24h 200–300mg/24h	Divided doses Divided doses	Anti-androgen Cover flare of initial gonadorelin therapy Long term palliative therapy where orchidectomy or gonadorelin analogues not indicated
Co-proxamol	p.o.	1–2 tabs	4–6 h max 12 in 24h	Paracetamol 325mg + Dextropropoxyphene 32.5mg. Some NMDA activity. Relatively low dose of paracetamol. May increase risk of bleeding with warfarin
Cyclizine	p.o. SC PR **CSCI**	25–50mg 25–50mg 25–50mg **100–150mg**	t.d.s. t.d.s. t.d.s. **24h**	Antihistamine. Useful for vomiting of GI cause, or raised intracranial pressure. SC route may cause skin reaction. Supps. available by special order.
Dexamethasone	p.o. i/m i/v **CSCI**	Up to 16mg Up to 16mg **Up to 16mg**	in 24 h in 24 h **24h**	2–4mg o.d. for appetite 8–16mg daily for raised intracranial pressure, SVCO, spinal cord compression. 2–6mg prevent chemotherapy emesis. Give a.m. to avoid excitation. Reduce dose ASAP. Watch glucose and proximal myopathy. Consider PPI prophylaxis in patients at risk of peptic ulceration. Prescribe PPI if taking NSAID. Separate syringe driver.

Diamorphine	**SC**	Titrated	4 h	Strong opioid analgesic. More soluble than morphine.
	CSCI	**Titrated**	**24h**	SC diamorphine is three times as potent as oral morphine. Modify dose in elderly patients and in patients with renal failure. SE: see pain section
	Topical	20mg		Mix in lidocaine gel (topical)
Diazepam	p.o.	2–10mg	o.d.–t.d.s.	Anxiety; agitation; night sedation; breathlessness; convulsions. Alternative
	PR	5–10mg	p.r.n. (Supps. or soln.)	is SC midazolam which is shorter acting.
Diclofenac	p.o.	25–50mg	t.d.s.	Bone pain and other inflammatory conditions if paracetamol and weak
	p.o.	75mg (m/r)	b.d.	opioids found to be ineffective. May enhance the anticoagulant effect
	i/m	75mg	stat	of warfarin and caution required in patients with asthma.
	PR	100mg	o.d.	If ineffective, try another NSAID. Contra-indicated with active peptic ulcer, GI bleeding or renal failure. Consider PPI prophylaxis in patients
	SC	**up to 150mg**	**24h**	at risk of peptic ulceration. Use separate syringe driver. SE: Local irritation.
Digoxin	p.o.	62.5–500 mcg (maintenance)	o.d.	Supraventricular tachycardia especially atrial fibrillation Reduce dose in elderly, and if reduced renal function. Avoid if hypokalaemia. SE: Anorexia, nausea, vomiting, diarrhoea. Abdominal pain, confusion. Do not give if ventricular rate is <60 beats per minute

Drug	Route	Dose	Frequency	Indications/Side-effects/Remarks
Dihydrocodeine	p.o. p.o. (m/r)	30–60mg 60–120mg	4–6h b.d.	Moderate pain. Similar efficacy to codeine orally—one tenth as potent as morphine. Increased risk of toxicity in renal failure requires dose reduction to 8h. Anticipate constipation.
Disodium pamidronate	i/v	30–90mg	In minimum 500ml sodium chloride 0.9% over 2–4h	Hypercalcaemia. Rehydrate first. max dose rate 1mg/min. Dose according to corrected plasma calcium concentration. Repeat after one week if poor initial response. Bone pain (especially breast cancer and multiple myeloma). Takes 7 days to produce maximal effect which lasts 2–3 weeks. Repeat every 3–4 weeks as long as benefit maintained.
Docusate sodium	p.o.	100–200mg	Daily	Softens stool. Weak stimulant. May help constipation in presence of partial bowel obstruction. Acts in 1–2 days.
Domperidone	p.o. PR	10–20mg 30–60mg	4–8h 4–8h	Antiemetic, bowel motility stimulant. Beware intestinal obstruction as may cause pain. Less extrapyramidal problems than with metoclopramide
Dosulepin	p.o.	50–150mg	nocte or b.d.	Tricyclic antidepressant Neuropathic pain. Lower doses start at 10mg nocte. Depression. Higher doses from 50mg SE: lowers convulsion threshold, dry mouth, urine retention, constipation, blurred vision

Epoetin	SC	150–300u/kg	Weekly	Recombinant human erythropoietin Anaemia associated with erythropoietin deficiency. Aim to elevate haemoglobin at a rate not exceeding 2g/100ml/month. If haemoglobin reaches 14 suspend until returns below 13g/100ml Contra-indicated in patients with chronic renal failure SE: Hypertension
Etamsylate	p.o.	500mg	q.d.s.	Useful for capillary bleeding
Fentanyl	transdermal	25, 50, 75, 100mcg/h over 3 days	72 h	Strong opioid for severe pain. Due to slow onset of action, patients may need extra analgesia for up to 24 h after fentanyl patch is started. Laxatives may be reduced, as causes less constipation than other opioids. On removal of patch it may take 17 h or more for plasma levels to drop by 50%. Unsuitable for unstable pain due to slow onset of action. **Conversion:** **Daily oral morphine mg** **Fentanyl patch delivery mcg/h** 50–130 25 135–224 50 225–314 75 315–404 100 405–494 125 Caution: when changing from transdermal fentanyl to morphine; use lower morphine dose.
Fentanyl	OTFC Lozenge	200, 400, 600, 800, 1200 mcg	For breakthrough pain	Dose of breakthrough analgesia with OTFC is not related to background analgesic dose so start with 200 mcg. Mouth needs to be moist

Drug	Route	Dose	Frequency	Indications/Side-effects/Remarks
Fluconazole	p.o.	50 mg	o.d.	Candidiasis. Give 7–14 day course
Fludrocortisone	p.o.	50–300 mcg	o.d.	Mineralocorticoid Postural hypotension Adrenal replacement with hydrocortisone
Fluoxetine	p.o.	20mg	mane	Enervating antidepressant. Long half life (5 weeks) SE: anxiety. GI symptoms usually settle within a few days
Gabapentin	p.o.	Starting dose 100–300mg Doses above 1800mg/24h need specialist attention.	Initially nocte then t.d.s.	Neuropathic pain. Anticonvulsant. Higher benefit/side-effect ratio than most other agents used for neuropathic pain. Use lower dosing in elderly and if renal failure present. Standard dosing regime not established. BNF recommends 300mg day 1, 300mg b.d. day 2, 300mg t.d.s. day 3, then titrate according to response in 300mg steps to max. of 1.8mg/day Avoid abrupt withdrawal. (Withdraw over 1 week.) SE: drowsiness, fatigue, ataxia
Gliazide i/r m/r	p.o. p.o.	40–80mg 30mg (equivalent to 80mg i/r)	o.d. o.d. max 120mg/24h	Sulphonylurea SE: Weight gain, hypoglycaemia, GI upset.
Glycopyrronium	p.o. **CSCI** SC	0.2–0.4mg **0.6–1.2mg** 0.2–0.4mg	4h **24h** t.d.s.	Dries secretions. Proven efficacy via continuous syringe driver route not from stat injections. Probably less central and/or cardiac side-effects than atropine or hyoscine.

(Zoladex, Zoladex LA)	(Long acting) Implant	3.6mg	12 weeks Every 4 weeks	early breast cancer. Implant in anterior abdominal wall with local anaesthetic. 'Flare' of androgen release when starting therapy can lead to increased activity of disease, and symptoms such as back pain need to be taken very seriously, if there are known spinal metastases, since spinal cord compression can be precipitated. (Flare can be covered with an anti-androgen, such as cyproterone acetate)
Granisetron	p.o.	1–2mg		Serotonin antagonist. Nausea/vomiting especially post RT or C/T SE: Constipation
Haloperidol	p.o. SC **CSCI**	0.5–10mg 2.5–10mg **3–10mg**	o.d.–b.d. 4h p.r.n. **24h**	Antiemetic. Small doses (e.g. 1.5mg b.d.) for nausea, particularly drug or metabolic induced. Higher doses in psychosis and agitation. Beware extrapyramidal side-effects and avoid in Parkinson's disease
Hydromorphone i/r	p.o.	Titrated	4h	Alternative opioid. Caps: i/r 1.3, 2.6mg × 7.5 potency of morphine: i.e. 1.3mg hydromorphone = 10mg morphine
Hydromorphone m/r	p.o	Titrated	b.d.	Caps: m/r 2, 4, 8, 16, 24mg (12 h) hydromorphone (mg) morphine (mg) 2 15 4 30 8 60 16 120 24 180
Hydromorphone inj	**CSCI** SC	Titrated	24 h 4 h	10mg/ml, 20mg/ml, 50mg/ml ×7.5 the potency of morphine Conversion factors from oral to SC hydromorphone range from equipotent to 3:1 Available as a 'special' from Martindale Pharmaceuticals

Drug	Route	Dose	Frequency	Indications/Side-effects/Remarks
Hyoscine butylbromide (Buscopan)	**CSCI**	**60–180mg (Intestinal obstruction)**	**24h**	Antimuscarinic, anticholinergic. Less sedating than hyoscine hydrobromide. Uses: intestinal colic, reduces bronchial secretions
		20–60mg (reduce bronchial secretions)		Very short half life
	SC	10–20mg	4h	
	p.o.	20mg	q.d.s.	Poor oral bioavailability
Hyoscine hydrobromide	SC	0.2–0.4mg	4–8h	Antimuscarinic, anticholinergic
	CSCI	**0.6–0.4mg**	**24h**	Antiemetic for refractory nausea
				Dries secretions second line to glycopyrronium
	SL	0.3mg	6h p.r.n.	SE: paradoxical agitation, sedation
	patch	1 patch	Change every 72h	
		1mg		
Ibuprofen	p.o.	200–600mg	t.d.s.	First line NSAID. Lower risks of side-effects than other NSAIDs. Topical preparations available. See diclofenac for contra-indications.
Ipratropium bromide	Neb.	0.25–0.5mg	6h	For breathlessness when there is bronchospasm, particularly if COPD present. Drying effect on secretions.

Ketamine				
	p.o.	25–100mg	t.d.s/q.d.s.	Under specialist supervision only. Neuropathic pain; build up dose slowly.
Ketamine	**CSCI**	**75–300mg** **(Higher doses have been reported)**	24h	May need prophylactic oral haloperidol 3mg nocte or a benzodiazepine to cover for psychomimetic side-effects. Oral solution available. May need to reduce opioids by 50%. Use separate syringe driver.
Ketorolac	p.o.	10mg	4–6 h (elderly 6–8 h)	Bone pain and other inflammatory conditions. Max 40mg p.o.
	SC	10–30mg	4–6 h	Max 90mg SC daily. See diclofenac warnings and cautions. Beware gastric bleeding.
Ketorolac	**CSCI**	**60–90mg**	**24h**	Use separate syringe driver With gastric protection (PPI)
Lactulose	p.o.	15–30ml	b.d.	Osmotic laxative. May cause abdominal bloating and wind. Requires a good fluid intake May take 48 h for full effect.
Lansoprazole	p.o.	30mg	o.d.	Proton pump inhibitor. Gastric and duodenal ulcer and oesophagitis Prophylaxis with NSAIDS and corticosteroids. Susp. available.

Drug	Route	Dose	Frequency	Indications/Side-effects/Remarks
Levomepromazine (methotrimeprazine)	p.o.	6.25–25mg (6.25mg = 1/4 Tab.)	o.d.–b.d.	Nausea and vomiting. Broad spectrum 'second line' antiemetic. SE: Sedation 6mg and 25mg Tabs.
Levomepromazine	**CSCI**	**6.25–50mg**	**24h**	SC route may cause skin reaction Dilute with sodium chloride 0.9% There is a 2:1 oral: SC conversion ratio
Levomepromazine	p.o.	6.25–200mg	o.d.–b.d.	Psychosis or severe agitation. Useful in terminal sedation. SE: May cause anticholinergic side-effects, hypotension and extrapyramidal symptoms
Levomepromazine	**CSCI**	**6.25–200mg**	**24h**	SC route may cause skin reaction. Dilute with sodium chloride 0.9%. Avoid in Parkinson's disease
Levomepromazine	SC	6.25–25mg	4–8 h	
Lidocaine (lignocaine)	Topical	5% ointment		Topical analgesia
Lithium (Carbonate/citrate)	p.o.	Dose adjusted to individual patient		Treatment and prophylaxis of mania, bipolar disorder, recurrent depression. Narrow therapeutic/toxic window. Target serum lithium concentration 0.4–1mmol/l, 12 h after a dose. Requires regular monitoring SE: GI upsets, tremor, renal impairment, oedema, blurred vision, drowsiness. Worse if sodium depleted, so beware if using diuretics. Drug interactions: Numerous—check each medicine.

Lofepramine	p.o.	140–210mg	Divided doses	Antidepressant Lower incidence of antimuscarinic side-effects than amitriptyline
Loperamide	p.o.	2–4mg max. 32mg/24h	t.d.s. or with each loose stool	Useful for diarrhoea and the pain of bowel colic. No CNS effects.
Loratadine	p.o.	10mg	o.d.	Non-sedating antihistamine
Lorazepam	p.o./SL	0.5–2mg	b.d.	Anxiety/panic attacks. Shorter duration of action than diazepam. Useful sublingually in acute anxiety and breathlessness.
Macrogol (polyethylene glycol) (Movicol)	p.o.	Dissolve sachet in 125ml water	1–3 sachets/day up to 8 sachets/day for faecal impaction	Licenced for faecal impaction.
Medroxyproge-sterone acetate	p.o.	400mg (double dose if poor response)	o.m.	Appetite stimulation in anorexia. Effect enhanced with concurrent NSAID Takes 2–3 weeks to produce maximal effect. Hot flushes after surgical or chemical castration
	p.o.	5–20mg	b.d.–q.d.s.	
Megestrol acetate	p.o.	40–160mg	o.m.	Appetite stimulation in anorexia. Effect enhanced with concurrent NSAID Take 2–3 weeks to produce maximal effect. Hot flushes after surgical or chemical castration

Drug	Route	Dose	Frequency	Indications/Side-effects/Remarks
Methadone	p.o	Titrated	b.d.–t.d.s	May be used for nociceptive and possibly neuropathic pain if no longer responsive to/tolerant of morphine.
	SC	Titrated	b.d.–t.d.s	Long half life.
	CSCI	**Titrated**	**24h**	Subcutaneously, use 50–70% oral dose. Can be used in renal failure.
				Prescribed differently from morphine, see pain chapter.
				SE: Long 1/2 life can lead to overdosing
Methotrimeprazine, see levomepromazine				
Methylphenidate	p.o.	5mg	o.d.–b.d.	Similar to dexamfetamine
				Uses: Opioid induced drowsiness.
				Mood while awaiting antidepressant to work
				SE: restlessness, confusion, sleep disturbance
Metoclopramide	p.o.	10–20mg	q.d.s.	Antiemetic, especially useful for drug related nausea, and also for cancer
	p.o.(m/r SC)	15mg	b.d.	related anorexia.
		10–20mg	q.d.s.	Increases gut motility and gastric emptying.
	CSCI	**30–90mg**	**24h**	Use cautiously in GI obstruction If makes GI cramps or diarrhoea worse stop.
				Extrapyramidal side-effects. (reversible with procylidine)
Metronidazole	p.o.	400mg	t.d.s.	Antibiotic for anaerobic infections.
	topical	1g	t.d.s.	Topically useful for fungating, odorous wounds
	PR		t.d.s.	SE: Nausea
Midazolam	SC	2.5–10mg	p.r.n.	Benzodiazepine. Shorter duration of action than diazepam
	Buccal			Single doses useful for quick, uncomfortable procedures, anxiety, agitation,
	intranasal			as replacement for anticonvulsants and sedation in the terminal phase.
	CSCI	**10–100mg**	**24h**	

Mirtazepine	p.o.	15–45mg titrate	Nocte	Some evidence of faster onset of action and promotion of appetite and sleep than other newer antidepressants. (Lower doses more sedating than higher, enervating, doses)
Morphine (i/r)				Pain/breathlessness 1/3 potent as subcutaneous diamorphine. Anticipate constipation.
	p.o.	Titrated	4 h	Oramorph 10mg/5ml, 100mg/5ml Single unit dose vials 10mg, 30mg, 100mg, all in 5ml. Sevredol Tabs.; 10mg, 20mg, 50mg.
	PR	Titrated	4 h	Supps. 10, 15, 20, 30mg.
Morphine (m/r)	p.o.	Titrated	12 h	MST continuous 5, 10, 15, 30, 60, 200mg. MST Susp. 20, 30, 60, 100, 200mg (sachets). Zomorph 10, 30, 60, 100, 200mg.
	p.o.	titrated	24 h	MXL 30, 60, 90, 120, 150, 200mg.
Morphine	SC	Titrated	4 h	As for diamorphine, but high doses will require larger volumes.
	CSCI		24 h	Conversion: p.o. to SC 2:1.
Nabilone	p.o.	0.1–0.2mg	q.d.s.	Cannabinoid Breathlessness, nausea. SE: Sedation/dysphoria may occur with higher doses. Oral solution can be made up
Naloxone	i/v	0.1–0.2mg	every 2mins.	Reversal of opioid induced respiratory depression. Beware return of severe pain.
	i/m/SC	0.1–0.2mg	every 2mins	Mix Amp. with 10ml of sterile water and give 1ml a minute titrating response. Beware that treating opioid induced respiratory depression may require repeated dosing and close monitoring for several hours.

Drug	Route	Dose	Frequency	Indications/Side-effects/Remarks
Naproxen	p.o. PR	250–500mg 500mg	b.d. b.d.	Bone pain and other inflammatory conditions. If ineffective, try another NSAID. Beware with warfarin and in patients who are asthmatic. Contra-indicated with active peptic ulcer or GI bleeding See diclofenac for warnings and cautions
Nifedipine	p.o. SL	5mg 5mg	t.d.s. t.d.s.	Smooth muscle relaxant; useful for hiccups, oesophageal spasm and tenesmus. SE: Hypotension, peripheral oedema, headache
Nitrous oxide 50% +oxygen 50%				For incident pain. Produces analgesia without loss of consciousness. Exponents claim useful for changing painful dressings, etc. Patient must control administration
Nystatin	p.o.	1–5ml 100,000 u/ml	q.d.s.	Oral Candidiasis
Octreotide	SC **CSCI**	0.1–0.2mg **300–1000mcg**	t.d.s. **24h**	Somatostatin analogue. Very short duration of action. Carcinoid symptom control. Reduces GI secretions and motility. Useful in intestinal obstruction, enterocutaneous fistulae and intractable diarrhoea. Not sedative.
Sandostatin LAR	Depot injection	20mg/month × 3 months then review results		Expensive; use when other treatments have failed. Use with caution if patient has diabetes mellitus
Lanreotide	Depot injection	30mg/2 weeks × 3 months then review results		

Olanzepine	p.o.	5–10mg	o.d.	New generation antipsychotic Moderate to severe mania SE: less than with older antipsychotics but postural hypotension, extrapyramidal effects. Caution: Glaucoma, hyperglycaemia, elderly stroke patients with dementia.
Omeprazole	p.o.	10–20mg	o.d.	Proton pump inhibitor (PPI) Gastric and duodenal ulcer and reflux oesophagitis
Ondansetron	p.o.	8mg	b.d.–t.d.s.	Serotonin antagonist. Uses: Vomiting caused by RT or C/T, ovarian intestinal obstruction, hepatic cholestatic itch. Relatively more expensive than other antiemetics. Max. 8mg daily in severe hepatic failure. SE: Constipation Melt forms available
	i/v	8mg	b.d.–t.d.s.	
	PR	16mg	o.d.	
	CSCI	**8–24mg**	**24h**	
Oxybutynin	p.o.	2.5–5mg	b.d.–t.d.s.	Antimuscarinic Detrusor instability Urinary incontinence (urge) SE: Antimuscarinic effects
Oxycodone i/r	p.o.	Titrated	4–6h	Moderate to severe pain. 5mg, 10mg, 20mg Caps. Liquid 5mg/5ml, 10mg/ml 20mg Oral morphine equivalent to 10mg oxycodone Oxycodone 30mg Supps. available. (Longer acting than morphine Supps.)
	PR	Titrated	8h	
Oxycodone m/r	p.o.	Titrated	12h	Modified release Tabs. 10mg, 20mg, 40mg, 80mg 12 h. 20mg oral morphine equivalent to 10mg oral oxycodone

Drug	Route	Dose	Frequency	Indications/Side-effects/Remarks
Oxycodone inj	SC	5–10mg	4h	10mg/ml
	CSCI	**Titrated**	**24h**	1ml and 2ml Amps.
				Twice as potent as oral oxycodone e.g. 20mg of oral oxycodone is equivalent to 10mg of injectable oxycodone.
Pamidronate (see Disodium pamidronate)				
Pancreatin (Creon 10,000)	p.o.	1–2 Caps. with meals		For fat malabsorption
				e.g. Creon 1–2 sachets with meals
				Preparations containing lipase 25000 and 40000 units available.
Paracetamol	p.o.	0.5–1g	4–6 h	Analgesic. Antipyretic.
	PR	0.5–1g	4–6 h Max. 4g in 24h	Available as Tabs, Caps., caplets, Susp., dispersible and 125 and 500mg Supps.
Parecoxib	i/m i/v	40mg initially then 20–40mg	12 h	Cox-2 NSAID injection SE: as per other NSAID drugs
Paroxetine	p.o.	20mg	o.m.	SSRI antidepressant/ anxiolytic. Short half life. Used for itch and sweating. Withdraw slowly SE: extrapyramidal effects noted

Phenobarbital	p.o.	60–180mg	Nocte	Anticonvulsant. Useful as replacement oral anticonvulsant and in terminal sedation.
	i/m	50–200mg	b.d.	
	CSCI	**200–600mg**	**24h**	Use separate syringe driver. Max. 600mg daily

| Pilocarpine | p.o. | 5mg | t.d.s. | Cholinergic |
| | 4% eye drops (orally) | | t.d.s. | Sialagogue for dry mouth |

Piroxicam	p.o.	20mg	b.d.	NSAID
	melt	20mg	b.d.	Inflammatory pain
				Melt useful when swallowing not possible.
				SE: as per diclofenac

| Pregabalin | p.o. | 75mg | b.d. | Neuropathic pain, epilepsy and anxiety. Similar mode of action to Gabapentin |

Dose regime:

	Normal Kidney Function			Impaired Kidney Function		
Time		Breakfast	Supper	Time	Breakfast	Supper
Step 1		75 mg	75 mg	Step 1	50 mg	50 mg
Step 2		150 mg	150 mg	Step 2	100 mg	100 mg
Step 3		300 mg	300 mg	Step 3	150 mg	150 mg

If necessary step 2 can be started after 3–4 days, and step 3 after a further 7 days

Common side-effects are sedation, dizziness, and headaches.

Potentiated by alcohol and oxycodone

Prochlorperazine	p.o.	5–10mg	t.d.s.	Neuroleptic.
	i/m	12.5mg	t.d.s. p.r.n.	Antiemetic. May be useful for metabolic/drug induced nausea.
	PR	25mg	t.d.s.	Too irritant to be given subcutaneously.
	buccal	3–6mg	b.d.	

Drug	Route	Dose	Frequency	Indications/Side-effects/Remarks
Procyclidine	p.o. i/m / i/v	2.5–5mg 5–10mg	t.d.s. p.r.n.	For management of extrapyramidal side-effects of neuroleptic drugs or dopamine antagonists. (max. 20mg daily)
Ranitidine	p.o.	300mg 150mg	nocte b.d.	Peptic ulceration. Steatorrhea due to bile duct obstruction. Less evidence of protection against NSAID induced gastric ulceration than PPIs.
Riluzole	p.o.	50mg	b.d.	Used to extend life (?) or the time to mechanical ventilation in patients with motor neurone disease. SE: Nausea, vomiting, abdominal pafin, circumoral paraesthesia, altered liver function tests
Risperidone	p.o.	0.5–2mg	b.d.	'Atypical antipsychotic' useful for psychoses in which both positive and negative symptoms are prominent. Extrapyramidal symptoms are less common than with traditional antipsychotics, but it is more expensive. In elderly start at 0.25 or 0.5mg nocte
Salbutamol	neb p.o. SC	2.5–5mg 8mg m/r 0.5mg	6–8h b.d. 4h	β agonist Bronchospasm Beware causes tachycardia and multiple doses can lead to agitation and anxiety.
Senna	p.o.	2–4Tabs.	nocte	Stimulant laxative. Acts in 8–12 h Avoid in bowel obstruction.
Sertraline	p.o.	50mg	o.d.	SSRI antidepressant. Caution in epilepsy as reduces fit threshold Reduce slowly SE: GI upset

Drug	Route	Dose	Frequency	Notes
Sodium valproate	p.o.	100–300mg	b.d.	Anticonvulsant Start at 100mg b.d. for neuropathic pain; 300mg b.d. for convulsions. Tabs., m/r Tabs., Supps. available by special order. SE: Nausea, blood dyscrasia, liver dysfunction
Spironolactone	p.o.	100–200mg Max. 400mg for ascites	o.d.	Potassium sparing diuretic. Sodium and fluid retention, malignant ascites. (Ascites dose regimes vary considerably). Trial with furosemide for few days. Avoid with ACE inhibitors, potassium supplements and potassium sparing diuretics as could cause hyperkalaemia. SE: Gynaecomastia
Sucralfate	p.o.	2g	b.d.	Protects mucosa from acid-pepsin attack in gastric and duodenal ulcers and also protects oral mucosa. Paste/Susp.
Tinzaparin	SC	175u/kg	o.d.	Low molecular weight heparin (LMWH). Treatment dose for pulmonary embolus (PE) and deep venous thrombosis (DVT)
	SC	50u/kg	o.d.	Prophylaxis In cancer patients LMWH is now the treatment of choice if anticoagulation is required
Tizanidine	p.o.	2mg titrate 3 day intervals, 2mg steps Max. 36mg/day	o.d.	Muscle relaxant for spasticity associated with multiple sclerosis or spinal cord disease. Regular LFT monitoring for first four months

Drug	Route	Dose	Frequency	Indications/Side-effects/Remarks
Tramadol				May be useful for nociceptive and neuropathic pain.
i/r	p.o.	50–100mg	q.d.s.	Tramadol 50mg equivalent to morphine 10mg
m/r	p.o.	100–200mg (max 400mg/24h)	b.d.	Less constipating than codeine
Tranexamic acid	p.o.	1–1.5g	b.d.–q.d.s.	Useful for capillary bleeding e.g. surface bleeding from ulcerated tumours. Cautions if: 1. Haematuria, as may encourage clot formation and ureteric obstruction. 2. History of thromboembolism
Venlafaxine	p.o.	37.5–75mg	b.d.	SNRI antidepressant Used also for hot flushes and neuropathic pain
Warfarin	p.o.	As per INR	o.d.	Coumarin anticoagulant Takes 48–72 h to be fully effective Used to treat DVT and PE Used for prophylaxis with indwelling i/v lines and atrial fibrillation. Usual adult induction *10mg o.d. for 2 days then depending on INR target daily maintenance. * Lower dose if abnormal liver function, cardiac failure. Caution: Paracetamol, NSAIDs, Cranberry juice.
Zoledronic acid	i/v 15 minute 'push'	4–8mg	4–6 weeks	Bisphosphonate Bone pain and hypercalcaemia Monitor calcium levels in bone pain, as may require Vit D or calcium

6 Scottish Intercollegiate National Guidelines Network (2000) *Control of pain in patients with cancer: a national clinical guideline.* Edinburgh: SIGN (www.sign.ac.uk).

Syringe drivers

Fig. 4.2 A syringe driver

Fig. 4.3 A syringe

Syringe drivers are used to aid drug delivery when the oral route is no longer feasible.

Indications for use:
1 Intractable vomiting
2 Severe dysphagia
3 Patient too weak to swallow oral drugs
4 Decreased conscious level
5 Poor alimentary absorption (rare)
6 Poor patient compliance

Morphine conversion

Diamorphine can be administered subcutaneously in a smaller volume than morphine, and in countries where diamorphine is available is the preparation of first choice.

	Oral morphine	:	Subcutaneous diamorphine
Ratio	3	:	1

When converting from opioids other than morphine, calculate the equivalent dose of oral morphine over 24 h and continue as above.

The following drugs may be mixed with diamorphine
- cyclizine
- haloperidol
- hyoscine hydrobromide
- metoclopramide
- octreotide
- granisetron
- glycopyrronium
- hyoscine butylbromide
- levomepromazine
- midazolam
- ondansetron

Drugs not suitable for subcutaneous usage:
- diazepam
- chlorpromazine
- prochlorperazine

Use separate syringe driver for:
- dexamethasone
- phenobarbital
- diclofenac
- ketamine
- ketorolac

Conversion of oral morphine (or oral morphine equivalent) to parenteral diamorphine

morphine 3mg p.o. = diamorphine 1mg SC

Method add the total daily oral dose of morphine (or oral morphine equivalent) and divide by three.

e.g.   morphine 10mg p.o. 4h
           or
       MST 30mg b.d.   } = morphine 60mg p.o. 24h
           or
       MXL 60mg o.d.
       morphine 60mg p.o. 24h = diamorphine 20mg SC 24h

General principles

- Care should be taken when mixing more than two drugs in a syringe and in ensuring that the diluent used is compatible with the drugs. The diluent of choice is water for injection except in the following where sodium chloride 0.9% for injection should be used:- diclofenac, granisetron, ketamine, ketorolac, octreotide and ondansetron
- If requiring more than three drugs in one syringe driver, re-assessment of treatment aims is required
- With combinations of two or three drugs in one syringe, a larger volume of diluent may be needed, e.g. 20ml or 30ml syringe

Preparation of syringe driver

The following is an example only, to illustrate the principle; local practices may differ. Training is essential.

Important—check type of portable Graseby syringe driver

Blue driver hourly rate	We strongly encourage the use of only the green Graseby MS 26, mm per 24 h syringe driver as having two different types can cause dangerous dose errors.
Green driver daily rate	

Draw up prescribed 24 h medication mixed with water for injection as diluent.(Use sodium chloride 0.9% as diluent with levomepromazine.)

Set the rate on the syringe driver.

(The rate of delivery is based on a length of fluid in mm per unit time).

For example:

MS 26—Green   (mm per 24 h, a **daily** rate)

$$\text{rate} = \frac{\text{measured 'length of volume' in mm}}{\text{delivery time in days}}$$

e.g.
$$48\text{mm} = 48\text{mm per day}$$
Rate on dial is 48

MS 16 A—Blue   (mm per h)

$$\text{rate} = \frac{\text{measured 'length of volume' in mm}}{\text{delivery time in h}}$$

e.g.
$$\frac{48 \text{ mm}}{24 \text{ h}} = 2\text{mm per h}$$
Rate on dial is 02

Problems

Infusion running too fast:	Check the rate setting and recalculate.
Infusion running too slow:	Check start button, battery, syringe driver, cannula and make sure injection site is not inflamed.
Site reaction:	Cyclizine and levomepromazine cause site reactions most commonly. Firmness or swelling is not necessarily a problem but the needle site should be changed if there is pain or obvious inflammation. If there is no alternative to subcutaneous administration of drugs it may be helpful to add dexamethasone 1mg to the mixture. A plastic/teflon needle may reduce local irritation if there is a nickel allergy

Precipitation

Check compatibility of drugs.

Check solution regularly for precipitation and discolouration and discard if it occurs. Cyclizine may precipitate at high doses, particularly in combination with high doses of diamorphine. Other combinations may also cause cloudiness in the syringe. On rare occasions a patient may need two or three separate syringe drivers to separate the drugs.

Light flashing

This is normal. The light flashes:

Blue—Once per second   Green—Once per 25 seconds

Flashing will stop when the battery needs changing. The syringe driver will continue to operate for 24 h after the light has stopped flashing.

Alarm

This always sounds when the battery is inserted. It can be silenced by pressing Start/Test button.

Check for—empty syringe—kinked tube—blocked needle/tubing—jammed plunger.

Drug compatibilities—usually max. 3 drugs in one syringe

Table 4.1 Examples of commonly used syringe driver preparations

Diamorphine	+Haloperidol	+Cyciizine**
Diamorphirie	+Haloperidbl	+Hyoscine Hydrobromide
Diamorphine	+Haloperidol	+Hyoscine Butylbromide
Diarnorphine	+Haloperidol	+Levomepromazine***
Diamorphine	+Haloperidol	+Midazolam
Diarnorphine	+Cyclizine**	+Hyoscine Hydrobrornide
Diamorphine	+Cyclizine**	+Levomepromazine***
Diamorphine	+Cyclizine**	+Midazolam
Diamorphine	+Midazolam	+Hyoscine Hydrobromide
Diamorphine	+Midazolam	+Hyoscine Butylbromide
Diamorphine	+Midazolam	+Levomepromazine***
Diamorphine	+Midazolam	+Glycopyrronium
Diamorphine	+Levomepromazine***	+Hyoscine Hydrobromide
Diamorphine	+Levomepromazine***	+Hyoscine Butylbromide
Diamorphine	+Levornepromazine***	+Glycopyrronium

**Cyclizine is incompatible with normal saline.

If needing to use a dose of cyclizine greater than 75mg/24 h in conjunction with a dose of diamorphine greater than 160mg/24 h, a 20ml b.d. syringe should be used. This will enable dilution to 14ml so that the medication remains compatible in the syringe.

***Levomepromazine can be irritant.

If skin site soreness becomes a problem, it is recommended to dilute it with sodium chloride 0.9% rather than water for injections. However, please note if diamorphine is combined with levomepromazine, sodium chloride 0.9% can only be used when diamorphine concentration is less than 40mg/ml. If the diamorphine concentration exceeds 40mg/ml, water for injections should be used. If skin site soreness is a problem in this instance, increase the size of syringe used. If other drugs are in the syringe, check these are compatible with saline.

Table 4.2 Common drugs, doses and ranges for palliative care use with a 24 h syringe driver

The following is a guide to drugs that may be used in a 24 h subcutaneous syringe driver. They may be used alone or in combinations. Advice should be sought when combining drugs or in exceptional circumstances

All drugs should be mixed with WATER unless otherwise indicated.

Drug class of drug/ (Amp. size)	Indications	Compatibility	Contra-indications	Possible side-effects	p.r.n. dose onset of action	24h infusion dose ranges
Cyclizine Antihistaminic, antimuscarinic antiemetic (50mg/1ml)	Nausea and vomiting associated with motion sickness, Anticipatory nausea, Pharyngeal stimulation, Mechanical bowel obstruction, Raised intracranial Pressure	Can precipitate with dexamethasone, diamorphine (in higher doses), metoclopramide, midazolam and saline	No absolute ones in patients with advanced cancer Do not give with metoclopramide Do not give with levomepromazine Do not give with buscopan	Drowsiness, dry mouth, blurred vision, hypotension Injection can be painful Can be sedating If syringe driver site is irritated try to dilute further.	50mg i/m / SC every 8 h Within 2 h	50–150mg usual dose
Dexamethasone Corticosteroid 4(mg/ml)	Antiemetic Pain relief Raised Intracranial pressure	Mixes with metoclopramide Precipitates with cyclizine,	Diabetes—may need supervision	Gastro-intestinal side effects, Impaired healing.	Discuss with oncology/palliative care team	4–16mg usual dose

	Spinal cord compression intestinal obstruction	midazolam, haloperidol, levomepromazine, Advisable to put in separate driver but can mix with diamorphine		weight gain, hirsutism, increased appetite	Not usually needed	
Diamorphine Opioid analgesic (5mg, 10mg, 30mg, 100mg, 500mg)	Pain Dyspnoea Cough Diarrhoea	With most drugs	None if titrated carefully against a patients' symptoms Modify dose in renal failure	Nausea Drowsiness Dry mouth Constipation Confusion Twitching	One sixth of total 24h infusion dose Within 10–30mins	Variable depending on total oral intake of morphine Conversion of oral morphine to subcutaneous diamorphine is 3:1
Diclofenac NSAID Non-opioid analgesic (75mg/3ml)	Pain (particularly associated with tissue inflammation or bone pain/movement related pain)	Incompatible with most drugs. Give in a separate syringe driver Use sodium chloride 0.9% for dilution **Do Not Mix**	Active peptic ulceration Urticaria Rhinitis Asthma Angioedema	Skin ulceration especially with prolonged use (SC)	75mg SC every 12 h (do not give as well as the infusion) Within 20–30 mins	75–20mg usual dose

Drug class of drug/ (Amp. size)	Indications	Compatibility	Contra-indications	Possible side-effects	p.r.n. dose onset of action	24h infusion dose ranges
Glycopyrronium bromide Quaternary ammonium antimuscarinic (0.2mg/ml, 0.6mg/3ml)	Death rattle Colic in inoperable bowel obstruction, Reduction of secretion May be effective if no response to hyoscine Anti-secretory effect Does not cross the blood brain barrier so does not cause drowsiness	With most drugs	2–5 times more potent than hyoscine hydrobromide	Tachycardia Dry mouth	0.2mg SC every 6–8 h Within 20–40 mins	0.6–1.2mg usual dose
Haloperidol Butyrophenone Antipsychotic (5mg/ml)	Nausea and vomiting Psychotic symptoms Agitated delirium Intractable hiccup	With most drugs	Parkinson's disease Possible CNS Depression with anxiolytics & alcohol	Extra-pyramidal symptoms, dry mouth, sedation, drowsiness, difficulty in micturition, hypotension, blurred vision	1.5–3mg SC daily to every 8 h Within 10–15mins	2.5–5mg usual dose for nausea and vomiting
Hyoscine butylbromide Antimuscarinic antispasmodic antisecretory	Obstructive symptoms with colic and antisecretory effects, Death rattle	With most drugs, except cyclizine	Narrow angle glaucoma (unless moribund), Myasthenia gravis.	Does not cross blood brain barrier so does not cause drowsiness	10–20mg SC every 8 h Within 3–5 mins	Bowel obstruction with colic: 60–120mg usual dose

Drug	Uses	Interactions	Cautions	Side effects	Dose	Dose
Hyoscine hydrobromide 0.4mg/1ml or 0.6mg/ml	Death rattle Colic Reduce salivation Some antiemetic action			Sedation	0.4mg	1.2–2.4mg
Levomepromazine Antiemetic phenothiazine antipsychotic (25mg/1ml)	Nausea and vomiting Insomnia Terminal agitation Intractable pain. Useful as antiemetic and sedation. Can be very sedating	Precipitates with dexamethasone Do not use with cyclizine	Parkinson's disease, Postural hypotension, Antihypertensive therapy, Epilepsy, Hypothyroidism Myasthenia gravis	Sedation, dose dependent postural hypotension	6.25–12.5mg i/m/SC every 4–6 h usual dose within 30 minutes	6.25–25mg usual dose for nausea & vomiting 25–150mg usual dose terminal agitation
Metoclopramide Prokinetic antiemetic (10mg/2ml)	Nausea and vomiting caused by gastric irritation Delayed gastric emptying Stimulation of the CTZ Obstructive bowel symptoms without colic Non-sedating	With most drugs	Concurrent administration with antimuscarinic drugs, Concurrent i/v administration of 5-HT$_3$ receptor antagonists Do not give in bowel obstruction if colic present	Dizziness Diarrhoea Depression Extra-pyramidal effects	10–30mg i/m/SC every 8 h	60–120mg

Drug class of drug/ (Amp. size)	Indications	Compatibility	Contra-indications	Possible side-effects	p.r.n. dose onset of action	24h infusion dose ranges
Midazolam Benzodiazepine (10mg/2ml) Anxiolytic	Sedation for terminal agitation, Multifocal myoclonus Epilepsy Intractable hiccup Muscle spasm	With most drugs	Drowsiness, Hypotension	Dizziness, drowsiness	2.5–10mg SC every 4 h Within 5–10 mins	10–60mg usual dose
Octreotide Somatostatin analogues FOR SPECIALIST USE ONLY 50mcg/ml 100mcg/ml 200mcg/ml 500mcg/ml	Intestinal obstruction associated with vomiting intractable diarrhoea Symptoms associated with hormone secreting tumours Bowel fistulae Injection can be painful (gently hand warm the vial)	Precipitates with dexamethasone	Caution in diabetes mellitus may potentiate hypoglycaemia	Dry mouth, nausea, vomiting anorexia abdominal pain, flatulence	50–100 mcg SC every 8 h Within 30 mins	Intestinal obstruction: 300–600 mcg usual dose

Further reading

Books

Dickman A. et al. (2005) The syringe driver: continuous subcutaneous infusions in palliative care. 2nd edn. Oxford: Oxford University Press.

Reviews

Scottish Intercollegiate Guidelines Network, (2000) *Control of Pain in Patients with cancer a National Clinical Guideline*. Edinburgh: SIGN.

Oncology and palliative care

The best sentence in the English language is not 'I love you' but 'It's benign'.

Woody Allen, *Deconstructing Harry*, 1998

The commonest cancers are of the lung, breast, skin, gastrointestinal tract, and the prostate gland.

Introduction

Cancer is an important cause of morbidity and mortality, particularly in industrialized countries. Currently in the UK one person in three will be diagnosed with cancer during their lifetime and one in five will die of their disease.

As 60 per cent of all cancers are diagnosed in those aged over 65 years, our rapidly increasing older population suggests that cancer will become an even more common problem in the coming decades.

Cancers may develop in all body tissues. The cells that form cancers can be differentiated from cells in normal tissues in a number of ways, including:

1 Cell division that has escaped the control of normal homeostasis
2 Abnormalities of cell differentiation—in general terms cancer cells tend to be less well differentiated than their non-malignant counterparts
3 Resistance to programmed cell death
4 The potential for cancerous cells to invade local tissues and metastasize

The development of cancer is associated with the accumulation of defects or 'mutations' in a number of critical genes within the cell.

Many cancers, for example, are associated with mutations leading to overactivity of growth promoting genes known commonly as oncogenes. Conversely cancers may also be associated with mutations leading to underactivity of genes which act to suppress growth.

Although our understanding of the genetic abnormalities underlying cancer has grown exponentially over the last decade, the factors that cause these changes are not clear for most cancers.

There is evidence that exogenous carcinogens may be closely linked to some cancers. Smoking, for example, is a causative factor in lung, cervix and bladder cancer.

In other cancers there is an inherited susceptibility to particular types of malignancy. In the majority of common cancers, however, the cause remains elusive. It is likely that for many of these cancers both environmental and genetic factors are implicated.

Organization of cancer care

Optimal care of the patient with cancer requires input from a number of medical disciplines. Typically a provisional diagnosis of cancer is made by a surgeon or physician and confirmed by a pathologist following biopsy or fine needle aspiration. A surgeon or an oncologist may then undertake definitive treatment. Support of the patient through treatment may well involve input from a wide range of surgical, medical, allied medicine health professionals and laboratory disciplines.

Several factors facilitate this care:

1 Good organization of cancer services
2 Cancer site specialization for surgeons and oncologists
3 Multidisciplinary team working
4 Well-established links with laboratory and clinical cancer research

The disease journey

A close working relationship between oncology and palliative care professionals is important. In the past, this relationship was not optimal due to misunderstandings of their different rôles and treatment aims. Increasingly now the goals are shared and closer working relationships are being forged, at different points along the patient's disease journey.

At time of original diagnosis

Oncological services, specialist and generalist palliative care services, including the General Practitioner and community health team, need to share information quickly so, at this point, when patient and family feel particularly vulnerable, informed support can be maximized.[1]

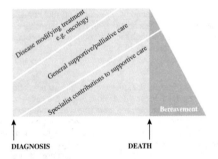

Traditionally palliative care services were only 'offered' to patients when 'there is nothing more that can be done'.

Increasingly palliative care is involved from the point of diagnosis with increasing input as the oncology needs decrease, maximizing at time of death and continuing on with bereavement support.

Through the period of staging and/or surgery

This can be a time of great uncertainty for patients, when communicating the often complex prognostic and treatment information is so important. Many find the issues very difficult to grasp, so vast are the associated life implications. An understanding of these issues and of the likely treatments by all those involved in the clinical and supportive care of patient and family can help to consolidate information transfer. It is often only a few days after a crucial oncology outpatient appointment that patients become receptive to important information.

If other healthcare professionals are hesitant or contradictory in their explanations of treatment options patient anxiety will be increased.

'When I was diagnosed with my bowel cancer I was simply devastated. You see, I had watched my father dying from lung cancer and I was sure I would go the same way. I could hardly get out of the hospital quickly enough to get my farm and affairs sorted out. The Doctor said something about treatment, but I knew from watching others with cancer that treatment was pointless, so I never went back for the cancer specialist appointment.

It was only after my own Doctor came out and we had a good chat that I even thought that they could do anything for me. In the end I decided to go and see what they were offering, still never believing that they could do any good.

I honestly believe if my own doctor hadn't taken the time to come and explain that there really was something they could do to help I would not been alive to enjoy these past six years.'

Through the period of treatment

While the majority of supportive care during this period tends to be linked through the oncology services, specialist and generalist palliative care teams need to be aware of the:
• Goals of treatment
• Side-effects of treatment
• Follow-up plans

The goals of oncology treatment

Before commencing any treatment it is important that both patient and carers are aware of the goals of treatment.

Frequently after what the consultant feels to have been a very full and frank discussion outlining these goals, a patient will ask a much more junior member of the team to clarify what has been said.

This may be because they do not wish to not fully understanding what was being discussed; alternatively they may feel able to ask more questions from a member of the team whom they find more approachable.

It is also possible, particularly if the outlook is not good, that patients will ask different members of the team hoping to find a more optimistic prognosis. Clearly it is not in the patient's interest to hear conflicting opinions about their prognosis and this should be avoided.

1 National Council for Hospice and Specialist Palliative Care Services (2002) *Definitions of Supportive and Palliative Care.* London: NCHSPCS (Briefing Bulletin 11).

Openness regarding realistic treatment outcomes is also important in maintaining staff morale. While the death of a patient is often difficult, particularly for the nurses who are most closely involved in care, this is especially so if unrealistic expectations of treatment are fostered.

Radical oncological treatment

Radical oncological interventions are curative in intent. They may involve surgery, radiotherapy or chemotherapy (or a combination of these modalities).

Because the potential benefits of treatment are great, a relatively high incidence of drug toxicity side-effects is more acceptable.

Providing patients with good symptom control and emotional support through radical treatment is important. They need to be encouraged to complete what is often a very demanding treatment course in order to benefit maximally.

Without such encouragement patients may miss the only opportunity they have of cure.

Increasingly there is an appreciation that such treatments may be associated with long term toxicities/side-effects (which may be especially relevant for children). Clearly in this potentially curative group care must be taken to minimize the potential for cumulative dose toxicities such as cardiotoxity caused by anthracyclines.

Adjuvant oncological treatment

Many patients suffer tumour relapse following apparently curative surgery for their primary tumour. This is believed to be due to the presence of micrometastatic disease that is not clinically apparent at the time of the primary treatment.

Anticancer treatment (usually chemotherapy) given at this stage has been shown to improve long-term survival for some tumours.

This approach has proven successful even for tumours where chemotherapy is not curative in the metastatic setting, and is presumably related to the increased chemosensitivity associated with microscopic volumes of disease.

The absolute gains in survival from adjuvant chemotherapy are generally small but real. (Adjuvant chemotherapy in premenopausal women with breast cancer, for example, is associated with an approximately 30 per cent relative improvement in 10 year survival). At present there are few predictive factors to identify patients most likely to benefit from adjuvant therapy. The decision to proceed is often based on the statistical likelihood of relapse, with those at highest risk benefitting most.

The fact remains that the majority of patients will not benefit from adjuvant therapies. Such treatments should therefore have manageable acute toxicities and a low incidence of long-term toxicities.

Palliative oncological treatment

Palliative treatment is indicated when curative treatment is not possible but where treatments may have sufficient anticancer activity to improve cancer-related symptoms. In many cases improvement of symptoms is accompanied by tumour shrinkage detectable clinically or by radiological methods such as

CT scan or MRI. Increasingly, however, it is recognized that there may be a palliative benefit even in the absence of tumour shrinkage.

As the primary object of therapy is to improve quality of life, such treatments should be well tolerated with a low incidence of acute side-effects. Long-term toxicities are generally not relevant.

In some cases the distinction between radical and palliative treatment may not be absolutely clear cut. Indeed the aims of treatment may change as the disease progresses.

Patients presenting with advanced ovarian cancer, for example, have largely incurable disease. However, the tumour is often chemosensitive and lengthy remissions are often seen following primary chemotherapy. In such patients a relatively high incidence of acute toxicity may be acceptable, with efforts being focused on managing chemotherapy-related symptoms. Conversely, a patient presenting with relapsed ovarian cancer following first line chemotherapy has a low expectation of benefit from further chemotherapy. Consequently only a low incidence of acute toxicity is acceptable with second line chemotherapy, from which expectation of benefit is very limited.

> For patients and carers who have been through radical or adjuvant therapy the switch to palliative treatment can be difficult to understand. Perhaps much of the 'bad press' that oncological care has received has been due to patients and relatives feeling that they were being given so called 'curative' treatments beyond the point when any cure was possible.
> In particular patients and carers can be bemused that unlike when they were receiving radical or adjuvant therapy there is little emphasis placed on assessment scans and X rays as the key question now relates purely to how the patient is doing symptomatically.

Managing patients receiving oncology treatments

Chemotherapy and radiotherapy is now given largely on an outpatient basis. Surgical patients also spend less time in hospital than in the past. This allows patients to spend more time at home, but inevitably places an increased burden of care on those providing support in the community, particularly where the cancer centre is a long distance from home. Thus a general understanding of the particular side-effects, and the appropriate treatment for such complications, is needed increasingly by healthcare professionals in the community and those providing on-call services.

It should not be assumed automatically that a new symptom developing in a patient undergoing treatment for cancer is related to the side-effects of treatment or to the cancer itself, although the high possibility of this must be considered. (*Chemotherapy does not prevent patients developing appendicitis!*) Thus the health professional needs to assess each new symptom independently, and be aware of the side-effects of commonly used oncological treatment regimes. (📖 See the sections on chemotherapy and radiotherapy.)

Supportive teams need to know the significance and *appropriate responses for individual patients* to such side-effects as:

Clinical anaemia

Nausea and Vomiting

Pain

Pyrexia and possible infection
  What are the risks of neutropaenia for this patient?

Increased drowsiness

Confusion
  Could this patient be opioid toxic, hypercalcaemic, or developing renal failure?

Hair loss

Altered sensation, back pain, incontinence
  Could this patient be developing spinal cord compression?

The appropriate response and management will differ according to what the patient and their family want, the disease process, and where the patient is on their disease journey.

Treatment planning

It is important that treatment plans are communicated adequately to patients, families, and professional carers to ensure that appropriate support is given.

A basic management plan should include:

- Details of proposed diagnostic and staging investigations
- Proposed treatment plan for surgery, chemotherapy and radiotherapy where appropriate. The plan should include details regarding the duration of treatment and timing of interval investigations to assess response to therapy. (Patients can be understandably anxious in the days preceding a scan aimed at assessing response to treatment.)
- Changes to treatment dosages or frequency including reasons for change
- Particular side-effects of treatment to watch out for, and specific advice on what to do if these signs or symptoms develop
- Clear instructions about how long treatments such as antibiotics or steroids should be administered or tailed off
- Treatment goals
- Details of significant conversations with patients and their carers relating to their understanding of their disease and their wishes for further treatment
- Clear details of who to contact in case of treatment complications

No single set of healthcare professionals can manage the many needs that patients have on their disease journey. Holistic, patient-centred, care requires a multi-professional and multi-disciplinary approach that places the patient and their family at the centre.

To facilitate improvements in communication many centres are now using patient-held records on which the different professionals record their findings and management plans, thus improving the continuity of care. With the increasing demand for transparency in care from patient groups, and the importance of ongoing care, such systems may well become normative in the UK.

Clinical trials

Clinical research is necessary in order to improve outcomes for patients with cancer. The link between the laboratory and the clinic is developing and increasingly patients are being recruited into trials.

There are three main types of clinical trial:

Phase I

Aim:
- To establish the human toxicity of a new drug through delivering carefully selected increasing doses to patients
- To establish the safe dose at which to start further trials with the drug
- To evaluate the body's handling of the drug by pharmacokinetic studies

Eligible patients
- Patients who have progressive disease despite standard oncological therapy or those for whom no standard therapy exists
- Patients must be aware that the primary objective of the studies is to assess toxicity. There is little expectation of benefit for themselves, with a response rate of approximately 5 per cent
- Patients recruited to Phase I trials usually have a high performance status and are highly motivated individuals, since involvement often requires intensive lengthy monitoring as an inpatient

Phase II

Aim:
- To establish the antitumour activity of the drug for a particular tumour type

Eligible patients
- Patients who have progressive disease despite standard chemotherapy or for whom no standard therapy exists
- Patients usually have a high performance status and are highly motivated
- Patients are closely monitored with toxicity and response assessments but not as intensively as those in Phase I studies

Phase III

Aim:
- To compare the new drug or drug combination with conventional therapy.

Eligible patients
- Patients for whom a standard therapy exists. (New drugs may also be compared with 'best supportive care' where no standard therapy exists.)

Important and common end points include disease free survival (in adjuvant studies), and overall survival (in palliative studies). Increasingly more clinically relevant end points such as improvements in pain, performance status and weight gain and quality of life are being used in Phase III trials of palliative agents.

Typically Phase III trials are much larger than Phase I/II trials and patients require less frequent monitoring.

Oncological surgery[2]

Surgery remains the modality of treatment most likely to cure patients diagnosed with solid tumours. It has most potential when the cancer is localized, though results are improving for patients with certain types of metastatic tumours.

Surgery has three main rôles in cancer management.

1 Diagnosis and staging
2 Curative treatment
3 Palliative treatment

Diagnosis and staging

In the past, many patients suspected of having cancer required surgery to confirm the diagnosis. The development of cross-sectional radiology and the ability to perform diagnostic biopsies using radiological guidance or endoscopy now often allows accurate diagnosis.

Patient morbidity has significantly reduced now that major diagnostic surgical procedures are no longer needed. The number of 'open and close' laparotomies for unresectable cancer, for example, has reduced to <5 per cent in recent years, largely due to these advances.

However surgical staging remains important in a number of common tumours:

- Axillary lymph node dissection for patients with breast cancer, for example, allows assessment of these nodes for involvement by tumour. Such information is important in determining prognosis and guiding decisions regarding adjuvant treatments
- Ovarian cancer spreads mainly via the transperitoneal route leading to tumour deposits in peritoneal surfaces and the omentum—sites poorly visualized on conventional imaging. A laparotomy for patients with ovarian cancer therefore allows a more accurate staging of disease than is currently possible with non-invasive means. Again such information is vital in determining prognosis and guiding further treatment

Curative surgery

Non-metastatic disease

Surgery is most commonly curative in intent for localized cancers and is generally dependent on complete resection of the tumour with a margin of normal tissue.

In some tumours with a propensity to spread to lymph nodes, resection of the draining lymph nodes may improve local control (e.g. vulval tumours). In other tumours the value of lymphadenectomy is uncertain and is the subject of ongoing clinical trials (e.g. endometrial cancer).

Unfortunately surgery still fails to cure many patients. There are a number of reasons for this:

1 Development of metastatic disease—this is due to the presence of micro-metastatic disease unidentifiable at the time of surgery. This is a common reason for failure of surgery to cure breast and bowel tumours
2 Development of local relapse—outcomes from surgery are often closely linked to the margin of normal tissue excised in continuity with

the tumour. The amount of tissue that can be resected may be limited by patient-related factors (e.g. only a partial lobectomy may be possible in patients with lung cancer due to the patients' underlying poor respiratory function) or by tumour related factors. (e.g. invasion by tumour of a vital structure such as the aorta.)

Metastatic disease

Although much less common, surgery may be curative in a limited number of tumours in the metastatic setting. The rôle for potentially curative surgery is best established in a small number of instances. These include:
- Pulmonary metastases from osteosarcoma
- Pulmonary metastases from soft tissue sarcoma
- Liver metastases from colorectal cancer
- Residual masses following chemothearpy for metastatic teratomas.

In each of these cases best results are seen with careful patient selection according to well defined criteria. In general terms the best long-term results are seen in patients who relapse after a long period from initial tumour diagnosis and who have low volume disease and a good performance status.

Palliative surgery

Surgery may provide very effective palliation in a number of situations. Given the specific problems of oncology patients in the palliative situation (limited life expectancy, poor performance status, rapid tumour progression), the decision to proceed with surgery must involve a careful weighing up of the benefit/harm of such procedures. These decisions are best made with a multidisciplinary approach by surgeons specialized in oncology and experienced in palliative management.

Bowel obstruction

Patients with colonic or ovarian cancer form the majority of patients with bowel obstruction referred for surgery. Surgery to relieve the obstruction is warranted even if disease is incurable (due to liver metastases or locally advanced disease for example) as such patients may live for many months. Where possible these patients should have the primary tumour excised and a primary anastomosis performed.

Patients with ovarian cancer commonly present with obstructive bowel symptoms. At initial presentation debulking surgery provides excellent palliation. Patients presenting with relapsed disease and obstructive symptoms often have multiple sites of obstruction due to widespread intraperitoneal dissemination of their disease. In this instance surgery is much less likely to be useful.

Fistulae

Fistulae may arise as a result of pelvic tumours or as a complication of radiotherapy. They are often associated with unpleasant symptoms. Optimum preoperative assessment requires imaging to delineate exactly the site of fistula formation and to guide surgical decisions. Surgery may provide excellent palliation but may not be useful in those with multiple

2 Cassidy J., Bissett D. et al. (2002) *Oxford Handbook of Oncology.* Oxford: Oxford University Press.

sites of fistulae or rapidly advancing intra-abdominal disease where life expectancy is limited.

Jaundice

Obstructive jaundice due to extrinsic pressure by lymph nodes on the biliary system, or due to intrinsic lesions such as cholangiocarcinoma, are commonly well palliated by radiological and endoscopic placement of stents.

The complications of stents include infection and blockage with consequent need for replacement.

Surgical relief of obstructive jaundice (e.g. by choledochoenterostomy) avoids problems associated with stents and may be indicated in a small minority of patients with an excellent performance status and slow-growing disease.

Pain

Surgical debulking of large slow-growing tumours can reduce pain and is justified in patients where the expected morbidity of the procedure is low. Neurosurgical approaches such as cordotomy are only infrequently considered.

Gastrointestinal bleeding

A wide range of endoscopic techniques have been developed to stop bleeding from benign and malignant causes. This may avoid the need for more major surgery in patients who have a limited life expectancy.

These include:
- Sclerotherapy
- Laser coagulation
- Radiological embolization

Bone metastases

Metastases to bones can cause major palliative problems. Specific problems include pain and pathological fracture. Factors that identify patients most at risk of pathological fracture include:
- Site—lesions in weight-bearing bones
- Extent of destruction—destruction of >50 per cent of cortex
- Symptoms—patients complaining of pain, particularly on weight bearing
- Type of lesion—lytic lesions > blastic lesions

Such patients may benefit (both in terms of reduced pain and reduced risk of fracture) from prophylactic fixation of a long bone. The type of internal fixation used depends on the site of fracture and the patient's performance status. In all cases internal fixation of the bone should be followed by radiotherapy to control tumour growth and promote healing.

Techniques such as vertebroplasty are available to manage pain in vertebrae.

Chemotherapy

> I am dying from the treatment of too many physicians
>
> Alexander the Great

Identification of agents

Chemotherapy generally refers to a group of agents used in the systemic management of cancer. A disparate group, they are linked by having demonstrated evidence of anticancer activity and a common range of side-effects.

The anticancer activity of these agents has been identified in a number of ways. For some the discovery of antineoplastic activity was serendipitous. Cisplatin was discovered because of using platinum electrodes in an antibiotic experiment.

For others this activity was identified during screening of a wide range of natural products (e.g. paclitaxel). Some of these agents have been biochemically modified to reduce their toxicity while retaining their anti-neoplastic activity (e.g. carboplatin).

Mechanism of action

Chemotherapy exerts its anticancer action by a wide variety of mechanisms which are, as yet, incompletely understood (see Table 5.1).

For many, DNA is believed to be the most important cellular target—irinotecan for example inhibits the topoisomerase I enzyme thereby causing double strand breaks in DNA. For other agents, microtubules, particularly those involved in formation of the mitotic spindle, appear to be the vital target—paclitaxel for example promotes tubulin polymerization and so arrests cells in metaphase.

A number of factors determine the likelihood of achieving a useful response to chemotherapy. Some tumours are inherently more sensitive to chemotherapy than others. In general terms chemotherapy tends to be most effective in tumours with fast cell turnover such as acute leukaemias and high grade lymphomas. Seminomas, however, a tumour with a long natural history, are also very chemosensitive. Clearly there are other factors, as yet poorly understood, that determine a tumour's chemosensitivity.

Patient-related factors are also important in determining likelihood of response. Patients with poor performance status, for example, respond less well than those with good performance status. The reasons for this are poorly understood but are probably due at least in part to a reduced tolerance to the acute toxicity of chemotherapy.

While chemotherapy may induce a partial or even complete response, the tumour may regrow with disease that has become chemoresistant. There is evidence in some cases that the tumour may have become more efficient at 'effluxing' the drug from the cell. Increasingly it is recognized that the ability of cells either to repair or tolerate the damage inflicted by chemotherapy may lead to chemoresistance. The causes of chemoresistance and the development of agents to overcome such mechanisms are active areas of research at present.

Tumours which divide rapidly with short doubling times respond best to chemotherapy.

Adverse effects of chemotherapy

Although the specific side-effect profile varies between agents, there are a number of side-effects common to most agents.

- *Alopecia* is a common and often distressing side-effect associated with many agents. Patients can be reassured that hair almost always regrows following chemotherapy although they may notice some changes. The hair may change colour and there can be a change in curliness
- *Nausea and vomiting* are common with many agents, although the degree to which this is a problem varies both between agents and between patients. The development of $5-HT_3$ antagonists (e.g. tropisetron, granisetron) has greatly aided the management of this troublesome side-effect. The efficacy of $5-HT_3$ antagonists can be improved by the addition of steroids
- *Myelosuppression* is another troublesome effect associated with chemotherapy. The white cells (in particular the neutrophils) are most commonly affected between 1 to 2 weeks following chemotherapy. Patients should be warned of the possibility of developing infection during this time and the urgency with which they should seek help, as they will require immediate treatment with broad spectrum antibiotics. The development of granulocyte colony stimulating growth factors has reduced this toxicity by shortening the duration of neutropaenia. This has allowed higher doses of chemotherapy to be given more safely in certain situations
- *Anxiety* The prospect of chemotherapy is a frightening concept for many patients—not least due to the (often mistaken) view of the difficult side-effects. It is important that the patient and their carers are fully educated about the type of side-effects they are likely to encounter during treatment and how best to deal with them. Most patients are extremely anxious during this difficult time and information may have to be repeated a number of times. It is very useful to have written information to supplement what has been said in consultations. It also useful if a relative or friend attends with the patient—they will often be able to help the patient review the information at a later date

Chemotherapy regimens

A wide and somewhat bewildering number of chemotherapy regimens are used in the treatment of patients with cancer. In general terms the tendency has been to combine drugs that demonstrate activity as single agents but which do not share the same side-effects.

More sophisticated techniques to examine synergy and pharmacokinetic interactions in a pre-clinical setting are now developing, and this will guide a logical approach to optimal combinations of agents.

Chemotherapy may be given in the following situations:

- Curative
- Adjuvant
- Neo-adjuvant
- Palliative

Curative

A small number of solid malignancies are curable by chemotherapy alone. Such tumours include germ cell tumours, lymphomas and certain childhood tumours.

In general terms chemotherapy regimens used in the treatment of these diseases are intensive and associated with a high incidence of acute toxicity. It is important that patients receive chemotherapy on schedule, with no delays, as there is evidence that dose reductions and prolonging treatment times may adversely affect outcome. Consequently treatment can exact a high physical and psychological toll on patients and their relatives.

Given that the long term aim of treatment is cure, patients and their carers need encouragement to persevere, which will be easier if physical symptoms are optimally managed. The palliative care team may well provide expert assistance at this stage of the patient's management.

Increasingly it is becoming clear that patients who are cured following chemotherapy are at risk of long-term toxicity from their treatment. Such problems include secondary leukaemias and solid tumours, fatigue, infertility and cardiomyopathy. These problems have only become appreciated in recent times. Undoubtedly as more people become long-term survivors of cancer, more problems will emerge. For this reason it is important that long-term survivors of cancer remain on long term follow-up.

Adjuvant

Many patients presenting with apparently localized cancer are known to be at high risk of developing metastatic disease. This is presumed to be due to the presence of micrometastases not apparent by current imaging modalities. Chemotherapy given following successful primary treatment for apparently localized cancer may reduce the risk of developing clinical metastatic disease.

Cancers where adjuvant chemotherapy is commonly used include breast and colorectal cancer where large multi-centre randomized controlled trials and subsequent meta-analysis have confirmed the survival gain.

At an individual level these gains are small, with absolute improvements in overall survival of 5–15 per cent after five years. At a population level, however, this represents a large number of lives saved in diseases as common as breast and bowel cancer.

Presently surrogate markers such as tumour size, grade and lymph node involvement are commonly used to assess risk of disease relapse and thereby identify those most likely to benefit from adjuvant therapy. Much current research is directed at developing predictive markers to identify more precisely those most likely to benefit.

Given that the majority of patients treated will not benefit from treatment as their disease will relapse anyway or because primary treatment has been curative, adjuvant regimens must therefore be well tolerated with a low incidence of serious acute side-effects and long-term side-effects.

Again, as with treatment in the curative setting, positive outcomes from treatment are closely linked to maintaining dose intensity and avoiding delays in chemotherapy. Where acute toxicities are a problem, involvement of the palliative care team may improve symptom management and facilitate delivery of treatment on schedule.

Neo-adjuvant

Chemotherapy may be used 'up front' in non-metastatic tumours prior to definitive treatment (usually surgery) for the tumour. This may be done in the case of a large inoperable primary tumour to shrink the cancer and facilitate surgery. Such an approach is standard practice for example in very large primary breast tumours or those with skin involvement.

Increasingly neo-adjuvant therapy is being utilized for tumours that are operable. Potential advantages of this approach include less extensive surgery in a tumour that has shrunk. From a research point of view a neo-adjuvant approach with biopsies before and after therapy may allow molecular markers that predict chemosensitivity to be identified.

Conversely there are a number of potential problems with neo-adjuvant chemotherapy. First, in a responding tumour there may be a loss of potentially useful prognostic information from the subsequently resected tumour specimen. There is also the risk that such an approach may allow interim tumour progression in a lesion that does not respond to chemotherapy. Finally performing less radical surgery in a tumour that has responded to chemotherapy may compromise local control.

This approach is being examined with particular interest in a number of tumours including oesophageal, gastric and breast tumours.

> Growth for the sake of growth is the ideology of the cancer cell.
> Edward Abbey 1927–1989

Palliative

The majority of solid cancers are not curable in the metastatic setting. Chemotherapy, however, may play a valuable rôle to play in the palliative treatment of such patients. Research now includes end points such as quality of life and toxicity, which is more clinically relevant in this setting than assessing overall survival as a sole entity.

Given that improvement or maintenance of quality of life is the most important aim of palliative chemotherapy, acute toxicities must be infrequent and easily managed.

Optimally a patient is best managed when chemotherapy is administered *in conjunction with* input from the palliative care team. Such input also facilitates the gradual handing over of care to the palliative care team as the patient's disease progresses. Such a team-based approach reduces problems of patients feeling neglected by their oncologist when chemotherapy is no longer useful.

Indications for palliative chemotherapy

'Treatment decisions are based on a consideration of the balance between the benefits expected and the toxicity and risks of chemotherapy which are different for each patient'.[3]

1 **Maintaining or improving quality of life:** This is the single most important aim of palliative chemotherapy. Chemotherapy may alleviate specific symptoms such as dyspnoea or chest pain in a patient with lung cancer. It may also improve or maintain general well-being with improvements in such factors as appetite and energy. The development of quality of life assessment tools, especially those with disease-specific elements, has greatly facilitated the assessment of the effect of chemotherapy on quality of life

3 McIllmurray M. (2004) Palliative medicine and the treatment of cancer. In D. Doyle, G. Hanks, and N. Cherney (eds). *Oxford Textbook of Palliative Medicine*, p 232. Oxford: Oxford University Press.

2 **Improving survival:** While this is a secondary objective in most cases, it is quite clear that chemotherapy given with palliative intent frequently prolongs survival. The extent to which it is expected that survival may be prolonged varies between diseases. Chemotherapy in pancreatic cancer is associated with an improvement in survival of only a few weeks, whereas patients receiving chemotherapy for ovarian cancer may have improved survival of many months or even years

3 **In emergency situations:** Potentially life-threatening tumour-related emergencies such as spinal cord compression or superior vena cava compression may be treated with chemotherapy where the primary tumour is very chemosensitive. Such tumours include lymphoma and small cell lung cancer

Chemotherapy within the palliative setting is increasingly common because of:

Earlier referral for palliative care services
Chemotherapeutic services and palliative care services will only be enhanced by a close working relationship with good lines of communication, early referral, and a seamless highway of care along which a patient can receive the specific form of care they need for the particular part of their journey. The journey from diagnosis to death is not linear but dynamic with different interventions governed not by the passage of time but by a patient's particular needs. With an integrated service and earlier referral patterns there will be an ever increasing number of patients in the palliative care setting who have just had, are having, or are just about to have, chemotherapy. In many cancer centres patients will be introduced to the palliative care team as part of their initial contact with 'the cancer service'.

Increasing indications for chemotherapy
Over the last decade there has been a huge increase in the number of drugs available to treat cancer patients and clinical trials have identified that these agents may provide palliative benefit in those for whom no treatment would have been available 20 years ago.

Patients undergoing clinical trials
Patients who have relapsed from their initial chemotherapy may well be involved in clinical trials of other agents if their overall fitness and clinical condition permits. As trials often involve treatments where conventional regimes have failed, such patients are often quite advanced in their disease, and in need of increasing palliative care input.

When is chemotherapy offered in the palliative care setting?
The decision to use chemotherapy with palliative intent is often a complex matter, and a number of factors must be taken into consideration:
• **Patient fitness**—Generally patients with ECOG performance status (see the box on p.xxxi) >2 tolerate chemotherapy very poorly—chemotherapy is contra-indicated in such patients. Possible exceptions include patients with very chemosensitive tumours that may be expected to respond quickly such as small cell lung cancer and lymphoma

- **Patient symptoms**—Chemotherapy in the palliative setting is generally delayed until the patient develops symptoms. The potential danger with this approach is that the patient may rapidly develop symptoms which render them unfit for chemotherapy. In some cases, therefore, oncologists may choose to monitor disease and institute treatment when there is evidence that disease, although asymptomatic, is progressing
- **Disease sites** —Generally large volume disease at life-threatening sites such as the liver requires urgent chemotherapy even in the absence of disease-related symptoms, unless the patient is imminently dying, as patients are likely to become symptomatic very quickly. Close relationships may build up between doctors and patients over many years. It may be difficult for doctors to withdraw toxic oncological treatment from a patient who continues to demand it, even if it has now become clearly inappropriate. Clear and open discussion with patients and their family about the potential benefits and risks of chemotherapy, the aims of treatment and, in particular, agreements for stopping treatment is important. The palliative care team may be helpful in supporting the oncology team with these discussions

How will chemotherapy affect the patient and family?'

Each individual patient and family will have their own particular response to chemotherapy in the palliative care setting. Certain themes may be common to many such individuals. The following are some of the scenarios encountered in GP surgeries, oncology services and palliative care units.

1 **'We've got to keep on trying.'** Having endured the rigours of their disease and its management, some patients reach the palliative setting protesting their capacity as 'fighters'. (There is now evidence that psychological disposition has no bearing on disease outcome.) They have coped with their disease by trusting in the system and in being 'active' in fighting their cancer. It is very hard to wean such patients off chemotherapy or to stop active treatment as to do so seems, in their eyes, to admit defeat. Such patients will ask to be put into trials and see their rôle as patients as being fulfilled only so long as they are participating in active treatment

2 **'It was not half as bad as I thought it was going to be.'** Increasingly due to improved symptom control measures and a more holistic approach, patients may be pleasantly surprised by their tolerance of chemotherapy. Most people have had a previous contact with someone going through chemotherapy and their expectations are often adversely affected by this

3 **'He has suffered enough.'** Other families come through their disease journey with very ambivalent attitudes towards the system and to chemotherapy. They arrive in the palliative care setting determined that further suffering should be kept to a minimum. They can be reluctant to consider any intervention at all, other than the administration of pain controlling medications. For such a family the prospect of chemotherapy entering into the palliative setting is anathema, and time may need to be taken to explain the benefits in certain situations, if appropriate

4 **'Her hair fell out, then she died.'** Many patients and families come with memories and histories of relatives who have received chemotherapy in the past. Memories seldom show clearly the distinction between problems caused by the illness itself and problems caused by side-effects. The two merge into a mess of suffering leaving the patient and the family convinced that there is only one thing worse than dying with cancer—and that is dying from cancer with the side-effects of chemotherapy. Doctors and nurses are not inured from such emotional responses

5 **'Whatever you say Doctor.'** Another group of patients cope with their disease by investing their trust in 'the doctor' looking after them. Such an approach runs contrary to non-patronizing modern trends but is still present particularly among older patients. To present such patients with a meta-analysis of the benefits of one form of chemotherapy or another and to ask the patient which one he wants to choose would be inappropriate

6 **'What about Mexican dog weed.'** Some patients and relatives may come into the palliative care setting clutching reams of printouts from the Internet about treatments from clinics around the world. They will often be very articulate and questioning of every intervention. Some will have an alternative medicine approach and be very sceptical of western medicine. Honest communication needs to include how health professionals interpret the clinical research literature and what they would be prepared to do in terms of agreeing to provide a treatment that is controversial, unproven and unlicenced. Boundaries need to be set and unrealistic expectations dispelled alongside not removing hope that a reasonable quality of life can still be achieved

7 **'I've had a good life.'** A section of patients come into the palliative setting without illness at the centre of their lives. Instead they are focused on their living and their dying, with its important stages and goodbyes. Such patients have accepted the inevitability of their death and have moved on to preparing for it. They have things that they want to do. When it comes to the possibility of chemotherapy for such people their main concern is, 'Will it interfere with what I still have to do?' They are strangely neutral about chemotherapy and it is almost as if they are humouring the professionals by agreeing to it, while they get on with the real business of living

8 **'I just can't face it.'** Some patients have been so worn down by their disease and treatment that the prospect of any more chemotherapy fills them with fear and dread. Sometimes the fears are justified and sometimes they are not. Sometimes their expression of fear about chemotherapy is a way of verbalizing fears about other matters which should be explored. They face the dilemma of risks and fears whether or not they accept chemotherapy and will need a lot of support in reaching a treatment decision

Cytotoxic drugs

Alkylating agents
Damage DNA by addition of an alkyl group eg. cyclophosphamide, ifosfamide, melphalan, busulphan.

Platinum agents
Damage DNA by addition of platinum adducts e.g. cisplatin, carboplatin, oxaliplatin.

Antimetabolites
Inhibit production of pyrimidine and purine metabolites e.g. fluorouracil, methotrexate, capecitabine, mercaptopurine, gemcitabine.

Antitumour antibiotics
Variable mechanism e.g. doxorubicin, epirubicin, mitoxantrone, bleomycin.

Vinca alkaloids
Bind to the tubulin blocking microtubule and therefore interfere with spindle formation at metaphase e.g. vincristine, vinorelbine, vinblastine.

Taxanes
Promote tubulin polymerization and arrest cells at metaphase e.g. paclitaxel, docetaxel.

Topoisomerase I inhibitors
Inhibit topoisomerase I leading to DNA damage e.g. irinotecan, topotecan.

Hormonal agents
Selective Oestrogen Receptor Modulators (SERMs)
Partial antagonists of the oestrogen receptor e.g. tamoxifen.

Aromatase inhibitors
Inhibit extragonadal oestrogen production e.g. anastrozole, letrozole.

Gonadorelin analogues
Inhibit gonadal production of oestrogen and testosterone e.g. leuprorelin, goserelin.

Anti-androgens
- Testosterone receptor antagonists
- Cyproterone acetate

Immunomodulatory
- e.g. Interferon

Novel agents
Many anticancer agents currently in development have been rationally developed to antagonize elements of the neoplastic process at a cellular level. While most of these agents are still in preclinical or early clinical testing, a number have already entered routine clinical practice. As a rule these agents are much better tolerated than conventional cytotoxic drugs with less myelosuppression, alopecia and emesis. Preclinical testing

suggests that many may act as cytostatics rather than cytotoxics and that there may be syergistic interactions with other drugs. The challenge in the future will be the rational design of clinical trials to investigate how these agents are best used.

Antibodies

- **Herceptin**—a monoclonal antibody to HER-2—a member of the epidermal growth factor receptors over-expressed in approximately 25 per cent of all breast cancers and associated with poor prognosis. Herceptin has demonstrated activity in HER-2 over-expressing tumours both alone and in combination with chemotherapy
- **Rituximab**—a monoclonal antibody to CD-20, a protein expressed in some lymphomas. Again rituximab is active both alone and in combination with chemotherapy

Tyrosine kinase inhibitors

Many of the signalling pathways within a cell involved in the cancer phenotype rely on enzymes called tyrosine kinases. Interruption of this activity may interrupt signalling pathways involved in cancer.

- **Iressa**—inhibits the tyrosine kinase activity of the epidermal growth factor receptor activity demonstrated as a second line agent in non-small cell lung cancer. Common side-effects include diarrhoea and skin rashes
- **Imatinib**—inhibits the tyrosine kinase activity of the S-kit proteins found in gastrointestinal stromal tumours and also of the BCR/ABL fusion protein found in chronic myeloid leukaemia

Table 5.1 Classification of anticancer agents

Class of agent		Mode of action	Examples in common usage
Cytotoxics	Alkylating agents	Damage DNA by addition of an alkyl group	Cyclophosphamide, ifosfamide, melphalan, busulphan
	Platinum agents	Damage DNA by addition of platinum adducts	Cisplatin, carboplatin, oxaliplatin
	Antimetabolites	Inhibit production of pyrimidine and purine metabolites	fluorouracil, metotrexate, capecitabine, mercaptopurine, gemcitabine
	Antitumour antibiotics	Variable	Doxorubicin, epirubicin, mitoxantrone, bleomycin
	Vinca alkaloids	Bind to tubulin blocking microtubule and therefore spindle formation at metaphase	Vincristine, vinorelbine, vinblastine
	Taxanes	Promote tubulin polymerization and arrest cells at metaphase	Paclitaxel, docetaxel
	Topoisomerase I inhibitors	Inhibit topoisomerase I leading to DNA damage	Irinotecan, topotecan
Hormonal agents	Selective oestrogen receptor modulators (SERMs)	Partial antagonists of the oestrogen receptor	Tamoxifen
	Aromatase inhibitors	Inhibit extragonadal oestrogen production	Anastrozole, letrozole
	Gonadorelin analogues	Inhibit gonadal production of oestrogen and testosterone	Leuprorelin
	Antiandrogens	Testosterone receptor antagonists	Cyproterone acetate
Immuno-modulatory	Interferon		
'Novel' agents	Antibodies	Opsonization, interrupt growth stimulatory pathways	Rituximab, trastuzumab
	Signal transduction inhibitors	Interrupt growth stimulatory pathways	Imatinib, iressa
	Vascular targeting agents	Target 'new' vessels associated with tumours—not in use outwith a clinical trial	Bevacizumab

Table 5.2 Commonly used anticancer drugs (new drugs are regularly being introduced)

Drug	Administration	Excretion	Side-effects	Indications
Bleomycin *Cytotoxic antibiotic*	i/v	Excretion: Urine	'Flu symptoms; Hyperpigmentation; Allergic reactions; Pulmonary fibrosis—common with doses >300 mg	Germ cell tumours Lymphoma
Busulphan *Alkylating agent*	p.o	Excreted in urine	Myelosuppression; Hyperpigmentation Pulmonary interstitial fibrosis; Hepato-venous occlusion	Leukaemia
Caelyx see doxorubicin				
Carboplatin	i/v	Renal	Myelosuppression especially thrombocytopaenia; Emesis	Ovarian cancer
Capecitabine *Antimetabolite*	p.o	Renal	'Hand foot' syndrome; Diarrhoea Stomatitis	Colorectal cancer Breast cancer
Cisplatin	i/v	Renal	Emesis; Renal Failure; Peripheral neuropathy Ototoxicity; Allergic reactions	Germ cell cancer Lung cancer
Cyclophosphamide *Alkylating agent*	p.o	Hepatic and renal	Myelosuppression; Alopecia; Emesis Haemorrhagic cystitis (reduced by mesna)	Breast cancer Lymphoma
Cytarabine *Antimetabolite*	i/v, i/t, SC	Hepatic and renal	Myelosuppression; Diarrhoea; Stomatitis	Leukaemia
Dactinomycin *Cytotoxic antibiotic*	i/v	Hepatic and renal	Myelosuppression; Mucositis; Diarrhoea Alopecia	Choriocarcinoma Ewing's sarcoma

Drug	Administration	Excretion	Side-effects	Indications
Docetaxel *Taxane*	i/v	Hepatic	Myelosuppression; Fluid retention Alopecia; Peripheral neuropathy	Breast cancer
Doxorubicin (Adriamycin) *Cytotoxic antibiotic*	i/v and intravesical	Hepatic	Emesis; Myelosuppression; Mucositis Alopecia; Cardiomyopathy—risk related to total cumulative dose.	Breast cancer Sarcoma
Doxorubicin Liposomal (Caelyx) *Cytotoxic antibiotic*	i/v	Hepatic	Palmar-plantar erythrodysaesthesia; Stomatitis	Ovarian cancer Breast cancer Kaposi's sarcoma
Etoposide	i/v	Renal	Myelosuppression; Emesis; Alopecia Secondary leukaemia	Lung cancer Germ cell tumour
Epirubicin *Cytotoxic antibiotic*	i/v	Hepatic	Similar to Doxorubicin but less cardiotoxic	Breast cancer
Fluorouracil *Antimetabolite*	i/v, topical cream	Liver and renal	Mucositis; Diarrhoea; Hand-foot syndrome; Myelosuppression; Gastrointestinal upsets; Cerebellar ataxia (rare); Gritty eyes and blurred vision	Colorectal cancer Breast cancer
Gemcitabine *Antimetabolite*	i/v	Renal	Myelosuppression; Flu like symptoms; Fatigue; Pneumonitis	Pancreatic cancer Bladder cancer Lung cancer

Drug	Route	Metabolism	Toxicity	Indication
Ifosfamide *Alkylating agent*	i/v	Hepatic and renal	Alopecia; Emesis; Haemorrhagic cystitis; Encephalopathy	Sarcomas
Irinotecan *Topoisomerase inhibitor*	i/v	Hepatic and renal	Cholinergic syndrome—associated with infusion; Delayed diarrhoea; Nausea and vomiting; Myelosuppression; Alopecia	Colorectal cancer
Mercaptopurine *Antimetabolite*	p.o	Peripheral tissues	Myelosuppression; Hepatic dysfunction; Stomatitis	Leukaemia
Methotrexate **(+ folinic acid)** *Antimetabolite*	p.o, i/v, i/m, i/t p.o.	Renal	Myelosuppression; Mucositis; Skin pigmentation; Nephrotoxicity	Osteosarcoma Breast cancer Leukaemia and lymphoma
Mitomycin *Cytotoxic antibiotic*	i/v or intravesical	Hepatic metabolism	Myelosuppression; Lung fibrosis; Nephrotoxicity Stomatitis; Diarrhoea; Haemplytic uraemic syndrome	Anal Bladder

Drug	Administration	Excretion	Side-effects	Indications
Mitoxantrone *Cytotoxic antibiotic*	i/v	Excretion: Bile > urine	Myelosuppression; Emesis; Alopecia; Mucositis; Cardiotoxicity	Lymphoma Leukaemia
Oxaliplatin	i/v	Renal	Peripheral neuropathy; Myelosuppression; Nausea and vomiting; Laryngeal spasm	Colorectal cancer
Paclitaxel *(Taxane)*	i/v	Hepatic	Myelosuppression; Alopecia; Hypersensitivity reactions; Peripheral neuropathy	Ovarian cancer Lung cancer Breast cancer
Temozolomide *Alkylating agent*	p.o.		Emesis; Myelosuppression	Astrocytomas Melanoma
Tioguanine *Antimetabolite*	p.o. (40 mg)	Renal	Myelosuppression; Mucositis; Diarrhoea; Hepatic dysfunction	Leukaemia
Thiotepa *Alkylating agent*	i/v	Excreted more in urine than bile	Myelosuppression	Leukaemia

Drug	Route	Metabolism/Excretion	Side effects	Uses
Topotecan *Topoisomerase inhibitor*	i/v	Liver metabolism Urine excretion	Myelosuppression; Emesis; Alopecia; Diarrhoea	Ovarian cancer
Vinblastine *Mitotic spindle inhibitor*	i/v	Hepatic	Myelosuppression constipation and stomatitis Rare: hair loss or peripheral neurotoxicity	Lymphoma Germ cell tumours
Vincristine *Mitotic spindle inhibitor*	i/v	Hepatic	Peripheral neuropathy; Autonomic neuropathy	Lymphomas Leukaemia
Vindesine *Mitotic spindle inhibitor*	i/v	Hepatic	Myelosuppression; Mild neurotoxicity; Autonomic neuropathy	Leukaemia
Vinorelbine *Mitotic spindle inhibitor*	i/v	Hepatic	Myelosuppression; Phlebitis; Peripheral neuropathy	Breast cancer Non-small cell lung cancer

Table 5.3 Hormone and anti hormone drugs

Drug	Administration	Side-effects	Comments
SERMs			
Tamoxifen	p.o.	Menopausal symptoms Thromboembolic event Endometrial hyperplasia and cancer	Used first line in adjuvant treatment of ER/PR +ve breast Cancer
Anti-androgens			
Bicalutamide	p.o.	Hepatotoxicity Gynaecomastia	Used in prostatic cancer sometimes in combination with gonadorelin analogues
Cyproterone acetate			
Flutamide			
Aromatase inhibitors			
Anastrozole	p.o.	Menopausal symptoms? Increased fractures	Used in post-menopausal breast cancer
Formestane	i/m		
Letrozole	p.o.		
Gonadorelin analogues*			
Buserelin	SC and intranasal	Gynaecomastia, impotence, nausea, fluid retention	Prostate cancer
Goserelin	implant	Menopausal symptoms	Breast cancer
Leuprorelin	i/m		
Triptorelin	i/m		

*Beware initial flare of symptoms when start use in men with prostate cancer. This should be 'covered' with the concomitant use of antiandrogens for the first few weeks of therapy.

Table 5.4 Emetic risk of common chemotherapy drugs

Cytotoxic agents	Risk
Cisplatin*	High
Cyclophosphamide >1000 mg/m²*	
Ifosfamide*	
Melphalan*	
Actinomycin	Moderate
Amsacrine	
Busulphan	
Carboplatin*	
Chlorambucil	
Cladribine	
Cyclophosphamide <1000 mg/m²	
Cytarabine >150 mg/m²	
Dacarbazine	
Daunorubicin	
Daunorubicin liposomal	
Doxorubicin	
Epirubicin	
Lomustine	
Methotrexate > 1G/m²	
Mitoxantrone	
Procarbazine	
Bleomycin	Low
Cyclophosphamide <300 mg/m²	
Cytarabine <150 mg/m²	
Etoposide	
Fludarabine	
Mercaptopurine	
Methotrexate <IG/m²	
Tioguanine	
Thiotepa	
Vinblastine	
Vincristine	

*Delayed emesis risk.

Radiotherapy

Radiotherapy is the most important type of non-surgical treatment for patients with common cancers. The proportion of these treated by radiotherapy at some time during their illness has risen steadily and is now well over 50%.

Tobias, UCH London

Introduction
Radiotherapy as a therapeutic modality developed shortly after the discovery of x-rays at the end of the nineteenth century. Clinical and technological advances subsequently have made it one of the most successful modalities in the treatment of patients with cancer, both in the curative and palliative settings.

Mechanism of action
Radiotherapy is the therapeutic use of ionising radiation to destroy cancerous cells. The critical cellular target is, in common with chemotherapy, the nuclear DNA. Double-stranded breaks in the DNA molecule appear to be the lesion responsible for cell death. Cell death takes place during subsequent mitotic cell division, hence the term mitotic cell death. Much less commonly, certain tissue types, such as lymphocytes and parotid acinar cells, undergo cell death without attempting mitosis, a process known as interphase cell death. Not all double-stranded DNA breaks, however, result in cell death, indeed most are repaired by the cell's DNA repair enzyme apparatus. The success or otherwise of the repair process determines the fate of the cell.

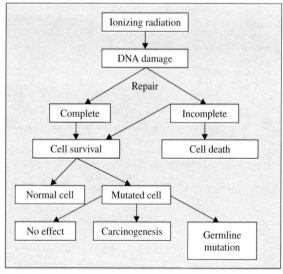

Fig. 5.1 The cell repair process after radiotherapy

Response of normal tissues to radiation

Different types of normal tissue respond differently to radiation. Homeostatic mechanisms control cell populations by balancing cell death with new cell growth through the proliferation of stem cells. If a proportion of these stem cells are destroyed by radiation, the rate of renewal of normal cells will be reduced. The time of appearance of this tissue damage is determined by the lifespan of the mature cells within that tissue. For certain tissues such as skin and mucosa, this lifespan is short as cells are quickly lost by desquamation, and hence tissue damage is manifest during the radiation course. For other tissues, cell turnover is much slower and radiation damage will only become apparent many months or years after radiation exposure. This gives rise to the distinction between the acute and late effects of irradiation.

Acute effects of radiation

This refers to the normal tissue reactions during a course of radiotherapy. The mucosa and haemopoetic system, i.e. tissues with a fast normal cellular turnover, display effects of irradiation earliest. For example, patients receiving radiotherapy to the head and neck area may develop severe oral mucositis, and those receiving radiotherapy to significant volumes of bone marrow, may develop bone marrow suppression.

Acute reactions are usually observed during the course of conventionally fractionated radiotherapy (1.8–2 Gy per fraction five times a week).

Late effects of radiation

These occur predominantly in slowly proliferating tissues (lung, kidney, heart, liver and CNS). By definition, late reactions occur more than 90 days after commencing a course of radiation.

In addition some of the tissues which develop their effects early, can also demonstrate late effects such as fibrosis or telangiectasia in the skin. This reflects the differing populations of cells (fibroblasts, endothelium etc.) which exist within a single organ.

Normal tissue tolerance

Not only do different tissues respond at different rates to irradiation, they also vary in their sensitivity. Certain tissues e.g. the lens, exhibit damage at very low doses while other tissues demonstrate marked resistance to the effects of radiation, e.g. uterine cervix. The situation is analogous among cancers. Lymphomas and seminomas show sensitivity to radiation while renal cell carcinomas and melanomas are radioresistant.

A number of treatment and patient factors influence tissue tolerance to radiation. These include:

- Total radiation dose given: higher doses are more toxic
- Fraction size: late responding tissues more sensitive to large fractions
- Overall longer treatment time: better tolerated by normal tissues
- Treatment volume: larger volumes are generally more toxic
- Quality of the radiation: neutrons are more damaging than photons or electrons
- Concomitant therapy: oncurrent chemotherapy reduces tolerance

Patient factors adversely influencing tissue tolerance:
- Older age
- Haemoglobin level
- Smoking
- Diabetes mellitus
- Connective tissue disorders
- Genetic syndromes (e.g. ataxia telangiectasia)

Tolerance doses for specific tissues

The following tissues suffer a 5 per cent incidence of toxicity at five years when conventional radiotherapy is given in fraction dose sizes of 1.8–2 Gy per fraction at the doses stated for each tissue type.

Table 5.5 Normal tissue tolerance

Tissue	Injury	Tolerance
Brain	Necrosis	60 Gy
Spinal cord	Myelopathy	45 Gy (<1% incidence)
Lens*	Cataract	10 Gy
Small intestine	Ulceration/perforation	45–50 Gy
Kidney*	Clinical nephritis	23 Gy
Lung*	Pneumonitis	18–20 Gy
Heart*	Pericarditis	40 Gy

*Whole organ.

Retreatment

Traditional teaching precluded retreating areas that had already received a maximal radiation dose. Recent studies have shown some tissues and organs have a greater capacity to recover from subclinical radiation injury than was previously thought. For example the large capacity of long-term regeneration of the CNS allows new possibilities for retreating recurrent neurological tumours with irradiation.

Table 5.5 Radiation effects within specific tissues (following standard radical doses)

Skin	Acute reaction—erythema begins week 3–4 Dry or moist desquamation later	Reaction settles within 2–4 weeks of completion of therapy
	Late reaction—fibrosis, atrophy, telangiectasia	
Oral mucosa	Acute reaction—erythema/oedema from wk 2–4 Patchy followed by confluent mucositis later	Reaction settles within 2–4 weeks of completion of therapy
Gastrointestinal tract	Acute reaction—mucositis causes nausea, anorexia, cramps, and diarrhoea	Reaction settles within 2–4 weeks of completion of therapy Treat symptomatically
	Late reaction—ulceration and fibrosis leading to strictures, fistulae, and malabsorption	Usually >6 months post RT
Brain	Acute reaction—lethargy common Occasionally cerebral oedema	
	Late reaction—somnolence syndrome at 1–3 months post RT Brain necrosis at 6 months to 3 years	Resolves spontaneously with/without help of steroids Indistinguishable clinically from recurrent tumour
Spinal cord	Late reaction—Lhermitte's syndrome 2–18 months after RT Radiation myelopathy at 6–12 months	Resolves spontaneously. Does not progress to myelopathy. Irreversible
Lung	Early/intermediate reaction—pneumonitis at 1–3 months Results in pulmonary fibrosis	Classical straight-edged appearance on chest x-ray
Kidney	Late reaction—proteinuria, hypertension, renal failure	May take up to 10 years to develop
Heart	Late reaction—pericarditis/effusion Most within 6 months of RT	Most resolve spontaneously; may develop into a constrictive process
	Cardiomyopathy	10–20 years post RT
	Coronary artery disease	10–15 years post RT

NB Patients undergoing radiotherapy usually experience lethargy as a general side-effect.

Types of radiation therapy

There are three main types of radiation therapy:
1 External beam radiotherapy, delivered by radiotherapy machines
2 Brachytherapy, solid radiation sources delivered directly into tumours
3 Unsealed source or radioisotope therapy, given by mouth, intravenously or into tissue spaces

External beam radiotherapy

External beam radiation consists of different energies, as shown in Table 5.7.

Table 5.7

Type of radiation	Energy	Use
Superficial X-rays	80–150 kV	Skin tumours
Orthovoltage X-rays (DXT)	200–400 kV	Thick skin tumours Superficial tumours e.g. ribs
Megavoltage radiation		
γ rays—cobalt 60	1.25 MV (mean)	Deep tumours
X rays—linear accelerator	4–25 MV	Deep tumours
Electrons	4–20 MeV	Skin tumours Superficial tumours

Superficial X-rays use relatively low energy x-ray photons in the range 80–400 kV. These x-rays are relatively non-penetrating, depositing the majority of their energy in the most superficial few millimetres of skin. They therefore deliver a high dose to the skin with rapid fall-off with increasing depth and are thus appropriate for the treatment of superficial skin lesions such as basal cell cancers.

Orthovoltage energy X-rays are slightly more penetrating and deliver sufficient dose at depth to treat adequately thicker skin or subcutaneous lesions such as rib metastases. (Both superficial and orthovoltage x-rays suffer the disadvantage of delivering a higher absorbed dose to bone compared to soft tissue, thus increasing the risk of osteoradionecrosis if a lesion is positioned too close to underlying bony tissue.)

Megavoltage X-ray photons possess energies 50–200 times those of superficial x-rays. (1–20MV) In contrast to superficial/orthovoltage x-rays, megavoltage photons are produced by the acceleration of electrons along a linear tube (wave guide) before striking a target. This is done within a machine called a linear accelerator. The interaction of these high energy electrons with the target material generates high energy x-rays.

High energy x-rays are very penetrating and give a much higher dose at a given depth within a tissue than superficial x-rays.

Megavoltage x-rays possess the advantage of relative sparing of the superficial skin tissues as the maximum absorbed dose occurs up to several centimetres below the skin surface. There is also no increased absorption of dose in tissues containing elements of high atomic mass such as bone.

Electron therapy

Electrons may be generated using a linear accelerator. In this situation the accelerated electron beam exits the linear accelerator without striking the target. Electron therapy is used to treat superficial tumours, most often of the skin. It is their characteristic deposition of dose with depth which makes electrons ideal for this purpose: >90 per cent of the dose is deposited in the first few centimetres of tissue with very rapid dose fall-off thereafter, thus sparing underlying structures.

Treatment planning

This is the essential prerequisite step before treatment delivery. During the process of treatment planning questions such as 'where to treat?', 'what to treat?', 'what not to treat?', 'how to treat and how much to treat?' are addressed. It is essentially an iterative process with changes being made at various stages to facilitate the design of an optimal treatment schedule. There are several rungs in the planning ladder (Fig. 5.2).

The complexity of treatment planning depends upon the tumour and the intent of therapy. Radical plans are generally more complicated and time-consuming than those with palliative intent.

Immobilization is relatively more important for those tumours positioned close to sensitive normal tissue structures and for radical, high-dose, treatments.

Patient positioning	Appropirate, comfortable and reproducible position makes therapy more tolerable and enables more reliable delivery
Immobilization	Immobilizaton will vary with the intent of treatment and the tumour site e.g. Perspex shells for head and neck cancers
Localization of the tumour	This may be clinical or using various imaging modalities e.g. fluroscopy, CT scanning
Target definition	The demonstrable tumour is outlined with additional margins allowed for microscopic extension and patient/organ movement
Generation of optimal dose distribution	Simple arrangement of x-ray beams used for palliative situations. Radical plans require more complex multiple beam configurations
Verification	Essential prior to treatment delivery to ensure target covered and critical normal organs protected

Fig. 5.2 The treatment ladder

The tumour is **localized** either by clinical examination e.g. skin tumours, or by imaging, most commonly fluoroscopy or CT scanning. Newer technology permits the fusing of various imaging modalities e.g. CT/MRI images, PET/CT images.

Once the tumour is localized the **target volume is defined**. This encompasses the tumour with a safety margin. This margin is added to allow for microscopic tumour extension, the so-called clinical target volume. Additionally, the margin will also accommodate movements in the organ containing the tumour, and uncertainties inherent in the treatment delivery system.

After the target has been delineated differing beam arrangements are generated. The arrangement is chosen which best covers the target volume and most successfully spares the normal tissue structures.

The final step in treatment planning is **verification**. This is an essential step to ensure that a plan generated on a planning computer actually fits the patient i.e. the tumour is accurately targeted and critical structures such as spinal cord are adequately spared. The verification process continues through treatment with dose measurements confirming appropriate dose delivery.

Radiotherapy dose prescription

Once the final treatment plan is decided upon, the radiation dose must be prescribed. There are several constituents that together make up the prescription:

- Total dose
- Number of fractions (fraction size)
- Overall treatment time

Total dose/number of fractions

Rather than deliver the entire dose of radiation in a single treatment, the dose is divided up into smaller quanta. This is the process of fractionation, each treatment dose being known as a fraction. Fractionation is performed to permit repair of normal tissue radiation damage. Fractionation will also permit repair to occur within tumour tissue, although this is relatively less efficient. In consequence, when a treatment course is fractionated, the total dose of radiation must be increased. Early studies showed that changing from a single dose to a six-week fractionated course of therapy required an increase in the total dose by a factor of three in order to achieve the same biological effect.

- The relationship between total dose and number of fractions is, however, complex and mathematical models are used to help predict the biological effects

Small numbers of fractions are convenient for the patient as travelling is kept to a minimum, however, the fraction size is in consequence larger; this increases the biological effectiveness of each fraction resulting in more severe damage to late-responding tissues. The total dose in such hypofractionated courses must be reduced to maintain an acceptable level of late tissue damage.

Hypofractionated treatment courses are often employed in the palliative setting on account of their convenience for patients and the relative unimportance of adverse long-term effects of radiation in patients with limited life expectancy.

Overall treatment time

Standard radical fractionation schedules involve treating once per day, Monday to Friday, for four to seven weeks. As treatment usually extends beyond four weeks, tumour cell repopulation becomes a problem.

As the number of tumour stem cells and mature functional tumour cells are depleted as a result of radiotherapy, the remaining stem cells sense this loss and begin to replicate actively to counteract this deficit. This is known as *tumour repopulation*. It appears that there is a lag period of approximately 3–4 weeks before this phenomenon occurs. Each fraction of radiotherapy delivered after the onset of repopulation is therefore relatively less effective, since part of the fraction must counteract this increase in the number of tumour cells resulting from repopulation.

A means of circumventing this effect of tumour repopulation is to *accelerate* the radiotherapy course so that the dose is delivered over a shorter time period, preferably less than the 3–4 weeks required for the onset of repopulation. A large randomized controlled clinical trial[4] of accelerated radiotherapy in non-small cell lung cancer has demonstrated that such an approach can be effective, with an increased rate of local tumour control and overall survival.

Brachytherapy

Here the radiation source is closely applied to the tumour. (Literally: therapy at a short distance, from the Greek βραχνS, brachys, short).

The underlying principle is the inverse square law, which states that the intensity of radiation, R, at a given distance, D, from a radioactive source, and therefore the absorbed dose, is inversely proportional to the square of that distance. Put simply, doubling the distance between the radiation source and the tissue reduces the dose absorbed by the tissue by a factor of four (rather than a factor of two as might be expected if the relationship was linear).

$$R \propto \frac{1}{D^2}$$

The beauty of brachytherapy lies in the ability to administer high doses of radiation to the tumour with relative sparing of neighbouring normal tissue because of rapid fall-off of absorbed dose with distance.

Brachytherapy is also known as **sealed source therapy** because the radioactive substance (often a metal) e.g. Iridium[192], is usually encased or sealed within a metal casing such that the radioactive substance does not actually physically touch the tissue even when inserted directly into the tumour (see below).

Brachytherapy takes three main forms:
- **Interstitial:** The radiation source is inserted directly into the tumour tissue
- **Intracavitary:** The radioactive source is inserted into a body cavity such as the uterus or the vagina when treating endometrial or cervical cancer
- **Intraluminal:** The radioactive source is positioned in the lumen of a hollow viscus e.g. bronchus, oesophagus

Brachytherapy, because it involves the placing of radioactive sources in close proximity to the patient, must of necessity make staff vulnerable to the risk of radiation exposure.

Decreasing the time during which exposure might occur, maximizing the shielding between source and staff, and most importantly increasing the distance from source to personnel all help to diminish risk.

In practice the brachytherapist places hollow tubes into the tumour, cavity or lumen, through which the source may subsequently be driven mechanically. Thus the radioactive source is brought into very close proximity to the tumour but staff experience no significant exposure.

Unsealed source therapy

This involves administering radioactive substances directly into the patient either in the form of liquids for ingestion or solutions for intravenous administration.

Unsealed source therapy is most often used as a palliative manoeuvre, although radioactive iodine[131] is employed as an adjuvant to curative surgery for well-differentiated thyroid cancer and indeed is often used to treat thyrotoxicosis, a non-malignant condition.

Radiation protection issues are to the fore as patients emit radiation for a variable period after administration of the radioisotope depending on the half-life of the isotope. They are carefully instructed regarding the precautions necessary to prevent excess exposure to others, most notably family members. Such precautions include double flushing of the toilet after micturition, and refraining from close contact with children and avoiding places of entertainment or work for a specified period of time post-treatment.

A number of radioisotopes are commonly used:

- **Strontium^{89}(Sr^{89}):** Often used for the relief of bone pain due to metastatic bone disease. A disadvantage is the relatively long half-life which poses radiation protection problems, especially if the patient dies within a short period after treatment. Some patients experience a flare up in their bone pain within a few days of treatment. This usually settles with appropriate analgesia. As strontium is absorbed into bone tissue, bone marrow toxicity may occasionally occur, and regular blood count monitoring after treatment is advised
- **Samarium^{153}(Sm^{153}):** Used less commonly than Sr^{89} but indicated likewise for the relief of pain from bony metastatic disease. It has the advantages of a shorter half-life and the production of photons as part of its decay pathway. These photons permit scintigraphy and thus bone scan images may be obtained. The propensity to pain flare and marrow toxicity pertain as for Sr^{89}
- **Iodine^{131}:** Both normal thyroid and well-differentiated thyroid cancer (papillary and follicular variants) selectively take up and concentrate iodine. This can be exploited therapeutically using I^{131}. Due to this concentrating effect within thyroid tissue, high doses can be selectively delivered to the normal or malignant thyroid tissue leading to its

destruction. In the case of normal thyroid tissue, hyperthyroid patients may be rendered euthyoid with a relatively low dose of I^{131}; in the case of malignancy, I^{131} is used as an adjuvant treatment following surgery to ablate the remaining normal thyroid tissue and any potential microscopic residual tumour

- **Phosphorus³²**: P^{32} has proved useful in the treatment of polycythaemia rubra vera although, because it may increase the risk of subsequent development of leukaemia, it is generally reserved for patients over 70 years of age

4 Saunders M., Dische S. et al. (1999) Continuous, hyperfractionated, accelerated radiotherapy (CHART) versus conventional radiotherapy in non-small cell lung cancer: mature data from the randomised multicentre trial. *Radiotherapy and Oncology*, **52**: 137–48.

Radiation therapy

Radiotherapy is used for about half of the 200,000 patients who develop cancer in the UK each year. It has a curative rôle in two-thirds, and a palliative rôle in the remainder.

Horwich, Royal Marsden

Radiotherapy may be administered in differing clinical situations and with varying intents.

Treatment can be:
- **Radical**—Curative intent
- **Adjuvant**—Postoperative
- **Palliative**—Symptom control

Radical radiotherapy

Radiotherapy may be administered with the intent of cure either as the preferred primary therapy (e.g. early stage Hodgkin's disease), or as an alternative to surgery.

In the latter situation it has the advantage of preserving normal anatomy e.g. anal canal cancer, bladder cancer. Additionally, acute morbidity is often less severe. However, as no surgical specimen is obtained, there can be no pathological data to permit accurate staging. Stage must therefore be assessed by clinical or radiological methods. Late effects of radiation, such as fibrosis, may also make subsequent assessment of the tumour site for local recurrence difficult.

Radical radiation is reserved for tumours which can be encompassed within a reasonable radiation treatment volume, i.e. localized, as opposed to widely metastatic disease; this presupposes accurate staging investigations.

Treatment is often complex, with effort given to rigid immobilization and the use of complicated beam arrangements to obtain a uniform dose distribution confined to the tumour with preservation of normal surrounding structures. A high dose of radiation is necessary for all but the most radiosensitive of tumours, and treatment is delivered in conventional (small) fraction sizes in order to reduce the late adverse effects of radiation.

Examples of radical radiotherapy include:
- **Head and neck tumours:** Many squamous cell tumours of the head and neck region can be cured by radical radiotherapy (often combined with synchronous chemotherapy) e.g. early stage cancers of the larynx are frequently cured with preservation of good quality phonation
- **Anal canal cancer:** A radical approach using concurrent chemo-radiotherapy has been shown to be effective management for epidermoid anal canal cancer. Additionally between 60–70 per cent of patients retain a functioning anal sphincter after treatment. A common alternative to such an approach is primary abdominoperineal excision of the rectum and anal canal, which results in a permanent colostomy

- **Lung cancer:** Radical radiotherapy is not infrequently employed as a second-best option in the management of lung cancer. The patients considered for such treatment are not deemed sufficiently fit to undergo radical surgery but may be fit for radiation treatment

Adjuvant radiotherapy

Adjuvant radiotherapy is administered as an adjunct to potentially curative surgery. The principle underpinning such treatment is the possibility of microscopic residual disease, either within the tumour bed, lymphatic channels or regional lymph node drainage. The aim of adjuvant radiotherapy is the eradication of this microscopic disease and thereby to reduce the rate of local relapse and improve overall survival.

Examples of adjuvant radiotherapy:

- **Breast cancer:** This is perhaps the best example and is certainly the most common exemplifier of adjuvant radiation. Up to 50 per cent of the workload of many UK radiotherapy centres is devoted to adjuvant breast irradiation. Local relapse rates following partial mastectomy may reach 30 per cent. Postoperative breast irradiation can reduce this figure by three to fourfold. Local control rates then conform to those achieved after mastectomy but with a superior cosmetic outcome
- **Head and neck cancer:** Surgery for squamous tumours of the head and neck is complex. Due to the close proximity of tumours to important structures, surgical margins may often be inadequate because compromise must be made to retain acceptable functional and cosmetic outcomes. Adjuvant irradiation is employed if margins are unsatisfactory or following radical neck surgery which demonstrates multiple involved lymph nodes. Classically adjuvant radiotherapy is administered after surgery has been performed

However, in some situations, although surgery remains the mainstay of treatment, radiotherapy may be delivered as a prelude to a surgical procedure.

True **neo-adjuvant radiation** is administered in order to shrink or downstage the tumour, thus facilitating subsequent surgery. In this case time must elapse between irradiation and surgery to allow tumour shrinkage. An illustration of this technique is preoperative rectal radiotherapy for tethered or fixed rectal adenocarcinoma. Treatment is delivered over 4–5 weeks after which there is a gap of about six weeks during which tumour shrinkage occurs. Surgery is then often made possible, when pre-radiotherapy it would not have been.

Short fractionation preoperative rectal radiotherapy, by contrast, is delivered over the week immediately prior to surgery. No time is permitted for tumour shrinkage. Trials have, however, confirmed a significant improvement in local control and overall survival with this approach.

Adjuvant radiation treatment courses typically extend over 4–6 weeks. The general principles applied to radical radiotherapy also hold for the adjuvant setting as treatment intent is curative i.e. immobilization, careful avoidance of critical organs at risk, and low dose per fraction. Total doses tend to be slightly lower since the target is microscopic residual disease. It must, however, be remembered that following surgery the vascular supply to tissues is disrupted resulting in areas of tissue hypoxia. **Radiation is relatively less effective in an environment that is poorly oxygenated**.

Palliative radiotherapy

When radiotherapy is administered in the palliative setting, the focus of interest is the control of distressing symptoms. The disease is, by definition, incurable. These factors impact upon treatment in a variety of ways:

- Only symptomatic sites of disease are targeted
- Sites at high risk of producing symptoms may receive prophylactic treatment
- Fractionation regimens are kept short
- Moderate doses of radiation are employed
- Palliative benefit must outweigh treatment-related toxicity

Palliative radiotherapy may produce prolongation of survival but this is not its primary aim, rather it is the quality of that survival which is the goal. Palliative radiotherapy often produces significant symptomatic gain.

There are several clinical scenarios in which palliative radiotherapy commonly proves useful.

Pain

Bone metastases, pain due to nerve compression or soft tissue infiltration will usually respond to radiation treatment and will respond to large single fractions of radiotherapy as effectively as more prolonged treatment schedules.

The former are more patient-friendly and may be repeated if necessary. If pain is diffuse, affecting many disparate sites within the skeleton, wide field—hemibody—irradiation often produces relief. An alternative is radioisotope therapy with Sr^{89} or Sm^{153}.

Osteolytic tumour deposits in weight-bearing bones are at risk of fracture and are best fixed prophylactically by orthopaedic intervention. This is often followed by postoperative irradiation, although good evidence of benefit is lacking. Rarely radiation is given without prophylactic surgical intervention.

Haemorrhage

Haemoptysis, haematuria, haematemesis, and rectal bleeding all respond to radiation. A hypofractionated treatment course often produces prompt sustained benefit (at least 70 per cent in carcinoma of the bronchus).

Obstruction

Any hollow viscus may undergo obstruction caused by a malignant process. Several organs may commonly be obstructed by cancer:

- Superior vena cava (SVC)
- Upper airways i.e. trachea, bronchus
- Oesophagus

Prompt, if not immediate, relief is frequently afforded by stent insertion under the care of the interventional radiologists for SVC or oesophageal obstruction. There is a rôle for palliative radiotherapy in some patients who are unsuitable for such procedures, or in the case of stent overgrowth by tumour.

Radiotherapy is most often used for bronchial obstruction due to lung cancer; laser resection or stent insertion are less commonly employed alternatives.

Radiotherapy probably remains the treatment modality of choice for SVC obstruction caused by radiosensitive tumours, for example, small cell lung cancer.

Neurological symptoms

- Spinal cord compression
- Brain metastases
- Cranial or peripheral nerve compression
- Malignant meningitis
- Choroidal or orbital metastases

Radiotherapy is the most common means of treating spinal cord compression. There are a number of important indications for surgical as opposed to radiotherapeutic intervention (e.g. uncertain pathology, unstable spine).

Radiotherapy often improves pain associated with the compression, but neurological recovery is less predictable and mainly depends on the degree of weakness prior to therapy and the particular histological tumour type.

Brain metastases are increasing in incidence as oncological management improves and patients survive long enough to develop relapse within the brain. Steroids can produce significant benefit if the effects are due to oedema or compression rather than tissue destruction. However, their beneficial effects tend to be short-lived. Prolongation of symptom control and a small gain in survival (1–2 months) can additionally be obtained with cranial irradiation, usually at the cost of alopecia and lethargy. Those with good pre-treatment neurological function and sensitive tumours stand to gain most.

Cranial or peripheral nerve compression most often occurs with breast or prostate neoplasms. Pain is often improved but nerve palsies seldom show significant recovery.

Fungating tumours

Locally advanced breast tumours, skin tumours, metastatic skin or lymph node deposits, can all lead to fungation. If surgical intervention is not possible or felt to be inappropriate, radiotherapy can reduce the tumour mass, serous ooze or haemorrhage, and promote healing.

Managing side-effects of radiotherapy

Skin

General advice

- Skin reactions tend to be worse in the skin folds i.e. inframammary fold, axilla, groin and perineum
- Deodorants should be avoided within the treatment area
- Avoid aftershave lotions or astringent cosmetics
- Mild soaps are permitted, and washing should be gentle (no vigorous rubbing) and the area patted dry
- Care must be taken not to remove skin markings delineating the treatment fields

Mild reactions

- Skin pink or slightly red
- Apply aqueous cream frequently

Moderate reactions

- Skin red, dry and scaly; some pruritus/tingling
- Apply aqueous cream frequently
- If itch is problematic, 1% Hydrocortisone cream q.d.s. useful

Severe reactions

- Skin inflamed patchy areas of moist desquamation
- Epidermis may blister and slough exposing the dermis leading to pain and serous ooze with increased risk of infection
- Hydrogel or alginate dressing to moist areas; Diprobase® cream to intact epidermis
- Swab if evidence of infection

Mouth and throat care

This is particularly important for patients receiving radiotherapy for head and neck lesions

General advice

- The patient needs a dental assessment and any dental treatment should be carried out before radiotherapy begins
- A good fluid and nutritional intake is very important and nutritional support by NG feeding is indicated if >10 per cent weight loss occurs.
- Cessation of smoking should be strongly encouraged
- Avoid alcohol and spicy foods
- The voice should be rested as the radiotherapy reaction becomes established

Treatment of mucositis

- Normal saline or bicarbonate mouth washes often help
- Antiseptic mouth washes, e.g. chlorhexidine, keep the mouth clean but can cause pain due to their alcohol content
- Oropharyngeal candida infection should be actively sought and treated

- Local analgesics include:
  - aspirin (which may be gargled)
  - paracetamol (which may be gargled)
  - benzydamine (Difflam®)
  - local anaesthetics (Xylocaine®)
  - topical steroids (Adcortyl in orobase®, Corlan pellets®)
  - coating agents (Sucralfate®, Gelclair®)

Dysphagia

Thoracic radiotherapy can lead to oesophagitis which needs explanation and symptomatic treatment. Smoking should be strongly discouraged; spirits and spicy food should be avoided.

An antacid e.g. Gaviscon®, soluble paracetamol or aspirin may all help. A non-steroidal anti-inflammatory drug either orally or by suppository may be used. The oesophagus can be coated with some effect by Sucralfate®.

Nausea and vomiting

Radiotherapy to the abdomen often causes nausea due to serotonin release. All patients should thus be considered for prophylactic antiemetic therapy, e.g. ondansetron.

Diarrhoea

This side-effect frequently accompanies radiotherapy to the abdomen or pelvis. Dietary modification i.e. reduction in dietary roughage, may sometimes relieve the diarrhoea. Anti-diarrhoeal drugs (e.g. loperamide) should be provided to all patients with clear instructions of when and how they should be taken. Proctitis often accompanies rectal or prostatic irradiation and should be treated with rectal steroids either by suppository or enema.

Pneumonitis

Acute radiotherapy-induced pneumonitis can develop one to three months after treatment and is associated with a fever, dry cough and breathlessness. The main differential diagnosis is pneumonia and this should be excluded where possible. The diagnosis can be confirmed by a chest x-ray, which shows lung infiltration confined within the treatment volume. Treatment is with a reducing course of steroids i.e. a starting dose of prednisolone 40 mg.

Cerebral oedema

This can occur during or after cranial irradiation, particularly if no surgical decompression of the brain tumour or metastasis has been undertaken. Oedema usually responds to an increase in the dose of oral steroids.

Somnolence syndrome

This occurs within a few weeks of completion of brain irradiation and may manifest itself with nausea, vomiting, anorexia, dysarthria, ataxia and profound lethargy. Recovery occurs spontaneously but can be accelerated with steroids.

New developments

Radiotherapy has advanced markedly since the early days of the nineteenth century. Progress is still being made to improve the quality and effectiveness of treatment for patients.

There are a number of areas of development:

Defining tumour volume

Improvements in imaging have enabled tumours to be targeted more accurately. This reduces the risk of missing the tumour, and also allows the treatment volume to encompass the tumour more closely. The dose of radiation can therefore be higher (giving improved tumour control) without risking additional toxicity to normal tissues.

Imaging

Refinements in CT scanning technology have led to the advent of the multi-slice CT scanner that provides multiple high quality images rapidly, from which tumour volumes may be defined not only in two but also in three dimensions.

Images can now be fused from different imaging modalities, e.g. MRI/CT image fusion. The new development of co-registered CT/PET scanning. combines functional data (through PET scanning) and high quality spatial information (through CT scanning) providing opportunity for optimal target volume definition.

Conformal therapy

Imaging improvements provide the ability to identify the tumour target more accurately. This reduces the risk of missing the tumour, but it also provides the opportunity of conforming the treatment more closely to the tumour volume and thereby lessening damage to surrounding normal tissues. Taken further, conformal therapy may permit dose escalation with resulting improved tumour control rates, but without increased toxicity. Multileaf collimators within the treatment unit can automatically shape the treatment field, conforming it to the desired target shape.

Intensity Modulated Radiotherapy (IMRT) takes this a step further. With IMRT the intensity of the treatment beams are modified in such a way that almost any three-dimensional volume may be generated. Even concave volumes may be created and so targets which envelop the spinal cord, e.g. thyroid, can be treated much more satisfactorily than with conventional techniques.

Fractionation/combined modality treatment

Advances in the understanding of the principles of fractionation have led to improved treatment outcomes for patients, e.g. CHART in non-small cell lung cancer. Further research with hypo/hyperfractionation and acceleration is ongoing in other tumour types.

The integration of chemotherapy with radiation treatment has provided benefit in a number of tumour sites, e.g. cervical cancer. Research seeks to refine this further and also to incorporate the newer molecular agents into radiation therapy.

Individualization of therapy

Two patients with ostensibly similar tumours receiving identical treatments may respond differently, one being cured and the other dying from cancer in a short time. There are clearly factors inherent within tumours which predict for response to radiotherapy. If such variables could be identified before a treatment course commences, the chance of response would be defined which would help clinicians in deciding whether or not radiotherapy would be a good treatment option. Furthermore, it might be possible, knowing the particular tumour characteristics, to adapt the treatment course accordingly perhaps by modifying the dose prescribed, altering the fractionation schedule such that the prospect of cure could be enhanced. Predictive assays are being developed to realize this possibility. New microchip technology may help elucidate the genes behind the differing responses to therapy, and more importantly, offer patients the possibility of treatment tailored to their individual needs.

Common cancers

Incidence

There are huge variations in cancer incidences across the globe, reflecting the impact of environmental and genetic factors on the causes of cancer.[5]

Table 5.8 The eight commonest cancer types affecting men and women worldwide

Cancer type	Ratio, high:low rate	High incidence	Low incidence
Oesophagus	200:1	Kazakhastan	Holland
Skin	200:1	Australia	India
Liver	100:1	Mozambique	UK
Nasopharynx	100:1	China	Uganda
Lung	40:1	UK	Nigeria
Stomach	30:1	Japan	UK
Cervix	20:1	Hawaii	Israel
Rectum	20:1	Denmark	Nigeria

Table 5.9 The eight commonest cancer types effecting men and women in the UK[5]

Men	Women
Lung	Breast
Colorectal	Lung
Skin	Colorectal
Prostate	Skin
Stomach	Stomach
Pancreas	Ovary
Oesophagus	Cervix
Leukaemia	Pancreas

In this Handbook it is not possible to outline oncological management of all cancer types. The following cancers are the commonest, and those for which the palliative care team has a particular rôle to play.

Table 5.10 Common cancers

Cancer Type	Page	Cancer Type	Page
Lung	132	Upper GI	154
Colorectal	138	Bladder and ureter	158
Breast	142	Brain	160
Prostate	146	Haematological	164
Gynaecological	150	Unknown primary	166

5 Souhami R. L., Tobias J. D. (2003) *Cancer and its Management.* 4th edition. Oxford: Blackwell Science.

Patients with lung cancer

Background
- Most common cancer in men and women in the UK and the US
- Eighty per cent due to smoking
- Eighty per cent are non-small cell subtype (squamous, adenocarcinoma or large cell)
- Twenty per cent are small cell subtype

Symptoms at presentation
- Cough
- Haemoptysis
- Chest pain
- Recurrent chest infection
- Hoarseness

Diagnosis and staging
Diagnosis
- CXR
- Sputum cytology
- Bronchoscopy with biopsy
- Bronchial brushings and washings
- CT guided biopsy

Staging
- Bronchoscopy
- CT scan of chest, liver and adrenals
- Mediastinoscopy
- Pleural aspiration, pleural biopsy
- Bone and brain scan if symptomatic

Small cell lung carcinoma (SCLC)

This is generally believed to be a systemic disease at the time of diagnosis; thus surgery generally plays no part in the management of this disease

Staging
- Limited stage disease—disease confined to one hemithorax
- Extensive stage disease—disease present beyond one hemithorax

Management
- Because of chemoresponsiveness and frequent dissemination at diagnosis combined chemotherapy is the treatment of choice.
- Many chemotherapeutic agents have demonstrated activity in this disease. Commonly used regimes include cisplatin/etoposide and cyclophosphamide/doxorubicin/vincristine
- For patients with limited stage disease, thoracic irradiation in addition to chemotherapy improves local disease control and prolongs survival when compared with chemotherapy alone. Prophylactic cranial irradiation reduces the incidence of brain metastases but has not been shown to prolong survival
- Further radiotherapy may be a useful palliative treatment for patients relapsing after or resistant to chemotherapy

Prognosis
Approximately 80 per cent of patients respond to chemotherapy but the majority relapse and only approximately 10 per cent of patients are alive two years following diagnosis.

Non-small cell lung carcinoma (NSCLC)
Non-small cell lung cancer metastasizes later in its course than small cell lung cancer and consequently surgery offers the best chance of cure. All patients being considered for surgical treatment must be carefully staged to determine tumour operability. The patient must also be carefully assessed preoperatively to assess fitness for surgery.

Postoperative mortality rate should be less than 5 per cent.

Table 5.11 TNM staging of lung cancer

T_1	Tumour <3 cm diameter; distal to main bronchus
T_2	Tumour >3 cm diameter; or involve main bronchus 2 cm distal to carina; or invading visceral pleura; or atelectasis extending to hilum
T_3	Tumour invading chest wall, diaphragm, mediastinal pleura or pericardium; or tumour in main bronchus <2 cm distal to carina or atelectasis of whole lung
T_4	Tumour invading mediastinum, heart, major vessels, trachea, oesophagus, vertebra or carina; or malignant pleural effusion
N_0	No regional node metastases
N_1	Ipsilateral peribronchial or peribronchial or hilar nodes
N_2	Ipsilateral mediastinal or subcarinal nodes
N_3	Contralateral mediastinal nodes; scalene or supraclavicular nodes

Table 5.12 Stage grouping

I	$T_{1-2} N_0$
II	$T_{1-2} N_1$ or $T_3 N_0$
IIIA	$T_{1-2} N_2$ or $T_3 N_{1-2}$
IIIB	T_4 any N M_0; or any $N_3 M_0$
IV	Any M_1

Management
Surgery
Surgical resection offers the best chance of cure in this disease. The aim of surgery is to resect the primary tumour with clear lateral and bronchial margins with draining peribronchial and hilar lymph nodes. Lobectomy is the most commonly performed operation but a bilobectomy or pneumonectomy may be performed for more extensive tumours.

Conversely in less fit patients with limited respiratory reserve only a partial lobectomy may be tolerated, although the results from this surgery in terms of the risk of tumour recurrence may be inferior.

NSCLC radiation therapy
Radical radiotherapy
Selected patients with stage I–III disease who are unfit for surgery may be suitable for radical radiotherapy. Five year survivals of 15–20 per cent have been reported in this highly selected patient group.

The benefit of adjuvant radiotherapy following surgery for high risk disease is uncertain but may reduce the risk of local disease relapse.

Palliative radiotherapy
Radiotherapy is a key component of symptomatic treatment for
- Haemoptysis
- Chest pain
- Dyspnoea
- Cough.

NSCLC chemotherapy
NSCLC is much less chemosensitive than SCLC. Cisplatin-based therapy, however, has recently been demonstrated to improve quality of life with some improvement in survival in the palliative setting. Commonly used regimens include cisplatin/paclitaxel and cisplatin/vinorelbine.

Chemotherapy may also be used in the neo-adjuvant setting to down stage a tumour prior to consideration of surgery. Adjuvant chemotherapy following surgery may also confer a small survival benefit.

Table 5.13 Prognosis

Stage	Five year survival(%)
I	60–80
II	25–40
IIIA	10–30
IIIB and i/v	<5

General issues
Lung cancer, because of its link with smoking, both active and passive, may be associated with emotional distress in the patient and their carers. Lung cancers often occur on top of a background of pre-existing lung disease which may alter the patient's perception of breathlessness and cough.

Specific pain issues
- **Pleuritic pain** may be associated with the tumour itself, metastases in ribs or local inflammation. This type of pain responds well to non-steroidal anti-inflammatory drugs (NSAIDs). It may also be helped by local nerve blockade
- **Pancoast tumour** can produce severe neuropathic pain which may only be partially opioid-responsive and will need adjuvant analgesics. Early referral for specialist help should be considered
- **Bone metastases** may occur, putting the patient at risk of pathological fractures and spinal cord compression. Management of subsequent pain may be difficult and specialist advice should be sought

Other complications
- **Breathlessness** is common and can be very distressing for carers
  (📖 see respiratory section). Treat reversible causes such as anaemia
  and pleural effusion, where appropriate. Give clear explanations of
  what is happening. Ensure that practical measures such as sitting
  upright, opening windows and using fans have been discussed with the
  family. Regular doses of short-acting oral morphine every 2–4 h
  may decrease the sensation of breathlessness. Other more specialist
  interventions such as palliative radiotherapy, endobronchial laser
  therapy and stenting may help some patients. Panic and anxiety are
  frequently associated with breathlessness and may be helped by simple
  relaxation techniques. A low dose of an anxiolytic such as diazepam
  may be helpful
- **Haemoptysis** is a frightening symptom. Palliative radiotherapy may
  be effective if the patient is fit enough. Oral anti-fibrinolytics such as
  tranexamic acid may help. Occasionally frequent small episodes herald
  a catastrophic haemoptysis. This is rare, but is a difficult situation to
  manage and early involvement of specialists should be considered.
  The risks of frightening a family with information about a possible
  risk of catastrophic haemoptysis need to be balanced against the
  potential distress that could be caused by leaving a patient and family
  unprepared
- **Cough** can exacerbate breathlessness and pain, and affect sleep and
  a patient's ability to eat. Its management will depend on the cause, but
  it is often appropriate to try and suppress the cough pharmacologically
  using codeine linctus or morphine. If not responding to simple
  measures refer for specialist assessment
- **Hypercalcaemia** may occur. It should be considered in any patient
  with persistent nausea, thirst, altered mood or confusion (even if
  intermittent), worsening pain and/or constipation. It should be treated
  with i/v hydration and bisphosphonates unless the patient is clearly
  dying, in which case treatment is not appropriate
- **Cerebral metastases** are common. Decisions about investigation and
  management may be complex and need to be made on an individual
  basis. Altered behaviour and personality, as well as problems of
  comprehension and communication, can be very distressing for
  relatives. Persistent headache, worse in the mornings and unexplained
  vomiting may be early signs of this diagnosis. There is a risk of epileptic
  fits and prophylactic anticonvulsant medication may be appropriate
- **Hyponatraemia** and other biochemical imbalances are particularly
  common in small cell lung cancer. Management can be complex and
  needs specialist input
- **Altered taste and anorexia** are common. Good oral hygiene, and
  effective treatment of oral candidiasis may help. Carers may find it
  helpful to talk through different ways of encouraging the patient to
  eat, such as freezing supplement drinks and making small meals
  frequently etc.
- **Superior vena cava obstruction (SVCO)** can occur, particularly
  in patients with right-sided lung cancers. Management includes
  consideration of vascular stenting, radiotherapy and high dose oral
  steroids in a single daily dose

Mesothelioma

General comments

This usually affects the pleura but can affect other mesothelial linings, most commonly the peritoneum. It is associated with exposure to asbestos, although unlike patients with asbestosis the history may be difficult to elicit, as the risk of mesothelioma appears unrelated to the length of exposure to asbestos and may occur many years after such exposure. It is a relentlessly progressive tumour.

It is important that the patient is aware that they may be entitled to *compensation* and should consult a specialist lawyer about this.

All deaths due to mesothelioma should be discussed with the coroner who will most probably carry out a post-mortem, unless the disease was clearly non-industrially related. The patient and family should be made aware that the coroner will be contacted (regardless of any compensation claims or litigation), to try and minimize distress at the time of death.

Diagnosis

- CXR
- CT scan of chest
- Pleural biopsy
- Thoracoscopic biopsy

There is a high incidence of false negative biopsies—in some cases these may need to be repeated a number of times to make a diagnosis.

Treatment

Surgery

Radical surgery is of uncertain value, with a high mortality and few long term survivors reported. Palliative surgery with parietal pleurectomy and decortication of the lung may offer excellent palliation with minimal morbidity.

Radiotherapy

The tumour may grow along the track of a biopsy or drainage needle to produce a cutaneous lesion. These areas can become painful, ulcerated and can be difficult to manage. Palliative radiotherapy is given prophylactically following the biopsy. It may also be used locally for established cutaneous spread.

Chemotherapy

The value of chemotherapy in this disease is uncertain. Recent reports however suggest that selected patients may respond to platinum-based regimes with some palliative benefit.

Specific problems in the management of mesothelioma

- **Pleural effusions** are common, frequently blood stained and become increasingly difficult to aspirate as the disease progresses. Surgical intervention to prevent re-accumulation of fluid may be helpful if carried out early enough
- **Breathlessness** can be severe due to pleural disease limiting the capacity of the lung as well as the occurrence of pleural effusions.

Give clear explanations of what is happening. Ensure that practical measures such as sitting the patient up, opening windows and using fans have been discussed with the family. Regular doses of short acting oral morphine every 4 h may decrease the sensation of breathlessness. Panic and anxiety are frequently associated with breathlessness and may be helped by simple relaxation techniques. A low dose of an *anxiolytic* such as diazepam may be helpful. Other treatment options are limited

- **Ascites** occurs with peritoneal mesothelioma. The ascitic fluid is frequently blood stained and becomes increasingly difficult to aspirate as the disease progresses.

Specific pain complexes

Mesotheliomas can produce severe neuropathic pain which may only be partially opioid responsive and may need adjuvant analgesics. Early referral for specialist help should be considered. Local nerve blockades can help in some cases.

Colorectal cancer

Background
- Fourth commonest cancer worldwide
- Approximately 50 per cent of tumours occur in the rectum or sigmoid colon
- Dietary factors are thought to be important
- 6–8 per cent of cases are familial
- Associated syndromes include Familial Adenomatous Polyposis Coli and Hereditary Non-polyposis Coli

Common presentations
- Iron deficiency anaemia
- Abdominal pain
- Altered bowel habit
- PR bleeding

Staging and diagnosis
- Barium enema
- Colonoscopy—all patients must have full evaluation of the colon prior to surgery
- Sigmoidoscopy
- CT/Ultrasound scan of abdomen
- MRI/endorectal ultrasound may be useful to assess local extent of tumour in the rectum

Table 5.14 TNM staging for colorectal cancer

T_1 Invades submucosa	Stage I—T_1/T_2, N_0 M_0
T_2 Invades muscularis propria	Stage II—$T_{3/4}$, N_0 M_0
T_3 Invades subserosa	Stage III—T_{1-4}, N_1/N_2 M_0
T_4 Invades through serosa	Stage i/v—T_{1-4} N_{1-2} M_1
N_0 N_0 lymph node involvement	
N_1 1–3 nodes involved	
N_2 4 or more nodes involved	
N_3 Central nodes involved	
M_0 No distant metastases	
M_1 Distant metastases	

Management

Surgery of primary disease
Surgery is the mainstay of therapy for colorectal cancer.

For colonic tumours a segment of colon with its blood supply and draining nodes is excised. Depending on the site of the tumour this may involve a right or left hemicolectomy or a sigmoid colectomy.

Traditionally surgery for rectal tumours has involved an abdomino-perineal approach. In the absence of radiotherapy local relapse rates of 25–30 per cent have been reported. Traditionally radiotherapy has been used postoperatively but increasingly a short course of radiotherapy is being used to 'sterilize' the area prior to surgery. Some surgeons now advocate more extensive local surgery in the form of a total mesorectal excision, where the rectum is excised en bloc with the adjacent perirectal tissue. This has reduced local relapse rates to less than 10 per cent.

Surgery for hepatic metastases

The majority of patients develop liver metastases as the first site of disease progression following definitive first line treatment.

A proportion of these patients may be suitable for metastatectomy. Up to 40 per cent five-year survival has been reported for carefully selected patients.

Chemotherapy

Adjuvant chemotherapy of colorectal cancer

Several large randomised controlled trials have demonstrated a small but definite survival advantage to fluorouracil-based therapy for patients with Stage III disease.

The value of adjuvant chemotherapy for patients with Stage I/II disease is uncertain and is being addressed in a number of ongoing trials.

Advanced colorectal cancer

Fluorouracil-based chemotherapy has also been demonstrated to confer a palliative benefit in patients with metastatic disease. There also appears to be a survival advantage to chemotherapy of at least six months. Combination regimes with fluorouracil and oxaliplatin or irinotecan may be superior to single agent fluorouracil.

Capecitabine, a recently developed orally available fluorouracil analogue has also been demonstrated to have activity in this disease.

Radiotherapy

Adjuvant treatment

Pelvic radiotherapy with concurrent chemotherapy reduces risk of pelvic relapse for patients with Stage II and III rectal cancer.

Pelvic chemoradiotherapy may also be useful for patients with large fixed rectal tumours to reduce tumour volume prior to consideration of surgical resection.

General comments

- **Liver metastases** often occur and may cause capsular pain. This usually responds well to non-steroidal anti-inflammatory drugs (NSAIDS) or steroids. Liver metastases may also lead to hepatomegaly, causing squashed stomach syndrome with delayed gastric emptying and a feeling of fullness. This may respond to a prokinetic agent such as metoclopramide
- **Perineal and pelvic pain** may be caused by advancing disease or be iatrogenic. There is nearly always a neuropathic element to the pain which will only be partially opioid sensitive. Tenesmus is a unique type of neuropathic pain which requires specialist assessment. It may respond to drugs that have an effect on muscle tone such as nifedipine, baclofen, or nitrates

- **Bone metastases** are rare but can occur with colonic cancer
- **Bowel obstruction**, unless it can be palliated surgically, should be managed medically using a syringe driver containing a mixture of analgesics, antiemetics and anti-spasmodics. Multiple levels of obstruction of the bowel, which is not infrequent, may make surgery inappropriate. Differentiating between a high blockage (where vomiting is a feature) and blockage lower in the bowel can be useful in targeting treatment strategies. Imaging techniques may also be helpful to delineate the level of obstruction
- **Fistulae** between the bowel and the skin or bladder may occur. These can be very difficult to manage and require a multidisciplinary approach with specialist input
- **Poor appetite** is not uncommon and can be helped with the use of steroids
- **Rectal discharge and bleeding** are unpleasant and difficult symptoms to manage. Referral to a clinical oncologist is appropriate as radiotherapy may be of benefit
- **Hypoproteinaemia** is common due to poor oral intake and poor absorption from the bowel and may lead to lower limb oedema
- **Cerebral metastases** are not common with colonic cancers

Breast cancer

Background

- Accounts for 20 per cent of all cancers
- Life time risk 1/12
- Factors which increase the risk of breast cancer include increasing age, a family history of breast cancer, nulliparity and use of HRT
- Incidence of breast cancer is increasing although overall mortality is decreasing
- Male breast cancer is rare—accounting for only 0.7 per cent of all breast cancers

Genetics of breast cancer

Five to ten per cent of breast cancers are believed to be hereditary. Many of these cancers are due to germline mutations in the tumour suppresser genes BRCA1 or BRCA2. For patients with proven mutations in the BRCA1 or BRCA2 gene prophylactic subcutaneous mastectomy reduces the incidence of breast cancer.

At present treatment for a breast tumour arising in a mutation carrier is the same as for non-mutation carriers.

Presentation

- Breast lump
- Nipple inversion or discharge
- Mammographically detected lesion—increasingly common mode of presentation

Diagnosis

- Mammogram
- Ultrasound
- Fine needle aspiration cytology
- Core biopsy

Pathology

Table 5.15 Pathology

Preinvasive lesions

Lobular carcinoma in situ (LCIS)—significance uncertain

Ductal carcinoma in situ (DCIS)—usually detected mammographically may progress to invasive disease

Invasive lesions

Ductal carcinoma—not otherwise specified—accounts for approximately 80% of all tumours

Lobular carcinoma

Tubular carcinoma

Medullary carcinoma

Presentation and staging

Breast cancer is diagnosed by a 'triple assessment'.

1 Clinical examination
2 Bilateral mammography
3 Fine needle aspiration cytology or core biopsy

This approach has >90 per cent sensitivity and specificity.

All patients with proven invasive disease should have axillary node dissection as a staging procedure to assess axillary node involvement. Staging investigations are more likely to reveal metastases in patients presenting with node-positive disease than in those with disease localized to the breast.

Prognostic factors

Include:

• Axillary node involvement—most important prognostic criterion
• Five years survival node +ve patients 20–30 per cent, node –ve patients 70–80 per cent
• Tumour size
• Tumour grade
• Oestrogen receptor (ER)/Progesterone receptor (PR) status. More favourable prognosis if ER/PR positive
• Patient age—<35yrs is an adverse independent prognostic factor, see Table 5.16 overleaf

Common problems

Bone pain due to bone metastases

• **Pathological fractures** may occur without obvious trauma
• **Spinal cord compression** requires prompt diagnosis, high dose oral steroids and urgent referral to the oncologist. The steroids should be continued at a high dose until a definitive plan has been made
• **Neuropathic pain** can be a particular problem especially if there has been spread into the brachial plexus
• **Liver metastases** are common and may require steroids or NSAIDs to reduce the pain of liver capsule stretch. Surgery may be appropriate
• **Hypercalcaemia** may occur. In many cases treatment should be considered with i/v hydration and i/v bisphosphonates on a monthly basis
• **Lymphoedema** can develop, at any point in the course of the disease, affecting the arm following surgery and/or radiotherapy. Early referral to a lymphoedema specialist provides the best chance of minimising the morbidity and distress caused. Management includes good skin care, avoiding additional trauma to the affected arm (including taking of blood tests and BP measurement) and appropriately fitting compression garments
• **Lung and pleural spread** are common causes of breathlessness and cough. These symptoms need to be investigated thoroughly. Drainage of a pleural effusion may be a useful symptomatic procedure and pleurodesis should be considered
• **Psychosocial problems.** A section of these patients will be mothers with young children for whom the trauma of disease is worsened by fears for their children. A multidisciplinary supportive approach at a pace dictated by the patient can help to reduce some of the distress for the patient and her family

Management

Table 5.16 Management

Non-invasive breast cancer DCIS and LCIS	Simple mastectomy OR Partial mastectomy and postoperative radiotherapy. Axillary dissection not indicated.
Early breast cancer T_{1-3}, N_{0-1}	**Surgery:** either simple mastectomy or partial mastectomy (lumpectomy) and axillary node dissection.
	Loco-regional radiotherapy: indicated for all patients with partial mastectomy and for mastectomy patients at high risk of local relapse (e.g. patients with > 4 nodes positive).
	Adjuvant endocrine therapy: Tamoxifen indicated for all ER- or PR-positive tumours. Approximately 30% relative reduction in mortality. Value of aromatase inhibitors is being examined in randomized controlled trials.
	Adjuvant chemotherapy: Combination chemotherapy reduces recurrence and improves overall survival. Anthracycline based regimens are probably slightly more effective than non-anthracycline based regimens but with a higher incidence of cardiotoxicity. Absolute 10 year survival benefit: 7–11% <50 years; 2–3% > 50 years. Commonly used regimens include Adriamycin/cyclophosphamide (AC), fluorouracil/epirubicin/cyclophosphamide (FEC), cyclophosphamide/methotrexate/fluorouracil (CMF). The benefit risk ratio for chemotherapy must be assessed on an individual patient basis.
	Neo-adjuvant therapy: Not yet fully evaluated. May have some advantage in allowing more patients to have breast conserving surgery. Trials to assess the value of a neo-adjuvant approach are ongoing.
Locally advanced breast cancer *(Presence of infiltration of the skin, chest wall or fixed axillary nodes)*	The presence of infiltration of the skin, chest wall or fixed axillary nodes requires a *neo-adjuvant* approach. Younger patients and those with ER/PR negative disease may need chemotherapy. Elderly patients with ER or PR positive disease may be treated with hormonal therapy alone. In this situation aromatase inhibitors increasingly appear to be superior to tamoxifen.

Metastatic breast cancer

The aim is palliation. Usual sites of metastases: lung, liver, bone, brain

Bone metastases often respond to hormone manipulation with e.g tamoxifen

Such patients may survive for many years

Endocrine therapy: indicated in those patients with ER- or PR-positive disease and slowly progressive disease. Responses tend to be slower in onset (3–6 months) than with chemotherapy but also tend to be more durable. Expected response rates of 40–60% to first line hormonal therapy in those with ER- and/or PR-positive tumours. Disease that responds to endocrine therapy and then progresses has a 25% response with second line treatment. Response to a third hormonal agent is 10–15%.

Chemotherapy: indicated in situations where a high response rate and rapid time to response are required. Anthracycline based regimens are used first line. Combinations such as FAC produce response rates of 40–60% with a median time to progression of 8 months. Taxanes are used in patients who have had prior exposure to anthracyclines—response rates 40–60%. In patients with HER-2 over expression addition of Herceptin (trastuzumab) to Taxotere (docetaxel) increases response rate and prolongs survival. In patients unfit for a taxane Herceptin may be used as a single agent. Other agents which may be used include capecitabine, vinorelbine and Caelyx (liposomal doxorubicin).

Radiotherapy: useful for palliation of painful bone metastases or of soft tissue metastases causing pressure effects.

Bisphosphonates: useful in the treatment of malignancy related hypercalcaemia. As a maintenance treatment in patients with bone disease, they have been demonstrated to reduce bone pain, skeletal events related to malignancy, and the incidence of hypercalcaemia.

Prostate cancer

Background
- Accounts for approximately 30 per cent of all cancers in men
- Second to lung cancer as a cause of cancer deaths in men
- Increasing age is major risk factor—70 per cent of men >80yrs have some evidence of prostatic cancer
- Appears to be linked to androgen exposure—rare in men castrated before 40yrs
- Incidence of prostate cancer is rising—in part this is due to increased detection of early disease by PSA screening
- Many PSA-detected cancers are clinically unimportant—more work needs to be done to distinguish patients with raised PSA levels who are at risk of developing metastatic disease

Presentation
- Urinary outflow symptoms
- Haematuria
- Back pain

Diagnosis and staging
- PSA assessment: PSA >4 ng/ml: clinical suspicion, requires transurethral ultrasound and needle biopsy
- PSA >50 ng/ml: often distant metastases
- Transurethral ultrasound and biopsy
- CT/MRI—may help to assess lymph node involvement
- Isotope bone scan

Table 5.17 TNM staging of prostate cancer

T_1—Clinically inapparent
T_2—Palpable tumour confined to prostate
T_3—Tumour extends through capsule
T_4—Tumour is fixed or invades structures other than seminal vesicles
N_0—N_0 regional nodes
N_1—Regional lymph node metastases
M_0—N_0 metastases
M_1—Metastases present

Management
Many prostate tumours are clinically insignificant and will not cause symptoms in the patient's lifetime. It is important, however, to recognize those patients whose tumours are likely to become clinically apparent.

Prognostic factors in patients with cancer confined to the prostate:
- Tumour grade—assessed by Gleason Score
- Tumour stage
- Patient age—younger patients are more likely to develop problems than older patients

Cancer confined to prostate gland

If aged <70 and fit, consider radical local therapy:

- Prostatectomy
- Radiotherapy

There are currently no trials directly comparing these approaches. In general terms fitter patients tend to be treated with surgery rather than radiotherapy.
Complications:

- Prostatectomy: 50 per cent impotence; 8–15 per cent long term incontinence
- Radiotherapy: 40 per cent impotence; rectal stricture/bladder irritation but no incontinence

If over 70 years:

- 'Wait and see' policy

Locally extensive disease (T_3/T_4) or Node N_1 disease

- Neo-adjuvant anti-androgen therapy
- Radical radiotherapy

Metastatic disease

The natural history is very variable, with a number of patients with metastatic bone disease living for >5years following diagnosis.

The majority of tumours are sensitive to androgens. Hormonal manipulation aimed at reducing the effect of androgens (mainly testosterone) at a cellular level will produce responses in around 70 per cent of men with bone metastases with a median response duration of 12–18 months.

Commonly used hormonal treatments include:

- Medical castration with gonadorelin analogues. (These can induce a flare of hormone induced activity on initiating therapy which needs to be suppressed with anti-androgens for the initial two weeks.)
- Anti-androgens (cyproterone acetate, flutamide, bicalutamide). These may be used alone or in combination with gonadorelin analogues. The value of the combination is, however, uncertain
- Oestrogens are only used by oncologists as third line therapy because of the high incidence of thromboembolic side-effects
- Bilateral orchidectomy—less popular due to availability of medical methods of castration

The side-effects of these hormone treatments include:

- Loss of libido and potency
- Hot flushes
- Change in fat deposition
- Osteoporosis
- Poor concentration
- Decreased energy and drive

Local radiotherapy may be useful as an additional palliative measure particularly for bone pain. Strontium[89] (i/v), a bone-seeking radio isotope, has proved an effective, though expensive, treatment for reducing bone pain.

Hormone refractory prostate cancer

The prognosis for patients whose disease has progressed through anti-androgen therapy is poor.

Therapeutic options at this stage include:

- Anti-androgen withdrawal—this results in a response in a small number of patients
- Chemotherapy—prostate cancer is relatively chemoresistant and no standard regimen has been established. Mitoxantrone however has been used in this disease with some evidence of useful clinical activity

Common palliation issues

- **Pathological fracture** may occur without obvious trauma. These may need orthopaedic intervention (pinning or joint replacement) and radiotherapy. Prophylactic orthopaedic intervention may also be required for bone lesions at high risk of fracture
- **Spinal cord compression** requires prompt diagnosis and treatment with high dose steroids and radiotherapy. A minority of cases may be suitable for surgical intervention. Such patients include those with a single site of disease and those in whom there is uncertainty regarding the diagnosis. These patients should be discussed with a neurosurgeon
- **Neuropathic pain** Local recurrence of tumour, pelvic spread or a collapsed vertebra may cause neuropathic pain. Such pain is partially opioid sensitive but adjuvant analgesics are usually required to supplement the effect of the opioid
- **Bone pain** Specialist advice should be sought about the appropriate use of radiotherapy and radioactive strontium as well as nerve blockade. Bisphosphonates such as pamidronate and zoledronate help to reduce bone pain and also reduce the number of cancer-associated skeletal events and incidence of hypercalcaemia
- **Bone marrow failure** may occur in patients with advanced disease. Typically the patient has symptomatic anaemia and thrombocytopenia. Support with palliative blood transfusions may be appropriate initially, but their appropriateness should be discussed with the patient and their family when there is no longer symptomatic benefit gained from transfusion
- **Retention of urine** Problems with micturition including haematuria may lead to retention of urine. This may be acute and painful or chronic and painless. If the patient is unfit for transurethral resection of the prostate (TURP) then consider a permanent indwelling urinary catheter. Chronic urinary retention can lead to renal failure
- **Lymphoedema** of the lower limbs and occasionally the genital area is usually due to advanced pelvic disease. It needs to be actively managed if complications are to be avoided
- **Altered body image** and sexual dysfunction can result from any of the treatment modalities, hormone manipulation, radiotherapy, or surgery. This may be exacerbated by apathy and clinical depression. Specialist mental and psychological health strategies may be required

Gynaecological cancer

Ovarian carcinoma

Background

- Fifth commonest cancer in women
- Median age at diagnosis 66yrs
- Approximately 5 per cent are familial
- 95 per cent of tumours are epithelial in origin
- Risk is reduced by factors that reduce the number of ovulatory cycles e.g. pregnancy, use of oral contraceptive pill

Presentation

Ovarian cancer spreads mainly intraperitoneally and may remain silent until late: 80 per cent of patients therefore, present with disease which has spread beyond the pelvis.

Commonly presenting symptoms include:

- abdominal distension
- abdominal pain
- altered bowel habit
- weight loss

Diagnosis and staging

Table 5.18 Diagnosis and staging

Stage	Description	Five year survival (%)
Stage I	Confined to ovaries but without pelvic extension	75
Stage II	Tumour with pelvic extension	45
Stage III	Tumour with peritoneal spread outside the pelvis, or involves small bowel; retroperitoneal or inguinal nodes	20
Stage IV	Distant metastases	<5

Preoperatively a diagnosis of ovarian cancer may be suspected if the marker CA 125 is raised (elevated in approximately 85 per cent of patients with stage III/i/v disease) and the presence of a pelvic mass or ascites on CT scan.

Confirmation of the diagnosis requires histology. Adequate staging and initial disease management requires total abdominal hysterectomy, bilateral salpingo-oophorectomy, omentectomy, lymph node sampling, and multiple peritoneal biopsies.

Management

Radical surgery has an important rôle in treatment and retrospective studies demonstrate significantly improved survival in patients whose disease has been optimally debulked (i.e. no tumour remaining measuring >1 cm in diameter). Where optimal debulking is not possible initially there may be a survival benefit to performing debulking surgery after three cycles of chemotherapy—so called interval debulking.

First line chemotherapy

A platinum/taxane combination is considered by most oncologist to be the optimum treatment for ovarian cancer, the most commonly used combination being carboplatin and paclitaxel (Taxol). Response rates are approximately 70–80 per cent, and median survival is 2–3 years with such treatment.

Although the introduction of paclitaxel has improved the median survival in this disease, the majority of patients develop progressive disease and 5 year survival is still less than 20 per cent.

Treatment at relapse

The vast majority of patients who relapse after first line therapy are incurable. Secondary surgical debulking may be useful in selected patients, but its value is uncertain. The choice of further chemotherapy depends on the interval between completion of previous chemotherapy and relapse.

Patients relapsing more than six months after completion of platinum-based therapy may respond to further chemotherapy and should generally be rechallenged with a platinum agent. The response rate depends on the 'time out' from treatment ranging from very low <6 months to 60 per cent >2 years.

Patients relapsing less than six months after completion of platinum-based chemotherapy are unlikely to respond to further platinum based therapy. Fit patients should be considered for Caelyx or topotecan.

Eventually all patients who relapse following primary chemotherapy will develop chemotherapy-resistant disease. The majority of these patients will have symptoms related to intra-abdominal disease, including abdominal pain and bowel obstruction. Management of these symptoms can be very challenging and requires a multidisciplinary approach with involvement of palliative physicians, surgeons and oncologists.

Carcinoma of the cervix

Background

- Strongly associated with Human Papilloma Virus (HPV) 16 (and also, but less strongly, with HPV 18 and 31)
- 30–40 per cent of patients with untreated cervical intraepithelial neoplasia progress to invasive squamous cell carcinoma with a latent period of 10–20yrs
- Commonest female cancer in South East Asia, Africa and South America
- In the UK incidence and mortality have fallen by approximately 40 per cent since the 1970s

Presentation

- Generally asymptomatic until late
- Post coital bleeding
- Intermenstrual bleeding

Staging

Table 5.19 Staging

	FIGO staging system
Ia	Micro-invasive disease (max. depth 5 mm, max. width 7 mm)
Ib	Clinical disease confined to the cervix
IIa	Disease involves upper 2/3 of vagina but not parametrium
IIb	Disease involves parametrium but not pelvic wall
IIIa	Disease involves lower 1/3 of vagina
IIIb	Disease extend to pelvic side wall
IVa	Spread of tumour to adjacent pelvic organs
IV	Spread of tumour to distant organs

MRI plays an increasingly important rôle in the preoperative staging of these tumours.

Management

Management depends largely on disease stage. Patients with stage Ia may be treated with simple hysterectomy or a conisation procedure in those patients wishing to preserve their fertility.

For Stage Ib or IIa disease, radical hysterectomy appears equivalent to radical pelvic radiotherapy. For patients with Stage IIb to IVa disease, recent evidence suggests that combined radical pelvic radiotherapy with platinum-based chemotherapy gives best results. Chemoradiotherapy may also be indicated for patients with Stage Ib and IIa disease with adverse prognostic factors, such as those with bulky tumours.

For patients with Stage IVb disease pelvic radiotherapy may be useful in palliating troublesome pelvic symptoms. Cervical cancer is only moderately chemosensitive with responses to single agents of around 20–30 per cent. Agents with some activity in this disease include cisplatin, ifosfamide and paclitaxel.

Palliative issues in gynaecological cancers

- Primary treatment often affects sexual function, fertility and body image, which may impact on coping strategies and need specialist counselling. Ovarian and vulval cancers often present late and specialist palliative care input from the point of diagnosis may be appropriate. Genetic counselling should be considered for close female relatives of patients with ovarian cancer, particularly if there is also a strong family history of breast cancer
- **Perineal and pelvic pain** is common in all three of the common gynaecological malignancies; cervical, ovarian and vulval carcinomas. There is nearly always a neuropathic element to the pain which may be only partially opioid-sensitive
- **Lymphoedema affecting one or both limbs** develops with uncontrolled pelvic disease. It can develop at any time in a patient's cancer journey and frequently affects both lower limbs. It needs to be actively managed if complications are to be avoided. Management includes good skin care, avoiding additional trauma to the affected leg(s), and appropriately fitting compression garments
- **Ascites** is particularly common with ovarian cancer and can be difficult to manage. Oral diuretics, particularly spironolactone in combination with a loop diuretic such as furosemide, may help a little. Repeated paracentesis may be needed. Consideration of a peritoneovenous shunt may be appropriate in some cases where prognosis is thought to be longer than three months
- **Complete or subacute bowel obstruction** is often not amenable to surgical intervention and should be managed medically using subcutaneous medication via a syringe drive. Nasogastric tubes are rarely needed, and hydration can often be maintained orally if the nausea and vomiting are adequately controlled
- **Renal impairment** can develop in any patient with advanced pelvic disease. It may be a pre-terminal event. Ureteric stenting may be appropriate depending on the patient's perceived prognosis, the patient's wishes and future treatment options. Renal impairment increases the risk of a patient developing opioid toxicity as renal excretion of opioid metabolites may be reduced
- **Vaginal or vulval bleeding** may respond to antifibrinolytic agents such as tranexamic acid, radiotherapy and/or surgery
- **Offensive vaginal or vulval discharge** can cause considerable distress to both patient and carers. Topical or systemic metronidazole may help as can barrier creams. Deodorizing machines may also help if the patient is confined to one room
- **Vesico-colic and recto-vaginal fistulae** need surgical assessment. These can be very difficult to manage and require a multidisciplinary approach with specialist input

Upper gastrointestinal tract cancer

Stomach cancer

Background

- Second most common cancer worldwide
- Sixth most common cancer in the UK
- More common in males than females (2:1)
- 90–95 per cent of gastric tumours are adenocarcinomas
- In the UK incidence of cancer of the distal stomach is falling but incidence of tumours of the cardia or gastro-oesophageal junction is rising

Presentation

- Anaemia
- Weight loss
- Dyspepsia

Diagnosis and staging

- Endoscopy and biopsy
- Endoluminal ultrasound to assess depth of invasion and lymph node involvement
- CT scan to assess lymph node involvement and distant metastases
- Laparoscopy—may be indicated to assess peritoneal disease if surgery is being considered

Treatment

Resectable disease

Surgery remains the only potentially curative modality of treatment. Partial or total gastrectomy (depending on tumour site and mode of spread) and regional lymphadenectomy is the most commonly performed operation. Factors determining outcome include:

- Tumour location—patients with distal tumours do better than those with more proximally located tumours
- Tumour extent—patients with tumours beyond the gastric wall have a worse prognosis
- Extent of lymph node involvement

Following surgery many patients remain at high risk of local and distant disease relapse. Recent trials have suggested that such patients may benefit from adjuvant chemoradiation.

Neo-adjuvant approaches are also being investigated.

Locally advanced/metastatic disease

Palliative operations can be performed to control pain or bleeding or to relieve obstruction for patients with advanced disease. The type of operation performed depends to a large extent on the status of the patient and anticipated disease course.

Chemotherapy has also been demonstrated to have a palliative benefit for patients with locally advanced or metastatic gastric cancer and may also improve survival by some months. Endoscopic procedures such as stenting or laser coagulation may also provide useful palliative benefits.

Radiotherapy may provide useful palliation for e.g. bleeding from locally advanced tumours. It may also be useful in palliating pain caused by metastatic disease, e.g. bone metastases.

Oesophageal carcinoma

Background

- Eighth most commonly occurring cancer in the UK
- More common in males than females (2:1)
- Tumours in the upper two-thirds of the oesophagus are usually squamous cell cancers
- Tumours in the lower third are usually adenocarcinomas
- Adenocarcinoma often arises in a Barrett's oesophagus—endoscopic screening may reduce the incidence

Symptoms

- Dysphagia
- Chest pain
- Dyspepsia

Diagnosis and staging

- Endoscopy and biopsy
- Barium swallow—demonstrate tumour length
- Endoluminal ultrasound—demonstrates extent of local invasion and lymph node involvement
- CT scan—assesses nodal involvement and distant metastases.

  Staging investigations include:
- Laparoscopy
- Mediastinoscopy
- PET scanning

Treatment

Resectable disease

Surgery remains the only potentially curative modality for tumours in the lower two-thirds of the oesophagus. Unfortunately, however, due to the tendency of the tumour to spread longitudinally via the submucosa, circumferentially to other mediastinal structures and to lymph nodes early in its course, the results are poor with five year survival of <30 per cent. Neo-adjuvant approaches examining preoperative chemotherapy or chemoradiotherapy are currently under investigation.

Tumours in the upper third of the oesophagus are inoperable but may be suitable for radical radiotherapy treatment.

Radiotherapy may also be used with radical intent in tumours in the lower two-thirds of the oesophagus in patients who are unfit for surgery.

Unresectable disease

Endoscopic placement of stents or radiotherapy may provide excellent palliation. Platinum-based chemotherapy may also be useful in palliating symptoms in patients who are fit.

Pancreatic carcinoma

Background

- Seventh most common cause of cancer death in the UK
- Seventy-five per cent arise from the head of pancreas, 15 per cent from the body, 10 per cent from the tail
- Risk factors include:
  - smoking
  - chronic pancreatitis
  - diabetes mellitus
- 90 per cent are adenocarcinomas

Presentation

- Insidious onset of symptoms
- Jaundice
- Weight loss
- Backache

Investigations

- CA19–9—elevated in majority of cancers but low sensitivity
- ERCP with brushings or biopsy
- Ultrasound scan or CT with FNA or biopsy of pancreatic mass
- CT chest abdomen and pelvis
- Laparoscopy—may be required to assess peritoneal involvement prior to surgery

Management

Surgery is the only potentially curative modality of treatment. Unfortunately less than 20 per cent of patients present with surgically resectable disease. A pancreaticoduodenectomy is the operation of choice. However even in those patients who are suitable candidates for this surgery five year survival is less than 30 per cent.

The majority of patients will present with advanced unresectable disease, although surgical bypass procedures may be possible. Primary treatment is aimed at relief of jaundice, which is generally achieved by endoscopic or percutaneous transhepatic placement of a stent.

Chemotherapy (e.g. gemcitabine) can provide a small survival benefit and should be considered in patients with unresectable disease and a ECOG performance status of less than three.

Palliative issues for patients with upper gastrointestinal tract cancer

Mild and non-specific symptoms often precede the onset of dysphagia for many months in oesophageal carcinoma. Stomach cancer often presents late and is frequently metatstatic at presentation.

- **Liver capsular pain** due to liver metastases is common. This is only partially opioid responsive but responds well to NSAIDs or oral steroids
- **Oesophageal spasm** may occur and can be difficult to manage. Specialist advice should be sought. It may be aggravated by oesophageal candidiasis, which needs systemic treatment with oral systemic. antifugals. Smooth muscle relaxants such as nifedipine may also help
- **Involvement of the coeliac plexus** causes a difficult pain syndrome with non-specific abdominal pain and mid back pain. Blockade of the plexus using anaesthetic techniques can be useful
- **Dysphagia** can occur in both oesophageal and stomach cancer. It may be helped by stenting. Oncological treatment of the tumour may provide temporary relief. Advice about appropriate diet and consistency of the food may also help. Feeding gastrostomies are sometimes used prior to aggressive treatment to improve functional status and the ability to tolerate such intervention. Gastrostomies can also improve nutrition and quality of life but should only be inserted after careful multidisciplinary discussion involving the patient and their family. Ethical dilemmas can arise towards the end-of-life when issues of avoiding the prolongation of an uncomfortable dying period (by reducing or stopping artificial feeding) may need to be discussed. There is no evidence that the insertion of feeding tubes in the dying either extends life or improves symptoms
- **Anorexia** is frequent and often profound. There may be a fear of eating because of pain. This may bring the patient and their carer into conflict about food and the 'need to eat'. Open and honest explanation can help to relieve anxiety and provide practical approaches to dealing with the situation
- **Weight loss and altered body image** can be profound with these cancers and can cause distressing problems for the patient and their family
- **Nausea and vomiting** can be persistent and difficult to control. Specialist advice is often needed and drugs may need to be given by routes other than oral. Small frequent meals may improve the frequency of vomiting
- **Haematemesis** may be one of the presenting symptoms but can also occur as the tumour progresses. Where possible local treatment may help and brachytherapy and laser therapy, where available, can reduce the incidence. There is risk of a major bleed. This is a difficult situation to manage and early involvement of specialists should be considered

Cancer of the bladder and ureter

Background
- Account for 1 per cent of all cancers
- 90 per cent are transitional cell carcinomas (TCC)
- Risk factors for TCC include:
  - smoking
  - occupational exposure to aromatic amines and azo dyes
- Squamous cell carcinoma of the bladder is less common and associated with schistosomiasis and bladder calculi

Presentation
- Haematuria
- Frequency
- Urgency

Diagnosis and staging
- Cystoscopy and biopsy
- CT/MRI

Treatment
- 70–80 per cent of all bladder cancers are 'superficial'—that is, they do not invade the muscularis mucosa

'Superficial' tumours
- Treated with transurethral resection of tumour
- Many will recur and follow-up with regular cytoscopy is required
- Factors which identify patients likely to develop invasive disease include:
  - high grade tumours
  - tumours have breached the basement membrane
  - multiple tumours

Such patients may benefit from intravesical chemotherapy or immunotherapy.

'Invasive' tumours
Disease which invades the muscularis mucosa of the bladder may be treated with radical cystectomy or radiotherapy. These modalities have not been directly compared and decisions regarding the choice of therapy tend to be based on performance status, with surgery reserved for the younger and fitter patients.

Bladder cancer is moderately chemosensitive—patients with locally advanced or metastatic disease may benefit from palliative chemotherapy. Active agents include cisplatin, gemcitabine and paclitaxel. No regimen is considered standard and these patients should be considered for entry into clinical trials.

Common problems
- **Bladder spasm** can be frequent and troublesome leading to urinary frequency as well as pain
- **Pelvic pain** is common in advanced disease due to tumour progression. This pain can be extremely difficult to control as it is often complex and includes neuropathic elements. Anaesthetic interventions, including intrathecal and epidural procedures, may be needed to gain pain control

- **Recurrent haematuria** is common and may be sufficient to cause anaemia, and urinary retention due to clot retention. Catheter blockage may be a problem
- **Urinary incontinence** may occur
- **Urinary tract infections** due to long term indwelling catheters are common but not necessary to treat unless symptomatic
- **Lymphoedema** of the lower limbs and genital area may occur and requires specialist management to prevent complications
- **Fistulae** may occur which are often suitable for surgery. If surgery is not possible the risks of skin breakdown are high
- **Renal failure** may occur. Stenting the renal tract may be possible but, may not be appropriate and needs full discussion
- **Altered body image** and problems with sexual function are understandably common
- **Depression** is common because of the long course of the disease, sleep disturbance, and damage to self-esteem

Tumours of the central nervous system

> To expect a personality to survive the disintegration of the brain is like expecting a cricket club to survive when all of its members are dead.
>
> Bertrand Russell

Background

- About a third of all brain tumours are metastatic from primary sites outside the CNS
- Primary brain tumours account for approximately 2 per cent of all cancers
- Primary brain tumours tend to remain localized to the CNS
- Primary brain tumours include:
  - astrocytomas—account for 80 per cent of gliomas most commonly occurring primary brain tumour grade is important in determining prognosis oligodendroglioma—account for 5 per cent of gliomas commonly occur in the frontal lobes longer prognosis
  - ependymoma—tend to occur in children and young adults may metastasise within the CNS
  - medulloblastoma—accounts for 25 per cent of all childhood tumours
  - cerebral lymphoma—increasing in incidence partly due to HIV-associated malignancy

Symptoms

- Headache
- Epilepsy
- Neurological symptoms

Investigations

- Contrast-enhanced CT scan
- Gadolinium-enhanced MRI scan
- If CSF spread is anticipated (e.g. for high grade ependymoma) a neuroaxis MRI +/– CSF cytology is required
- Biopsy is usually required to confirm diagnosis

Primary brain tumours

Surgery

Where possible surgical resection for some low grade tumours may be curative. For higher grade lesions decompression of the tumour may provide palliation and facilitate postoperative radiotherapy.

Radiotherapy

For high grade gliomas postoperative radiotherapy prolongs the effectiveness of surgery and increases median survival. For tumours with a propensity for leptomeningeal spread, such as high grade ependymoma or medulloblastoma, cranio-spinal irradiation improves prognosis.

Chemotherapy

Chemotherapy has a limited rôle to play in the treatment of most brain tumours and its use remains to be clearly defined.

As a general rule in patients with brain tumours poorer prognosis is related to:

- High tumour grade
- Neurological deficit at presentation
- Older age at presentation

Secondary brain tumours

Brain metastases

Cerebral metastases account for approximately a third of all brain tumours. The commonest primary cancer sites include lung, melanoma and breast. Autopsy reveals that metastases are commoner than revealed clinically (60 per cent in small cell lung carcinoma and 75 per cent in melanoma). Carcinoma of the prostate, bladder and ovary rarely metastasise to the brain. Only 5–10 per cent of all patients with cerebral metastases will develop clinical problems.

Assessment—clinical history

Neurological examination of higher cortical function, cranial nerves, musculoskeletal system, sensation, cerebellar function and gait.

Clinical features

Symptoms and signs can evolve over days to weeks. Multiple deposits are present in over two-thirds of patients and clinical signs depend on the anatomical site.

- Focal neurological disturbance consists of motor weakness including hemiparesis (30 per cent), dysphasia and cranial nerve palsies
- Epileptic seizures (15–20 per cent)
- Raised intracranial pressure e.g. headache (50 per cent), nausea, vomiting and lethargy
- Change in mood, cognitive function or behaviour

Investigations

CT scan or MRI scan (better for tumours situated in the posterior fossa or brain stem) show the location of metastases, surrounding oedema and mass effect.

Management

Surgery may be suitable for a very small percentage of patients who are young, fit, with no disease elsewhere, a long treatment-free interval and with a solitary metastasis that will not respond well to radiotherapy, such as adenocarcinoma of the colon or renal carcinoma.

Patients who might benefit from radical treatment should be identified, including those with chemosensitive tumours such as the haematological malignancies, small cell lung cancer and possibly breast cancer.

Palliative radiotherapy with corticosteroids is the most usually appropriate treatment and may improve neurological symptoms and function in over 70 per cent (with a median survival 5–6 months), enabling a gentle reduction and sometimes withdrawal of steroids 4–6 weeks following treatment. Benefit may not be gained in those patients with poor prognostic factors which include poor performance status, over 60 years of age, non-breast primary site, multiple lobe involvement, short disease-free interval and overt uncontrolled metastases elsewhere. Decisions regarding treatment should be, as ever, tailored to the problems of the individual patient.

Cranial irradiation may cause some degree of scalp and upper pinna erythema and irritation. Temporary alopecia is universal in a population whose prognosis is unlikely to allow regrowth of hair within the remaining lifespan. The start of treatment may induce an increase in cerebral oedema which may require steroid dose readjustment. Other effects include transient somnolence, occurring within a few weeks, and longer term impairment of memory and cognition. These are significant problems in very few people and most patients do not survive long enough for late radiation changes in the CNS to develop.

Corticosteroids

High dose corticosteroids (dexamethasone 16 mg/day initially) reduce cerebral oedema and associated symptoms of headache and vomiting may be helped rapidly. In certain situations, particularly if metastases are in the posterior fossa, hydrocephalus may be present, in which case a ventricular shunt may be required for symptom control.

The short prognosis for most patients means that the issue of long term side-effects of steroids may not be a problem. It is best practice, however, gradually to reduce the dose to the lowest possible over a few weeks to minimize potential side-effects since difficulties may build up insidiously.

A stage may be reached when the dose necessary to control the cerebral oedema causes significant side-effects. Disabling problems such as obesity (and associated problems with immobility management), body image problems, proximal myopathy, mood swings, fragile skin and diabetes may then develop. There should be open dialogue (particularly while the patient is *compos mentis* and can join in discussions) about the ongoing use of steroids in the event that quality of life becomes adversely affected. Patients and families may view the steroids as agents to control the disease and resist attempts to reduce the dose, fearing the return of symptoms of raised intracranial pressure.

On the other hand, patients may have recognized that their quality of life is deteriorating despite continuing steroids and may then be happy for (or request that) steroids should be withdrawn. This should generally be done slowly while controlling the symptoms of raised intracranial pressure by other means.

When patients become moribund and can no longer swallow, steroids can generally be stopped but this may then depend on the particular clinical circumstances and may need negotiation with the patient/family. There should be adequate medication provision (subcutaneous) for analgesia, antiemetics, anticonvulsants and sedatives as necessary.

Multiple complex physical and psychological problems including poor mobility, heavy care needs, swings in mood, and confusion can completely exhaust even the most caring family who need the expert support of an experienced multi-disciplinary team (MDT).

Prognosis

Although some patients, particularly with metastases from breast cancer, may survive relatively longer, most patients with brain metastases from solid tumours have a survival in the order of a few weeks or months at best.

Metastatic disease of the leptomeninges (meningeal carcinomatosis)

Five per cent of patients with tumours may develop clinical signs and symptoms of leptomeningeal disease, although the autopsy rate is higher (10 per cent). It is most commonly seen in lymphoma and leukaemia although it may occur in breast cancer, small cell lung cancer and melanoma.

Clinical features

The presenting features may be varied and fluctuating and the diagnosis should be considered in any unexplained neurological disturbance in a patient with cancer. The most frequently encountered are cranial nerve problems (75 per cent), headache (50 per cent), radicular or back pain (40–45 per cent) and weakness in one or more limbs (40 per cent). Other presentations include meningism, altered consciousness, confusion, sphincter disturbance and seizures. Abnormal physical signs are more prominent than symptoms, with lower motor neurone lesions predominating.

Investigations

- Lumbar puncture if there is no evidence of raised intracranial pressure (90 per cent will have positive cytology and increased protein on CNS analysis)
- MRI scan

Management

This may include intrathecal chemotherapy, depending on the tumour type and radiotherapy. The aim is to halt progression of disease and relieve symptoms but is essentially palliative except for a curable sub-group of leukaemia or lymphoma. Steroids and NSAIDs may help symptoms.

Prognosis

Without treatment patients may survive for several months, depending on the tumour type, with relentless progression of neurological symptoms. Even with treatment, prognosis is usually less than six months and is worst in small cell lung cancer, widespread disease, poor performance status and where there are widespread neurological signs.

Chronic leukaemia and myeloma

General comments

The clinical course tends to be very variable, but is characterized by a *protracted cycle of relapses and remissions*. This can cause considerable distress as the patients and their carers have to live with uncertainty about the future. Both patient and professionals involved with their care may find it hard to accept that a patient is entering the terminal phase.

Infection is a frequent and unpredictable complication of both the disease process and its treatment. It can be fatal and this makes the prognosis even more uncertain.

Chemotherapy may continue in advanced illness because of the possibility of a further remission and/or useful palliation.

Specific pain complexes

• **Bone pain** is very common. The pain is often worse on movement or weight-bearing, which makes titration of analgesics very difficult. The pain often *responds well to radiotherapy and/or oral steroids*. NSAIDs may help but must be used with caution because they may interfere with platelet and renal function

• **Pathological fractures** are particularly common in myeloma due to the lytic bone lesions. These often require *orthopaedic intervention* and subsequent *radiotherapy*. Prophylactic pinning of long bones and/or radiotherapy should be considered to prevent fracture and reduce the likelihood of complex pain syndromes developing

• **Spinal cord compression** requires prompt diagnosis, high dose oral steroids in a single daily dose and urgent discussion with an oncologist. The steroids should be continued at a high dose until a definitive plan has been made. They may then be titrated down in accordance with the patient's condition and symptoms

• **Wedge and crush fractures of the spinal column** can lead to severe back pain which is often associated with nerve compression and neuropathic pain. Such pain is partially opioid sensitive but adjuvant analgesics in the form of antidepressants and/or anticonvulsant medication are usually required to supplement the effect of the opioid. Specialist advice is frequently needed to maintain symptom control

Other complications

Bone marrow failure is usual. Recurrent infections and bleeding episodes can leave the patients and carers exhausted. Patients often feel dependent on the administration of blood and platelet transfusions, unable to consider reducing the frequency of life-sustaining treatment. Difficult decisions about reducing regular transfusions or stopping them if they are providing no further benefit may need to be faced with patients and families.

Night sweats and fever are common, imposing a heavy demand on carers, particularly as several changes of night and bed clothes may be needed. Specialist advice may help in relieving the symptoms, as there are a number of drugs that appear to be effective. (📖 See Chapter 6d, p. 289.)

Hypercalcaemia may occur, especially in myeloma. It should be considered in any patient with persistent nausea, altered mood or confusion (even if this is intermittent), worsening pain and/or constipation. Treatment with i/v hydration and i/v bisphosphonates should be considered. Resistant hypercalcaemia may be a pre-terminal event when aggressive management would be inappropriate

Palliative care of patients with carcinomatosis of unknown primary

Background

Approximately 3 per cent of patients present with metastases from an unknown primary site. As a group the prognosis for these patient is poor, with median survival of 3–4 months.

Investigations

- Serological tumour markers including CA19–9, CEA, CA125, αFP, βHCG, PSA, and paraproteins
- Biopsy—thorough pathological assessment with immunohistochemistry may provide clues to the primary site
- CT scan of chest, abdomen and pelvis

In some instances the site of metastatic disease may suggest a probable primary site, e.g. adenocarcinoma in axillary nodes suggest a breast primary.

Particularly in young patients it is important to rule out the possibility of a potentially curable germ cell tumour. This may be suggested by elevated αFP or βHCG.

In a substantial number of patients a primary site is not identified. In this instance exhaustive investigations are not appropriate.

Treatment

In some patients where the clinical presentation suggests a primary, even if a tumour cannot be detected in that organ, it may be appropriate to treat the patient in the usual manner. For example, a patient presenting with ER-positive adenocarcinoma in an axillary node could reasonably be treated as if breast cancer was the primary.

For patients in which there is little evidence of a primary site (e.g. those presenting with liver metastases) the choice is much more difficult. As the primary is unknown it is impossible to give patients an idea of the likelihood of a treatment response or of how durable such a response is likely to be. Any potential benefit of treatment must be carefully balanced against possible toxicity and a decision to proceed with chemotherapy should only be undertaken following a very full discussion with the patient and carers, outlining the uncertainties and limitations of treatment and overall limited prognosis.

Anxiety is common in this group of patients. Not knowing the site of the primary tumour causes considerable distress. Extensive investigations may raise false expectations and may exhaust the patient. Equally patients and carers may feel cheated of the chance to have effective treatment if the primary is not looked for.

Carers may find coming to terms with the patient's death due to an 'unknown primary' difficult, and are perhaps at greater risk of an adverse bereavement reaction.

Key points

- Anxiety
- Anger
- Risk of over investigation
- Adverse bereavement reaction

Further reading

Cassidy J., Bissett D. *et al.* (2002) *Oxford handbook of oncology*. Oxford: Oxford University Press.

Kirkham S. (1988) The palliation of cerebral tumours with high dose dexamethasone: a review. *Palliative Medicine*, 2: 27–33.

Souhami R. L., Tobias J. D. (2003) *Cancer and its management*. 4th edition. Oxford: Blackwell Science.

Thomas K. (2003) *Caring for the dying at home: companions on the journey*. Oxford: Radcliffe Press.

The management of pain

> To Each his sufferings, all are men,
> Condemned alike to groan;
> The tender for another's pain,
> Th'unfeeling for his own.

> Thomas Gray, *Ode on a Distant Prospect of Eton College* (1747).
> London: R. Dodsley.

The intricacy of the human condition and the constantly changing interface between the external and the internal allows pain to be experienced in myriad different modalities. This ever-fluxing dynamic interaction between external stimuli and the individual's capacity to deal with those stimuli can greatly increase the complexity of pain management. What may be experienced as terrible pain by one individual may be brushed aside by another. Further, even individuals presented with the same painful stimuli at different times in their lives may be affected in a completely different manner. Stories abound of soldiers wounded in battle being able to ignore pain which, had it resulted from an accident at home, would have completely incapacitated them.

Pain is experienced by people and families not by nerve endings.

Experts in torture have used the huge and varied capacity to experience pain in plying their evil arts. Conversely, as the capacity to experience pain is so varied, so the methods used to alleviate pain need to be multidimensional.

A mother kissing away the pain of her child who has just had a fall, and an anaesthetist inserting a spinal catheter are both involved in the process of pain alleviation. Ensuring that the intervention used is appropriate for individuals and their families is crucial, but so also is ensuring that other causes, contributory factors and healing potentials are not ignored.

In the centre of Kathmandu there is a tree shrine to the God of toothache, to which sufferers go to hammer in a coin to help alleviate their pain. The tree is covered with thousands of coins. In a city which until very recently had only a handful of dentists, such an approach to pain control may not be as simplistic as it might first appear to western eyes which have had the benefits of modern anaesthetics and dentistry for a few generations.

The arrogance of healers who believe that their approach to pain alleviation is the only effective method does not stand up to the experience of life, and the reality that there are many ways in which pain is experienced and dealt with.

For health workers involved in dealing regularly with patients' pain there is a tension between two extremes of care.

The scientific clinician can be so specialized in synapse research that his model of pain control can sound mechanistic, simplistic and unbelievable.

The holistic clinician on the other hand can view patients' pain with such a wide angle lens that appropriate analgesic intervention with enough focused attention to relieve the symptoms is not achieved.

Of necessity this section will look at aspects of pain control in isolation, but quality pain management always involves both a holistic approach to patient care and a scientific approach with meticulous attention to diagnostic and management detail.

He was around 25 and obviously embarrassed to be at the surgery.

'It's these pains in my gut doctor, they are really bad'. A pause, a whiff of a hidden agenda hung in the air.

'How long have you had this problem?'

'Only these last two weeks, it's really bad in the morning, and if I don't eat.'

A shifty look is followed by a blank stare at the floor.

'Have you any idea what might have brought the pain on?'

No answer, just an uncomfortable silence.

'Have you been worried about anything recently?'

A look combining fear and hope crosses his face, 'It's hard to talk about.'

'Often problems like this come from stress and worry, so what you're experiencing is not all that unusual. Anything that we discuss will, of course be totally confidential'.

The story unfolds of sudden onset impotence following a relationship with a new partner while still harbouring strong feelings for his previous girl friend. Explanation and reassurance transform the man's demeanour, and he bounces out of the surgery relieved and unburdened.

I patted myself on the back for my ability to see beyond the offered reason for consulting to the deeper hidden meaning ignoring the fact that the doctor who treats 'just' the covert cause of pain is at similar risk as his colleague who focuses on 'just' the overt cause. Both lull themselves into the false sense of security that they have met the patient's real need.

Two weeks later the patient makes telephone contact.

'How are things?'

'Couldn't be better. I'm right back on form. It really made a difference talking with you, but, …'

'Yes?'

'But this pain in my stomach is still really bad. The only thing that seems to help is taking some of my mum's Zantac. Could you give me a script Doctor?'

Table 6a.1 Definition of pain terms[1]

Allodynia	Pain caused by a stimulus which does not normally provoke pain
Analgesia	Absence of pain in response to stimulation which would normally be painful
Causalgia	A syndrome of sustained burning pain, allodynia and hyperpathia after a traumatic nerve lesion, often combined with vasomotor dysfunction and later trophic changes
Central pain	Pain associated with a lesion in the central nervous system (brain and spinal cord)
Dysaesthesia	An unpleasant abnormal sensation which can be either spontaneous or provoked
Hyperaesthesia	An increased sensitivity to stimulation
Hyperalgesia	An increased response to a stimulus that is normally painful
Hyperpathia	A painful syndrome characterized by increased reaction to a stimulus, especially a repetitive stimulus, as well as an increased threshold
Neuralgia	Pain in the distribution of a nerve
Neuropathy	A disturbance of function or pathological change in a nerve
Neuropathic pain	Pain which is transmitted by a damaged nervous system, and which is usually only partially opioid sensitive
Nociceptor	A receptor preferentially sensitive to a noxious stimulus or to a stimulus which would become noxious if prolonged
Nociceptive pain	Pain which is transmitted by an undamaged nervous system and is usually opioid responsive
Pain	An unpleasant sensory and emotional experience associated with actual or potential tissue damage or described in terms of such damage
Pain threshold	The least experience of pain which a subject can recognize
Pain tolerance level	The greatest level of pain which a subject is prepared to tolerate

1 Mersky H., Bogduk N. (1994) *Classification of Chronic Pain*. 2nd edn. Seattle: IASP Press.

Pain is a common symptom

> For frequent tears have run
> The colours from my life.
>
> Elizabeth Barrett Browning 1806–61: *Sonnets from the Portuguese* (1850)

- 'Pain is an unpleasant sensory and emotional experience associated with actual or potential tissue damage or described in terms of such damage. In other words, pain is a somatopsychic phenomenon.' (Robert Twycross)
- Pain is a complex physiological and emotional experience and not a simple sensation

Pain involves
- Unpleasant sensory experience
- Unpleasant emotional experience
- Social and spiritual components

Incidence of pain in cancer
- One quarter of patients *do not experience pain*
- One third of those with pain have a single pain
- One third have two pains
- One third have three or more pains

Causes of pain in patients with cancer
- Caused by cancer itself (85%)
- Caused by treatment
- Related to cancer and debility
- Unrelated to cancer

Perception of pain is modulated by
- The patient's mood
- The patient's morale
- The meaning of the pain for the patient

Patients with palliative care needs most commonly have *chronic malignant pain*. However, patients with *acute pain* or *chronic non-malignant pain* sometimes require the help of palliative care services. For these reasons it is important to assess each specific pain and to identify the likely cause.

Common causes of pain in patients with cancer
Cancer-related
- Bone
- Nerve compression/infiltration
- Soft tissue infiltration
- Visceral
- Muscle spasm
- Lymphoedema
- Raised intracranial pressure

Treatment-related
- Surgery: postoperative scars/adhesions
- Radiotherapy: fibrosis
- Chemotherapy: neuropathy

Associated factors–cancer and debility
- Constipation
- Pressure sores
- Bladder spasm
- Stiff joints
- Post-herpetic neuralgia

Unrelated to cancer
- Low back pain
- Arthritis
- Angina
- Trauma

The experience of pain can
- Induce depression
- Exacerbate anxiety
- Interfere with social performance
- Negatively impact on physical capability
- Prevent work
- Decrease income
- Encourage isolation
- Impair the quality of relationships
- Create family disharmony and stress
- Challenge existential beliefs

These secondary effects are constantly affecting the patient's experience of pain.

Assessment of pain

When sorrows come, they come not single spies,
But in battalions.

William Shakespeare1564–1616: *Hamlet* (1601)

Assessment of a patient's pain is a crucial skill, which requires a structured approach, a closely listening ear and a sharp eye. Accurate assessment is also helped by experience, and is not a 'one-off' event—but needs to be constantly re-evaluated by the healthcare team as more information is gathered.

Assessment questions

There are many approaches to assessing pain, and each professional will develop his/her own approach to taking a *pain history*. The specifics of pain history questions are not crucial. What is important is that there is a logical outline scheme which works. Having good assessment technique is the basis for effective palliative care, and for prompt appropriate management of a patient's pain.

Pain History Principles

1 Seek to establish a relationship with the patient
2 Encourage the patient to do most of the talking
3 Begin with a wide angle open question before clarifying and focusing with more specific ones
4 Watch the patient for clues regarding pain
5 Avoid jumping to conclusions.

Remember, as you are assessing patients, they are assessing you.
- Eye to eye level contact
- Clear introduction
- Avoid over familiarity
- Explain what you plan to do
- Summarise back to the patient 'Have I heard things correctly'
- Avoid patronizing
- Use language and terms appropriate to patient

The most extreme agony is to feel that one has been utterly forsaken.

Bettelheim, Bruno (1979). *Surviving and Other Essays.* New York: Knopf.

Table 6a.2 One scheme of pain assessment questions

Is the patient currently in distress due to pain?	Before embarking on a full assessment it is important to achieve sufficient comfort for the patient to go through the assessment.
Is the pain related to movement?	Fractures/inflammation/peritonitis/pleurisy?
Is the pain periodic?	Colic: due to gastrointestinal or renal tract problems?
Is the pain worse on eating?	Mouth, oesophagus or stomach problems?
Is the pain associated with passing urine or stool?	Constipation, haemorrhoids, tenesmus, infection?
Is the pain associated with skin changes of colour, temperature or swelling?	Pressure sore/infection/ischaemic limb/DVT/skin tumour?
Is the pain associated with altered sensation?	This implies nerve damage: *neuropathic pain* which may occur in a dermatome (an area supplied by a peripheral nerve) *sympathetic pain* which occurs in the same distribution as the arterial blood supply.
Is the pain persisting?	Fear or depression, poor compliance with medication, inappropriate treatment or a new pain?
What relieves the pain?	What has already been tried which worked? e.g. change in position, distraction, medication?

Adapted from Thompson and Regnard.[2]

2 Thomson J. W., Regnard C. (1995) Pain. In C. Regnard, J. Hockley (eds) *Flow Diagrams in Advanced Cancer and Other Diseases*, pp. 5–10. London: Arnold.

Pain assessment tools

Symptom monitoring by patients can be used to enhance understanding of the symptoms and improve assessment of the effectiveness of management strategies. As an example of symptom monitoring, pain assessment charts and scales have been used extensively.

Used appropriately such evaluation tools provide a very useful quantifiable measure which both patient and healthcare professional can use to chart the effectiveness of pain reducing interventions.

However, for those patients who may ruminate about their 'pain scores', the use of such a method of assessment exacerbates pain, and pain awareness. Other patients who are in the advanced stages of illness will find the completion of pain charts an unnecessary burden.

From the health professional viewpoint, the collection of such data can be very useful, depending on the quality of the data collection, and can enhance understanding of how the patient perceives pain. However filling forms may draw the professional's attention away from the patient.

Pain is a multidimensional experience and as such requires a multidimensional assessment tool. The European Pain Group recommends two, the Brief Pain Inventory (BPI) and the McGill Pain Questionnaire (MPQ), as both have been well validated in a number of different languages.[3]

While such assessment tools cannot provide objective evidence of pain management, if applied appropriately they can provide clear evidence of trends experienced by individual patients.

A number of self report tools have been tested for use in palliative care to measure pain intensity in a reliable and valid way.

These include:

Visual analogue scales (VAS)

The VAS is an unmarked line with extremes marked as no pain and worst pain. Patients are asked to mark the point in the line that describes their pain.

No pain_____Worst pain

Categorical verbal rating scales (VRS)

A VRS involves a sequence of words describing different intensity levels of pain such as:

None   Mild   Moderate   Severe

Categorical numerical rating scales (NRS)

The NRS is similar to the VAS but uses numbers or gradations that indicate the severity of the pain experience

0____1____2____3____4____5____6____7____8____9____10
no pain   worst pain

---

3 Caraceni A., Cherny N., Fainsinger R., Kaasa S., Poulain P., Radbruch L., *et al.* (2000) Pain measurement tools and methods in clinical research in palliative care: recommendations of an expert working group of the European Association of Palliative Care. *Journal of Pain and Symptom Management.*

Brief Pain Inventory

Date: ___/___/___

Name: _____
        Last   First   Middle Initial

Phone: (___)_____   Sex: ☐ Female ☐ Male

Date of Birth: ___/___/___

1) Marital Status (at present)
    1. ☐ Single   3. ☐ Widowed
    2. ☐ Married   4. ☐ Separated/Divorced

2) Education (Circle only the highest grade or degree completed)
    Grade   0   1   2   3   4   5   6   7   8   9
             10 11 12 13 14 15 16 M.A./M.S.
                    Professional degree (please specify) _____

3) Current occupation_____
    (specify titles; if you are not working, tell us your previous occupation)

4) Spouse's Occupation_____

5) Which of the following best describes your current job status?
    ☐ 1. Employed outside the home, full-time
    ☐ 2. Employed outside the home, part-time
    ☐ 3. Homemaker
    ☐ 4. Retired
    ☐ 5. Unemployed
    ☐ 6. Other

6) How long has it been since you first learned your diagnosis? _____ months

7) Have you ever had pain due to your present disease?
    1. ☐ Yes   2. ☐ No   3. ☐ Uncertain

8) When you first received your diagnosis, was pain one of your symptoms?
    1. ☐ Yes   2. ☐ No   3. ☐ Uncertain

9) Have you had surgery in the past month? 1. ☐ Yes   2. ☐ No

10) Throughout our lives, most of us have had pain from time to time (such as minor headaches, sprains, and toothaches). Have you had pain other than these everyday kinds of pain during the **last week**? 1. ☐ Yes   2. ☐ No

IF YOU ANSWERED YES TO THE LAST QUESTION, PLEASE GO ON TO QUESTION 11 AND FINISH THIS QUESTIONNAIRE. IF NO, YOU ARE FINISHED WITH THE QUESTIONNAIRE. THANK YOU.

11) On the diagram, shade in the areas where you feel pain. Put an X on the area that hurts the most.

12) Please rate your pain by circling the one number that best describes your pain at its worst in the last week.
    0   1   2   3   4   5   6   7   8   9   10
    No   Pain as bad as
    Pain   you can imagine

13) Please rate your pain by circling the one number that best describes your pain at its least in the last week.
    0   1   2   3   4   5   6   7   8   9   10
    No   Pain as bad as
    Pain   you can imagine

14) Please rate your pain by circling the one number that best describes your pain on the average.
    0   1   2   3   4   5   6   7   8   9   10
    No   Pain as bad as
    Pain   you can imagine

Fig. 6a.1 Brief pain inventory. Reproduced with permission from Doyle et al. (2005) *The Oxford Textbook of Palliative Medicine*, 3rd edn. Oxford: Oxford University Press.

15) Please rate your pain by circling the one number that tells how much pain you have right now.

| 0 | 1 | 2 | 3 | 4 | 5 | 6 | 7 | 8 | 9 | 10 |
No
Pain
Pain as bad as
you can imagine

16) What kinds of things make your pain feel better (for example, head, medicine, rest)?

_____

17) What kinds of things make your pain worse (for example, walking, standing, lifting)?

_____

18) What treatments or medications are you receiving for your pain?

_____

19) In the last week, how much relief have pain treatments or medications provided? Please circle the one percentage that most shows how much relief you have received.

| 0% | 10% | 20% | 30% | 40% | 50% | 60% | 70% | 80% | 90% | 100% |
No
Relief
Complete
Relief

20) If you take pain medication, how many hours does it take before the pain returns?

☐ 1. Pain medication doesn't help at all   ☐ 5. Four hours
☐ 2. One hour   ☐ 6. Five to twelve hours
☐ 3. Two hours   ☐ 7. More than twelve hours
☐ 4. Three hours   ☐ 8. I do not take pain medication

21) Circle the appropriate answer for each item.
I believe my pain is due to:

☐ Yes ☐ No   1. The effects of treatment (for example, medication, surgery, radiation, prosthetic device).

☐ Yes ☐ No   2. My primary disease (meaning the disease currently being treated and evaluated).

☐ Yes ☐ No   3. A medical condition unrelated to primary disease (for example, arthritis).

22) For each of the following words, check yes or no if that adjective applies to your pain.

Aching	☐ Yes ☐ No	Exhausting	☐ Yes ☐ No
Throbbing	☐ Yes ☐ No	Tiring	☐ Yes ☐ No
Shooting	☐ Yes ☐ No	Penetrating	☐ Yes ☐ No
Stabbing	☐ Yes ☐ No	Nagging	☐ Yes ☐ No
Gnawing	☐ Yes ☐ No	Numb	☐ Yes ☐ No
Sharp	☐ Yes ☐ No	Miserable	☐ Yes ☐ No
Tender	☐ Yes ☐ No	Unbearable	☐ Yes ☐ No
Burning	☐ Yes ☐ No		

23) Circle the one number that describes how, during the past week, pain has interfered with your:

A. General Activity

| 0 | 1 | 2 | 3 | 4 | 5 | 6 | 7 | 8 | 9 | 10 |
Does not
Interfere
Completely
interferes

B. Mood

| 0 | 1 | 2 | 3 | 4 | 5 | 6 | 7 | 8 | 9 | 10 |
Does not
Interfere
Completely
interferes

C. Walking ability

| 0 | 1 | 2 | 3 | 4 | 5 | 6 | 7 | 8 | 9 | 10 |
Does not
Interfere
Completely
interferes

D. Normal work (includes both work outside the home and housework)

| 0 | 1 | 2 | 3 | 4 | 5 | 6 | 7 | 8 | 9 | 10 |
Does not
Interfere
Completely
interferes

E. Relations with other people

| 0 | 1 | 2 | 3 | 4 | 5 | 6 | 7 | 8 | 9 | 10 |
Does not
Interfere
Completely
interferes

F. Sleep

| 0 | 1 | 2 | 3 | 4 | 5 | 6 | 7 | 8 | 9 | 10 |
Does not
Interfere
Completely
interferes

G. Enjoyment of life

| 0 | 1 | 2 | 3 | 4 | 5 | 6 | 7 | 8 | 9 | 10 |
Does not
Interfere
Completely
interferes

Pain Research Group, Department of Neurology, University of Wisconsin-Madison

Pain and function

Surveys across different cultures show that the relationship between pain and physical performance is non-linear. Impairment in function becomes markedly worse above a pain severity rating of four on a ten point scale. This suggests that we have the capacity to deal with a certain amount of pain but once this capacity is exhausted, function quickly becomes impaired.[4]

This has important implications in the management of pain, as reducing some of the secondary effects of pain, such as anxiety or financial worries, may decrease the overall experience of pain to a point where function is markedly improved. Improvement of function can have a very positive effect reducing the experience of pain and restoring morale; some of the symptom control success achieved in inpatient palliative care units must be attributed to a reduction in secondary pain effects.

The pain threshold will vary from person to person and within the individual. It also varies according to multiple physical and psychosocial factors which are constantly changing. Models that help us understand pain need to take account of this constantly changing nature of pain perception. Such a model understands pain perception as a 'plastic phenomenon' which is constantly in flux.

This is supported by the growing understanding of the rapidly altering neurochemical environment of the central and peripheral nervous system. Changes in concentrations of neurotransmitters and of neuroreceptors impact on the transmission of painful stimuli.

Tom had been admitted to the hospice for symptom control from his local area hospital. Despite receiving nearly 1000 mg of diamorphine subcutaneously per day he persisted in scoring his pain at 8 or above.

Tom was a self made man of 55 who had built up a chain of shoe shops after leaving school at 16. When his oesophageal carcinoma was diagnosed he had a chain of shops all over the area.

He was not expecting his diagnosis of cancer and the news that curative intervention was not possible came as a devastating blow to a man used to controlling his own life and business.

Suddenly his life had been invaded and his inner resources for dealing with the situation overrun.

One week later Tom went home from the hospice requiring MST 20 mg b.d. and diazepam 5mg nocte to control his symptoms.

Tom achieved his improved pain control by having his underlying anxiety addressed and treated, and by gaining back some control over his life, the lack of which had caused him deep anguish.

'The space and peace in the hospice gave me time to get my head around things'.

4 Serlin R. C., Mendoza T. R., Nakamura Y., Edwards K. R., Cleeland C. S. (1995) When is cancer pain mild, moderate or severe? Grading pain severity by its interference with function. *Pain*, 61, 2: 277–84.

Pain classification

Pain is traditionally classified into four different modalities:
1 Physical,
2 Psychosocial,
3 Emotional, and
4 Spiritual.

It is imperative that patients' anxieties and frequent misconceptions related to these factors are explored. Pain will not be adequately controlled unless patients feel a degree of control over their situation. To ignore such psychological aspects of care may often be the reason for seemingly intractable pain. Having prescribed analgesics, the patient's pain should be under constant supervision and the response to treatment reviewed *regularly*.

Having identified the *cause* of the pain, it is useful to *classify* the pain into predominantly *nociceptive* or *neuropathic* categories in order to determine the correct management.

Nociceptive pain

This refers to pain resulting from stimulation of peripheral nerves transmitted by an undamaged nervous system. Pain impulses enter the spinal cord through the dorsal horn, where they ascend to higher centres in the brain. Inhibitory impulses block transmission at the dorsal horn in the spinal cord, preventing further transmission of the pain impulse. It is usually opioid responsive.

Fig. 6a.2 Nociceptive pain

Neuropathic pain

Neuropathic pain refers to pain arising from damage in the peripheral or central nervous system. Clinically it may present with hyperalgesia and allodynia, with patients describing sensations such as burning or stabbing. It may be only partially opioid responsive.

Fig. 6a.3 Neuropathic pain

Peripheral pain
Peripheral neuropathic pain is caused by damage within the peripheral nervous system. There is often an associated area of altered sensation around the site of nerve injury.

Central pain
Central pain refers to neuropathic pain caused by damage within the central nervous system. There is usually an area of altered sensation incorporating the area of pain. A cerebrovascular accident or spinal cord damage may be associated with central pain.

Sympathetically-maintained pain
Sympathetically-maintained pain is due to sympathetic nerve injury. Essential features are pain (often burning) and sensory disorder related to a vascular as opposed to neural distribution. In patients with cancer such pain is more common in the lower limbs, and is usually associated with disease in the pelvis.

Such pain is also associated with reduced sweating and dry shiny skin within the affected area.

Practical pain control

Fig. 6a.4 The analgesic ladder[5]

Step 1: Non opioid ± adjuvants
Start treatment with paracetamol 1g every 4 h REGULARLY (Max. daily dose 4g). If this is not adequate in 24 h, stop and proceed to step 2.

Step 2: Weak opioid + non opioid ± adjuvants
Start treatment with a combined preparation of paracetamol with codeine or dihydrocodeine. Use of dextropropoxyphene and paracetamol (co-proxamol) is being phased out in the UK in 2005. Many combined preparations are available and are some of the most widely used medicines in the community. NB Studies have shown that there is no additional analgesic benefit from preparations which contain only 8mg of codeine combined with paracetamol as opposed to paracetamol alone. It is important to stipulate the dose of codeine required in the preparation e.g. 'paracetamol 500mg/codeine 30mg'. Patients need also to be clearly advised to take these tablets regularly and not to assess efficacy after only a couple of doses.

5 World Health Organization (1996) *Cancer pain relief: with a guide to opioid availability.* 2nd edition. Geneva: WHO.

Step 3: Strong opioid + non opioid ± adjuvants

Two tablets of co-codamol contain 60mg of codeine which is already approximately equi-analgesic to oral morphine 5mg every 4h. (See conversion table). If changing to morphine, it will therefore be necessary to use a minimum of morphine 5mg but 10mg may be needed. Caution should be exercised in patients who are elderly or in renal failure, since active morphine metabolites are excreted by the kidney. The formulation of morphine may be immediate release (i/r) tablets or solution, depending on patient preference. If the pain seems responsive to opioids and there are no undue side-effects, continue to titrate the dose upwards by no more than 30–50 per cent every 24 h until pain is controlled. It is not necessary to wake the patient at night to give medication, but if pain during the night or first thing in the morning is a problem, it may be helpful to increase the last evening dose by 50 per cent.

Step 4: Adjuvant drug (co-analgesic)

This is a drug which is not an analgesic in its prime function but in combination with an analgesic can enhance pain control.

Examples of use of adjuvant drugs			
Corticosteroid:	pain caused by oedema	Night sedative:	when lack of sleep is decreasing pain threshold
Antidepressant:	neuropathic pain		
Anticonvulsant:	neuropathic pain	Anxiolytic:	when anxiety is contributing to pain
Muscle relaxant:	muscle cramp pain		
Antispasmodic:	bowel colic	Antidepressant:	when depressed mood is contributing to pain
NSAID:	inflammatory pain		
Antibiotic:	infection pain		

Breakthrough pain

Breakthrough pain is a flare in pain of rapid onset, moderate to severe intensity and of short duration. It may be precipitated by activity but it can also happen spontaneously. If pain starts to occur regularly before the next dose is due, this is probably an indication to increase the regular background dose.

- Analyse and avoid precipitating activities if possible. Predict pain and give analgesia 20 minutes prior to activity e.g. prior to changing dressings or movement

Treatment options to consider:
- Immediate release oral morphine or other opioid according to background analgesia (or diamorphine SC/ i/v if unable to swallow) at 50–100 per cent of the equivalent regular background 4 h dose
- Oral transmucosal fentanyl citrate lozenges (OTFC) or other fentanyl-like drugs
- Midazolam 2.5–5mg SC/lorazepam 0.5mg sublingually to allay anxiety
- NSAID SC e.g. parecoxib 40mg

Other therapies include:
- Visualization techniques, hypnotherapy, reassurance and a calm professional manner, distraction etc.

NB Nitrous oxide gas (Entonox) inhalation is now rarely used prior to painful procedures. For this means of analgesia to be effective, the patient needs to be able to inhale deeply, whilst holding the mask to the face. It is therefore not very useful with the weak , infirm or older patient. It *must* be administered with the demand valve and this *must* be held to the face by the patient alone. If the patient is made drowsy by the Entonox, the mask automatically falls away from the face and the patient breathes air again and recovers, before there is any risk of losing protective reflexes. Entonox should *never* be used on patients who have any air where it should not be e.g. pneumothorax, or pneumoperitoneum. Nitrous oxide rapidly enters these areas, causing potentially dangerous expansion.

Opioid-resistant cancer pain
Pseudo-resistant?
- Underdosing
- Poor alimentary absorption of opioid (rare, except where there is an ileostomy)
- Poor alimentary intake because of vomiting
- Ignoring psychological aspects of patient care

Semi-resistant?
- Bone pain
- Raised intracranial pressure
- Nerve trunk compression
- Neuropathic pain
- Activity-related pain

Resistant?
- Muscle spasm
- Abdominal cramps
- Spiritual pain (📖 Chapter 9)

As stressed earlier, patients with chronic unremitting pain from a deteriorating condition are particularly at risk of spiritual pain which needs to be addressed. Referral for psychological/spiritual support is important, and/or use of a complementary therapist. Using Hay's seven model assessment[6], 'spiritual pain' can be broken down into:
- Spiritual suffering—interpersonal or intra-psychic anguish
- Inner resource deficiency—diminished spiritual capacity
- Belief system problem—lack or loss of personal meaning system
- Religious request—a specifically expressed religious need

---

6 Hay M. W. (1989) Principles in building spiritual assessment tools. *The American Journal of Hospice Care*, **6**: 25–31.

Opioid analgesic therapy

Paracetamol and weak opioids

Codeine

Five to ten per cent of caucasians are CYP2D6 poor-metabolizers, an hepatic enzyme necessary to convert codeine to morphine. These patients will not obtain equivalent analgesia using codeine-containing analgesics. This bioactivation is markedly inhibited by antipsychotics (chlorpromazine, haloperidol, levomepromazine, and thioridazine), metoclopramide, and tricyclic antidepressants (amitriptyline etc.). If hepatic metabolism is decreased in patients taking these drugs, or with liver disease, the analgesic action of codeine may also be compromised.

Co-proxamol

Systematic reviews suggest that co-proxamol (dextropropoxyphene and paracetamol) is no more effective as an analgesic than paracetamol alone. Dextropropoxyphene has a longer elimination half-life than paracetamol and will therefore accumulate to higher blood levels during repeated dosing.

Compound analgesics containing sub-therapeutic doses of opioids should not be used for pain control in cancer patients.[7] The UK Committee of Safety of Medicines decided in January 2005 to withdraw co-proxamol use in the UK over a 12 month period because of its efficacy and safety profile.

Morphine

> We are all strong enough to bear the misfortunes of others.
> Duc de la Rochefoucauld 1613–80: *Maximes* (1678)

Morphine is the strong opioid of first choice for moderate to severe cancer pain. Alternative opioids may be as effective, and are appropriate for certain patients.

Starting a patient on morphine

- Start with immediate release (i/r) morphine liquid or tablets
  - Adult, not pain controlled on regular weak opioids: 10mg 4-h morphine
  - Elderly, cachectic, or not taking regular weak opioids: 5mg 4-h morphine
  - Very elderly and frail: 2.5mg 4-h morphine
- Although 4-h morphine gives greatest flexibility for initial dose titration, patients with less severe pain, difficulties with compliance and especially outpatients, can be started on 12-h modified release (m/r) morphine:
  - Adult, not pain controlled on regular weak opioids: 15–30mg 12-h morphine m/r
  - Very elderly and frail: 10mg 12-h morphine m/r
- Always prescribe a laxative concurrently
- Consider prescribing a regular antiemetic for those with a history of nausea/vomiting, e.g. haloperidol 1.5mg nocte: this can usually be stopped after a week. If not prescribed prophylactically, warn the patient to report any nausea so that an antiemetic can be prescribed as soon as possible
- Explain to patients that any drowsiness will usually wear off after a few days

---

7 Scottish Intercollegiate Guidelines Network (2000) *Control of pain in patients with cancer.* Edinburgh: SIGN.

- Advise patients not to drive, for at least one week after starting morphine, or after any increase in dose. Patients should continue to avoid driving even after this time of drowsiness persists

Titrating dose of morphine
- Increase the dose as needed by increments of 25–50 per cent rather than by a fixed amount. The increment percentage tends to decrease a little as the dose increases.
5–10–15–20–30–40–60–80–100–130–160–200mg. There is no pre-set maximum dose of opioids as long as increasing the dose gives further analgesia. Very few patients will require more than 600mg daily
- When pain is reasonably well controlled consider converting to modified release morphine 12-h for convenience of b.d. administration

Morphine preparations
Morphine (immediate release, 4-h)
- Mixture 10mg/5ml *(Oramorph/Sevredol)*
- Mixture 20mg/ml *(Oramorph concentrated/Sevredol concentrated)*
- Tabs. 10, 20, 50mg—scored Tabs. *(Sevredol)*

Morphine Unit Dose Vials
- Vials. 10, 30, 100mg all in individual 5ml vials *(Oramorph Unit Dose Vials)*

Morphine preparations, (modified release, 12-h)
MST and Zomorph can be used interchangeably.
MST Continus (Morphine m/r)
- Tabs. m/r 5, 10, 15, 30, 60, 100, 200mg
- Susp. 20, 30, 60, 100, 200mg
  Sachets to prepare Susp.

Zomorph caps. (Morphine m/r)
- caps. m/r 10, 30, 60, 100, 200mg
  Can be broken and administered via a **NG/PEG** tube, or sprinkled on food. Bioequivalent to *MST*

Morphine preparations—modified release (24-h)
MXL (Morphine m/r)
- caps. m/r 30, 60, 90, 120, 150, 200mg

Morcap m/r (Morphine m/r)
- caps. m/r 20, 50, 100mg
May not be bioequivalent to MST

Morphine preparations—rectal (4-h)
Morphine Supps.
- Supps. 10mg 15mg 20mg, 30mg
- Equianalgesic dose by oral and rectal routes

Converting to 12-h morphine
Divide daily morphine intake by half to give 12-h dose (e.g. morphine 10mg 4-h → 30mg morphine m/r 12-h).
  Ensure the patient has access to immediate release morphine for breakthrough pain. A dose of morphine of 50–100% of the 4-h dose equivalent may be taken for breakthrough pain.

Diamorphine

Diamorphine is more soluble in water than morphine, and is commonly used as the injectable strong opioid in a syringe driver for subcutaneous infusion.

To convert from oral morphine to SC diamorphine, divide the total dose of oral morphine by 3

e.g. 10mg 4-h morphine
$\cong$ 60mg oral morphine in 24h
$\cong$ 20mg diamorphine by CSCI over 24h
e.g. morphine 3mg p.o. $\cong$ Diamorphine 1mg by SC injection

Increments in dose should be between 25–50 per cent as for oral morphine. Additional SC doses for 'breakthrough' pain should be 50–100 per cent of the equivalent 4-h dose.

If vomiting or no longer able to swallow medication, convert to a subcutaneous infusion of diamorphine via a syringe driver by dividing the 24-h total dose of oral morphine by three.

Breakthrough doses

Use 50–100 per cent of the equivalent 4-h dose currently being used e.g.

A. for a patient on morphine m/r 270mg 12-h:
$\cong$ 540mg oral morphine in 24h
$\cong$ 90mg morphine p.o. 4-h
i.e. use breakthrough dose 45–90mg morphine p.o. 4-h p.r.n.

B. for a patient on 180mg diamorphine SC in 24h
$\cong$ 30mg diamorphine SC 4-h
i.e. use breakthrough dose of 15–30mg diamorphine SC 4-h

Intravenous use for pain emergencies

Various different protocols have been described for intravenous titration of opioids for severe pain 'emergencies'.

- monitor respiratory rate and conscious level regularly
- draw up diamorphine diluted to 10ml with water
  - If opioid naive dilute 5mg of diamorphine in 10ml of water
  - If on regular opioid use equivalent 4-h dose based on previous opioid use in last 24h (see 'Breakthrough doses' above) diluted in 10ml water
- give appropriate diamorphine dilution i/v at 1ml/minute (total over 10 minutes)
- stop if pain <5/10 or toxicity develops
- repeat the above after a further 10–20 minutes if required
- calculate the total dose of diamorphine administered and multiply by 6
- start maintenance infusion with CSCI, or regular oral morphine equivalent dose over 24h

NB It is unusual to give diamorphine intravenously in a hospice setting. Subcutaneous administration is most commonly used (takes 10 to 20 minutes to work) unless the pain is very severe and immediate relief is needed.

Diamorphine preparations
Inj. 5mg, 10mg, 30mg, 100mg, 500mg

Alternative strong opioids

A number of alternative strong opioid analgesics are available which have their place in palliative care:

Table 6a.2a Alternative strong opioids

Morphine and similar drugs	Morphine
	Diamorphine
	Hydromorphone
	Oxycodone
Fentanyl and similar drugs	Fentanyl
	Alfentanil
	Sufentanil
Methadone	Methadone
Intermediate weak–strong opioid	Tramadol
Other opioids occasionally used	Buprenorphine
Not recommended	Pethidine

Differences between these drugs are not fully understood, but include patient factors and drug factors. In clinical practice they may be divided into:

Morphine-like opioids

Oxycodone and hydromorphone, like morphine and diamorphine, are available in a wide range of doses in immediate (4-h) and modified release oral preparations. They can be used by CSCI.

Although there may be small intrinsic differences between the side-effect profiles of these drugs (e.g. oxycodone and hydromorphone may cause less toxicity than morphine in patients with renal failure, but neuroexcitatory side-effects are still reported), inter-individual variability seems to be a greater factor in determining the clinical picture. Substituting one opioid for another may reduce side-effects in up to 75 per cent of selected individuals.

Fentanyl and its analogues

Fentanyl and its analogues (alfentanil, sufentanil and remifentanil) are *selective* μ receptor agonists, unlike morphine. They may cause less sedation, cognitive impairment and constipation than morphine-like drugs in some patients. They are largely inactive orally because of high first-pass hepatic metabolism, but can be used by transdermal patch, oral lozenge (buccal absorption) or CSCI.

Fentanyl does not appear to accumulate and cause toxicity in renal failure.

Methadone

Methadone is an agonist at the μ- and δ-opioid receptors, and also an NMDA receptor antagonist and monoamine reuptake inhibitor. These actions make it a useful treatment for neuropathic and other pain states not fully responsive to morphine. However, it has a long and variable elimination half-life, making it difficult to use safely, and should be reserved for neuropathic, ischaemic or inflammatory pain, or use as a third- or fourth-line opioid.

Tramadol

Tramadol may be classed somewhere between the weak and strong opioids. It has additional pharmacological actions to its opioid effects. It is not classed as a 'controlled drug' which has some practical prescribing advantages.

Tramadol is a synthetic analogue of codeine that binds to μ-opioid receptors and also inhibits norepinephrine and serotonin reuptake. It is rapidly and extensively absorbed after oral doses and is metabolized in the liver. Analgesia begins within one hour and starts to peak in two h. In studies comparing equianalgesic doses of oral tramadol (up to 300 mg/day) and oral morphine for moderate cancer pain, constipation, nausea, neuropsychological symptoms, and pruritus were reported more frequently with morphine. Slow release formulations have also been shown to provide effective relief of moderate cancer pain.

Tramadol preparations

- caps. 50mg; Sachets effervescent powder 50mg; Sol. Tabs. 50mg
- Tabs. m/r (12-h) 75mg, 100mg, 150mg, 200mg
- caps. m/r (12-h) 50mg, 100mg, 150mg, 200mg
- Tabs. m/r (24-h) 150mg, 200mg, 300mg, 400mg

Starting dose: 50mg q.d.s. p.o. or 100mg b.d. p.o. (12-h m/r)
    Inj. 100mg/2ml

Buprenorphine

For many years palliative care physicians have been concerned about the use of buprenorphine because of potential problems encountered when patients taking regular morphine were given buprenorphine with consequent exacerbation of pain. Although buprenorphine is a very potent analgesic that strongly binds to opioid receptors displacing other opioids, it is a less effective analgesic.

The introduction of buprenorphine patches has caused such opinions to be revisited. Other opioids can be used in conjunction with buprenorphine patches if pain breaks through.

Side-effects of buprenorphine are similar to those of other strong opioids. Care needs to be taken with patients who are sweating heavily to ensure that the patch is sticking well to the skin.

- For opioid naïve patients the starting dose recommended by the manufacturers is 35mcg/h
- No more than two patches should ever be applied at the one time
- The maximum dose is 140 mcg/h
- The patch should be changed every three days

Buprenorphine preparations

- Patch strength 35, 52.5, 70 mcg/h

Applied every three days. Packs of 5 patches:

- Tabs. (sublingual) 200mcg

Other opioid analgesics

Pethidine has a short duration of action, and, when given regularly, active metabolites accumulate and can cause convulsions. It causes more dysphoria than morphine and is best avoided in palliative care.

Indications for starting with an opioid other than morphine:
- Patient choice
- Subacute/partial intestinal obstruction. A less constipating opioid such as fentanyl may be appropriate
- Patient reluctant to take 'morphine' despite appropriate counselling
- Patient reluctant to take oral medication regularly
- Renal failure

Indications for changing to alternative opioids

This practice is known as opioid rotation or opioid substitution.
- Patient choice
- Unacceptable side-effects with current opioid
- Renal failure
- Route of administration needs to be changed from oral as cannot swallow

Choice of alternative opioid

Rationale
- Hydromorphone, oxycodone and fentanyl are useful alternatives to morphine and diamorphine
- Methadone is difficult to use safely, and should be reserved for neuropathic, ischaemic or inflammatory pain, or used as third- or fourth-line opioid under specialist supervision
- Few strong opioids other than morphine have the range of doses and preparations needed to be suitable for routine use in cancer pain
- There is little to choose between oxycodone and hydromorphone, but oxycodone is chosen in preference because:
  - a liquid immediate release preparation is available
  - an injectable form is readily available in the UK
  - doses are simpler to calculate
  - there is less variation in the reported equianalgesic ratios
  - the manufacturer's recommended conversion of 7.5:1 for morphine to hydromorphone is higher than the more commonly used ratio of 5:1. This makes the tablet doses of 1.3mg even more complicated
- Fentanyl may cause less side-effects in some individuals (sedation, cognitive impairment, constipation, myoclonus and pruritus)
- Transdermal patch or CSCI are the only methods of administering fentanyl regularly for chronic pain as fentanyl has a short half life

Dose titration for unstable pain should not be attempted using a fentanyl patch

Oxycodone

Oxycodone is a strong opioid analgesic similar to morphine. It is available in 4-h immediate- release, and 12-h release preparations. It is a useful, though more expensive, alternative opioid in selected patients who develop side effects with morphine. The receptor affinity of oxycodone is not fully clear. It is partially metabolized to potent oxymorphone. Oxycodone is approximately 1.5–2 times as potent as morphine orally.

Side-effects

The side-effects are similar to morphine though vomiting, itch, and drowsiness may be less common in some individuals.[8]

Indications

Alternative opioid when morphine causes unacceptable side-effects.

Using oxycodone

Oxycodone should be used in the same way as morphine (remember to prescribe a laxative).

Comparison with morphine

In comparative studies with morphine, there are inconsistent reports of side-effect profiles. More vomiting has been reported with morphine, whereas constipation was more common with oxycodone. Other studies have shown no difference.

When selectively substituting morphine for oxycodone in patients with side-effects, improvements in almost all side-effects have been reported: less nausea, hallucinations, drowsiness, sweating and pruritus, but especially confusion/delirium. These reports do not necessarily reflect an overall difference between the drugs, but may reflect inter-individual variation.

Hepatic metabolism

Oxymorphone, a potent analgesic metabolite of oxycodone, is formed by the hepatic enzyme CYP2D6, which is under polymorphic genetic control. The rôle of oxymorphone in the analgesic effect of oxycodone is not yet clear. Oxycodone conversion to oxymorphone may be important for analgesic effect in some patients, and genetically 'poor-metabolizers' may not obtain the expected analgesia from oxycodone.

Synergy between opioids

In animal models, a combination of sub-analgesic doses of oxycodone and morphine showed synergy producing analgesia.

Oxycodone
- caps. 5mg, 10mg, 20mg (*OxyNorm*)
- caps. m/r (12-h) 10mg, 20mg, 40mg, 80mg (*OxyContin*)
- Liquid 5mg/5ml, 10mg/1ml

Manufacturers recommended conversion from oral morphine to oxycodone: divide morphine dose by 2.

- Injection: 10mg/ml 1ml and 2ml Amp

Manufacturers recommended conversion from oral oxycodone to subcutaneous oxycodone: divide dose by 2.

---

8 Heiskanen T, and Kalso E. (1997) Controlled-release oxycodone and morphine in cancer related pain. *Pain*, **73**: 37–45.

Hydromorphone

Hydromorphone is a strong opioid analgesic very similar to morphine, although it is a more selective μ-receptor agonist. It is used widely in North America as an alternative to diamorphine, which is not available. It is available in 4-h immediate release, and 12-h modified release preparations, but the injection is not routinely available in the UK.

It is a useful alternative opioid in selected patients who develop side effects with morphine. Hydromorphone has been used successfully and without toxicity in renal failure, but it has also been reported to cause neuro-excitatory effects in some patients (📖 see renal failure later).

Indications

- Alternative opioid if morphine causes unacceptable side-effects, especially—
  - Opioid-induced pruritus

Using hydromorphone

- Hydromorphone should be used in the same way as morphine (remember to prescribe a laxative)
- The capsules can be broken open and sprinkled on soft cold foods

Cough and dyspnoea

Information about the efficacy of alternative opioids for symptoms other than pain is limited. Hydromorphone may help cough and dyspnoea in lower doses than those used for analgesia.

Conversion ratios with other opioids

Conversion ratios between hydromorphone and other strong opioid analgesics seem more variable and uncertain than for other opioids, perhaps representing greater variability in metabolism and bioavailability (10–65 per cent) between individuals.

- When converting from oral morphine to oral hydromorphone, the manufacturers recommend a ratio of 7.5:1 (i.e. morphine 10mg ≈ hydromorphone 1.3mg)
- It is suggested that the lowest potency ratio is used for any conversion, with the expectation of titrating up the dose rapidly if needed

Side-effects

Hydromorphone and morphine generally have the same side-effects. Pruritus, nausea and vomiting, sedation and cognitive impairment, which may be less common with hydromorphone. There may also be individual variation in side-effect profile between patients.

Drug preparations-Hydromorphone

- caps. 1.3mg, 2.6mg (*Palladone*)
- caps. m/r (12-h) 2mg, 4mg, 8mg, 16mg, 24mg (*Palladone SR*)

Manufacturers recommended conversion from oral morphine: divide morphine dose by 7.5

- Inj. 10mg/1ml 20mg/1ml 50mg/1ml
  Injections available in UK as a special order from Martindale. See BNF for contact details.

Fentanyl

Fentanyl is a selective μ-receptor agonist (morphine acts on μ and κ receptors). It has been promoted as causing less constipation, sedation, and cognitive impairment than oral opioids. Fentanyl may be associated with a slightly higher incidence of nausea than morphine.

As it has inactive metabolites and is metabolized mainly in the liver, it is less likely to cause adverse effects in uraemic patients.

As it is more selective than morphine, fentanyl will not relieve pain that is resistant to morphine, but may help patients with morphine-responsive pain who develop intolerable side-effects to morphine.

Fentanyl is available as a transdermal patch, oral lozenge (buccal absorption), or can be given CSCI. CSCI is better than a patch for establishing effective blood levels rapidly, and should be used when speed is important, or when more flexibility is desired.

Converting a patient from morphine to fentanyl can lead to a modified withdrawal syndrome of shivering, diarrhoea, bowel cramps, sweating and restlessness, even though pain relief is maintained. These symptoms can be relieved with morphine given p.r.n. for a few days.

Fentanyl toxicity may be clinically more subtle than morphine toxicity and may present as vagueness, drowsiness or 'not feeling well'.

Indications

Alternative opioid when morphine causes unacceptable side-effects.
- Starting a strong opioid in a patient with:
  - a history of subacute bowel obstruction (less constipating than morphine)
  - renal failure (which can lead to myoclonus or confusion with morphine due to metabolite accumulation)
  - biliary colic/obstructed bile duct (see additional notes below)
- Patient acceptability/compliance

Transdermal fentanyl patch—only when pain is stable
- Start with 25mcg/h, or convert dose from morphine
- It takes 12–24h to achieve therapeutic blood levels, and approximately 72h to reach steady-state:
  - CSCI of fentanyl or alfentanil will achieve more rapid blood levels
- If converting from morphine, give last dose of 12-h modified release morphine when applying patch except when accumulation of opioids in renal failure has occurred
- If converting from morphine, remember the possibility of withdrawal symptoms and use immediate release morphine p.r.n. until symptoms settle
- Up to 25 per cent of patients need a patch change every 48h
- Use either oral morphine or oral transmucosal fentanyl for breakthrough pain
- Fever may increase drug absorption due to vasodilation
- Sweating may decrease drug absorption because it prevents the patch from sticking to the skin
- After removal of the patch, blood levels decrease by only 50 per cent in 18h

- Mild to moderate skin erythema or pruritus in the location of the patch have been reported in <5 per cent of patients

Fentanyl patches

Absorption rate from a fentanyl transdermal patch is roughly proportional to the surface area in contact with the skin. Various techniques have been used to allow only half of the area to contact with the skin—to approximate to a 12.5mcg/hour dose delivery. Tegaderm or Opsite dressings, with the fentanyl patch placed half on skin/half over the dressing, have been used, but note that these dressings are semipermeable. Others have folded the patch in half and covered with adhesive tape. *Although the delivered analgesic effect may theoretically be less, the side-effect profile does not alter. Neither method is recommended by the manufacturers.*

Some patients develop itching and irritation at the site of transdermal patches—reports suggest that spraying the skin with aerosol corticosteroid spray may be effective (use beclometasone dipropionate aerosol inhaler 50mcg/dose).

Subcutaneous fentanyl

- Calculate dose as equivalent to transdermal patch e.g. 25mcg/h = 600mcg/24h; for convenience (and considering the widely variable absorption from a patch) use 500mcg/24h CSCI as equivalent to a 25mcg/h patch
- Large volumes are needed for high doses: consider substituting alfentanil (see next section)
- Compatible with most commonly used drugs in palliative care

Oral transmucosal fentanyl citrate (OTFC)

Fentanyl lozenges (on a stick) are rapidly absorbed through the buccal mucosa, leading to onset of pain relief within 5–10 minutes. The maximum effect is reached within 20–40 minutes with a duration of action of 1–3h. Bioavailability is about 50 per cent. One comparative study suggests they may give better results than immediate release oral morphine.

Indication

Breakthrough pain in patients on regular strong opioid therapy.

Use

The optimal dose is determined by titration, and cannot be predicted by a patient's regular dose of opioid. Approximately 25 per cent of patients fail to obtain relief even at the highest dose, or have unacceptable adverse effects.

- Lozenge should be placed in the mouth and sucked, constantly moving it from one cheek to the other
- Should not be chewed
- Water can be used to moisten the mouth beforehand
- The lozenge should be consumed within 15min
- Partially consumed lozenges should be dissolved under hot running water, and the handle disposed out of reach of children

Dose titration
- Initial dose is 200mcg, regardless of dose of regular opioid. This dose is probably approx. equivalent to morphine 2mg i/v
- A second lozenge of the same strength can be used if pain is not relieved after 15 minutes
- No more than two lozenges should be used to treat any individual pain episode
- Continue with this dose for a further 2–3 episodes of breakthrough pain, allowing the second lozenge when necessary
- If pain still not controlled, increase to the next higher dose lozenge
- Continue to titrate in this manner until dose is found that provides adequate analgesia with minimum adverse effects
- No more than four doses per day should be used (regular strong opioid dose should be increased)

Inflammatory and neuropathic pain
A few observations suggest that fentanyl (and similar analogues) may be less effective than morphine for inflammatory or neuropathic pain. This may be explained by the additional effects of morphine (e.g. at kappa or delta receptors).

Dose equivalence
Manufacturer's recommended dose conversion from oral morphine to transdermal fentanyl patch is based on a ratio of 150:1 (i.e. 15 mg morphine p.o 4-h ≅ 25mcg/h patch). Manufacturers information sheets should be consulted.

Bile duct obstruction
Many opioid μ-receptor agonists, including morphine and diamorphine, have been shown to increase the common bile duct pressure. Fentanyl or sufentanil have no discernable effect on common bile duct diameter and may be preferable.

Topical use of fentanyl
Fentanyl has been used topically for painful skin ulcers.

Drug preparations-Fentanyl
- Patches 25, 50, 75, 100mcg/h (*Durogesic*)
  Starting dose: (25mcg/h) patch every 3 days
- Inj. 50mcg/1ml, 100mcg/2ml, 500mcg/10ml
  Starting dose: 500mcg/24h CSCI
- Lozenge with applicator 200, 400, 600, 800, 1200, 1600mcg (*Actiq*)
  Starting dose: 200mcg lozenge regardless of regular opioid dose

Alfentanil

Alfentanil is a selective μ-receptor opioid agonist, similar to fentanyl. It is mainly metabolized in the liver to inactive compounds. It has been given by CSCI in a syringe driver, and appears to mix with most other commonly used drugs in palliative care. It should be diluted with water.

Compared to fentanyl, an equianalgesic dose can be used in a much smaller volume, making CSCI of large doses possible. It is thus a useful substitute for fentanyl if CSCI use is desired.

Alfentanil is rapidly eliminated and elimination appears unaffected by renal failure. Its onset is more rapid than for fentanyl.

Its short-lasting effect means it has been used for incident pain (dressing change), but should not be used for breakthrough pain as it quickly wears off.

Drug preparations-Alfentanil
• Inj. 1mg/2ml, 5mg/10ml, 5mg/1ml

Starting dose: 500mcg/24hCSCI (equivalent to diamorphine 5mg CSCI)

Sufentanil

Sufentanil is a synthetic opioid very similar to fentanyl, but with more rapid onset and shorter duration of action. It can be used as an alternative to alfentanil if the fentanyl dose necessitates too large a volume for the portable syringe driver in use. It has also been used sublingually. The clinically-derived sufentanil to fentanyl relative potency is approximately 20:1.

Methadone

Methadone is a strong opioid analgesic, with several non-opioid actions. It differs from morphine/diamorphine in a number of ways:
- δ-opioid receptor agonist
- NMDA receptor antagonist
- serotonin re-uptake inhibitor
- long and variable elimination half-life
- potential for numerous and complex drug interactions
- inactive metabolites (lower toxicity in renal failure)

The first three of these actions may help account for reports of its effectiveness in managing neuropathic pain.

The pharmacology of methadone is complex and very variable, so it must be used with specialist supervision. The commonest mistake is to underestimate its duration of action, since up to 10 days may be required to reach steady state plasma levels. The greatest tendency to accumulate the drug is in the elderly or those with liver failure.

Drug interactions
Methadone metabolism is increased by a number of other drugs, which when started could cause opioid withdrawal symptoms. Other interactions which inhibit metabolism can lead to overdose and toxicity.

Table 6a.3 Interactions which interfere with methadone metabolism

Decrease methadone levels	Increase methadone levels
Phenytoin	Fluconazole
Phenobarbitalno	SSRIs
Carbamazepine (not sodium valproate or gabapentin)	
Rifampicin	

Subcutaneous methadone
Subcutaneous methadone has been used but there is a problem with skin reactions, partly because methadone in solution is acidic. If necessary to use, dilute as much as possible. In conversion of oral to subcutaneous or intravenous dosing, halve the dose of methadone.

Use of methadone
Indications
- Pain only partially responsive to morphine e.g. inflammatory, ischaemic or neuropathic pain
- Alternative opioid when side-effects develop with morphine (or other opioid)
- Renal failure
- Morphine tolerance—patients requiring ever increasing doses of morphine with no overall improvement in pain
- Use with special caution in the elderly, COPD or asthma

Guidelines for use
Note: Patients are rarely started on methadone for pain outside a specialist unit.

The efficacy of methadone in comparison with morphine increases with chronic dosing and with higher dose. This is in part due to a long elimination half-life, and in part due to its non-opioid action. Many studies have shown the difficulty in converting doses between opioids and methadone. Several guidelines have been published.

Morley and Makin guidelines are most commonly used in the UK, and are recommended for general use, and especially for patients switching opioid because of lack of effect.

Guidelines (Morley and Makin 1998 Pain Reviews)
- Stop all other opioids abruptly, i.e. do *not* reduce gradually
- Loading dose of methadone. 1/10 of the 24h p.o. morphine or equivalent up to a maximum of 30mg
- This same dose can be given as needed but not more frequently than 3-h
- On day six, add the total dose of methadone given in last 48h, divide by four, and give at 12-h intervals, with provision for a similar or smaller dose q3h as required
- Subsequent dose changes are by percentage increments as for morphine, every 4–6 days. [example 10mg b.d. → 15mg b.d.; 30mg b.d. → 40mg b.d.]
- Re-assess carefully as accumulation can occur up to 10 days after methadone begun or dose changed

Side-effects
All the typical opioid side-effects can be expected, although hallucinations and myoclonus are rare. Compared to morphine, methadone may cause less constipation, sedation and nausea. Methadone causes histamine release and can exacerbate asthma. It also has an antidiuretic effect.

Drug preparations-Methadone
- Mixture 10mg/ml
- Mixture 1mg/ml
- Tabs. 5mg; Linctus 2mg/5ml (for cough)

Topical opioids
Opioids can act peripherally as analgesics, and there are a number of reports of their use on ulcerated skin, relieving pain and possibly inflammation. Morphine and diamorphine have been used most commonly, but fentanyl has also been reported. There have been no reports of systemic toxicity, and standard doses have been used, regardless of doses of systemic opioids taken simultaneously.

Morphine or diamorphine 10mg may be mixed with sterile aqueous gel, a hydrocolloid gel (e.g. intrasite), or metronidazole gel, as appropriate. Apply once daily, and increase frequency if needed up to three times daily.

Summary

1 Subcutaneous diamorphine is 3 times as potent as oral morphine.
2 Subcutaneous oxycodone is twice as potent as oral oxycodone.
3 Transdermal Fentanyl patches deliver 25,50,75 or 100mcg/h over three days.

  Peak plasma concentrations are achieved after 12–24h and a depot remains in the skin for some 24h after the patch is removed.

  Breakthrough doses of opioid will be necessary during the first 24h of application. One in ten patients who have had their pain controlled by morphine may experience a withdrawal reaction when converted to fentanyl. They may require oral morphine on a p.r.n. basis to manage the withdrawal symptoms for a day or two.

  A reduction of laxative may be necessary when converting from morphine to fentanyl.

4 Transdermal Buprenorphine delivers 35, 52.5 and 70 mcg/h over three days. No more than 140 mcg/h (two patches) should be used. Opioids other than buprenorphine can be used for breakthrough pain.
5 Transdermal Fentanyl and Buprenorphine should only be used where opioid requirements are stable.
6 Oral Transmucosal Fentanyl Lozenges (OTFC). For breakthrough pain in patients already on regular strong opioid therapy for chronic pain. Start titration at lowest dose (200 mcg) regardless of background opioid dose.
7 Topical opioids have been mixed with both metronidazole and hydrocolloid gels for the pain of skin wounds.

Table 6a.4 Equivalent opioid doses for step two and step three of the analgesic ladder

Opioid	Oral medication					
	Step 2 mild to moderate pain	Step 3 moderate to severe pain				
Codeine	30–60mg q.d.s.	Not applicable				
Morphine i/r	2.5–5mg 4-h	10mg 4-h	20mg 4-h	30mg 4-h	40mg 4-h	60mg 4-h
Morphine m/r	5–15mg b.d.	30mg b.d.	60mg b.d.	90mg b.d.	120mg b.d.	180mg b.d.
Oxycodone i/r	1.5–3mg 4-6 h	5mg 4-h	10mg 4-h	15mg 4-h	20mg 4-h	30mg 4-h
Oxycodone m/r	5mg b.d.	10–20mg b.d.	30mg b.d.	40–50mg b.d.	60mg b.d.	90mg b.d.
Hydromorphone i/r	Not applicable	1.3mg 4-h	2.6mg 4-h	3.9mg 4-h	5.2mg 4-h	6.5mg 4-h
Hydromorphone m/r	Not applicable	4mg b.d.	8mg b.d.	12mg b.d.	16mg b.d.	20mg b.d.
Tramadol i/r	Not applicable	50mg 4h	Not applicable			
Tramadol m/r	50mg b.d.	100–150mg b.d.	Not applicable			
Approximate 24 h oral morphine	**10–30mg**	**60mg**	**120mg**	**180mg**	**240mg**	**360mg**

In all opioid conversions there is uncertainty. If is safer to err on the side of underestimating analgesic requirements when converting between opioids but ensure that the patient has ready access to appropriate breakthrough analgesia. If in doubt about a conversion seek specialist advice if you are unfamiliar with the particular opioid.

Table 6a.5 Equivalent opioid doses for step two and step three of the analgesic ladder

Opioid	Transdermal medication			
	Step 2 mild to moderate pain	Step 3 moderate to severe pain		
Fentanyl	Not applicable	25 mcg/h every three days	50 mcg/h ever three days	75 mcg/h every three days	100 mcg/h every three days
Buprenorphine	35 mcg/h every three days	52.5 mcg/h every three days	70 mcg/h every three days	2×70 mcg/h every three days	Not applicable
Approximate 24 h oral morphine	15mg	60mg	120mg	180mg	240mg	360mg

In all opioid conversions there is uncertainty. It is safer to err on the side of underestimating analgesic requirement when converting between opioids but ensure that the patient has ready access to appropriate breakthrough analgesia. If in doubt about a conversion always seek specialist advice if you are unfamiliar with the particular opioid.

Table 6a.6 Equivalent opioid doses for step two and step three of the analgesic ladder

Opioid	Subcutaneous medication					
	Step 2 mild to moderate pain	Step 3 moderate to severe pain				
Alfentanil CSCI (24h)	0.5–1mg 24h	2mg 24h	4mg 24h	6mg 24h	8mg 24h	12mg 24h
Diamorphine SC 24h p.r.n.		2.5–5mg 4-h	5–7.5mg 4-h	10mg 4-h	15mg 4-h	20mg 4-h
Diamorphine CSCI (24h)	5–10mg 24h	20mg 24h	40mg 24h	60mg	80mg	120mg
Morphine SC (4h p.r.n.)	2.5mg	5mg	10mg	15mg	20mg	30mg
Morphine CSCI (24h)	15mg	30mg	60mg	90mg	120mg	180mg
Oxycodone SC (4h p.r.n.)		2.5mg 4-h	5mg 4-h	7.5mg 4-h	10mg 4-h	15mg 4-h
*Oxycodone CSCI (24h)	5mg 24h	15–20mg 24h	30mg 24h	50mg 24h	60mg 24h	90mg 24h
Approximate 24 h oral morphine	**30mg**	**60mg**	**120mg**	**180mg**	**240mg**	**360mg**

In all opioid conversions there is uncertainty. It is a safer to err on the side of underestimating analgesic requirement when converting between opioid but ensure that the patient has ready access to appropriate breakthrough analgesia. If in doubt about a conversion seek specialist advice if you are unfamiliar with the particular opioid.

* The manufacturer of oxycodone states clearly that the conversion factor between oxycodone SC and diamorphine SC is 1:1. While most clinicians are comfortable with this ratio when converting from oxycodone SC to *diamorphine* SC, when converting from *diamorphine* SC to oxycodone SC some would advocate a 2:1 ratio with provision for breakthrough medication. As in every dose conversion the clinician must assess each individual patient and clinical situation.

Opioid side-effects and toxicity

> Thou hast the keys of Paradise,
> Oh just, subtle, and mighty opium!
>
> Thomas De Quincey 1785–1859: *Confessions of an English Opium Eater* (1822)

Patients should be warned of the possible side-effects of morphine such as nausea and drowsiness, which are usually short-lived, and are not often a problem. If drowsiness continues after a few days other possible causes, e.g. uraemia, hypercalcaemia or toxicity from other medication, should be excluded—otherwise seek advice. Constipation is predictable and most patients need prophylactic laxatives.

If unacceptable toxicity occurs, reduce morphine dose. The patient may need to miss several doses and restart at a lower dose.

Warning signs of morphine toxicity

- Drowsiness
- Hallucinations (auditory or visual)
- Confusion
- Vomiting
- Myoclonus
- Pin point pupils

Always ensure opioid doses are carefully titrated ('fine-tuned') to maximize analgesia and minimize side-effects.

Opioid toxicity may be increased by:

- dehydration or renal failure
- other change in disease status e.g. hepatic function, weight loss
- pain relieved by other methods
- co-administration of amitriptyline increases the bioavailability of morphine

General management

A number of different approaches may be used to manage persistent opioid-related side-effects:

- treat the side-effect
- use an alternative opioid
- use an alternative analgesic method, such as spinal opioids, which may cause less systemic or central side-effects

Drowsiness and cognitive impairment

Initial mild drowsiness on initiating opioid therapy will often abate over a few days as the body adjusts. It is often appropriate to continue opioids and wait for the drowsiness to wear off.

For persistent drowsiness or subtler cognitive impairment:

- Parenteral rehydration, if appropriate, may help neuropsychiatric toxicity (e.g. hallucinations, sedation, myoclonus)

- Alternative opioid
- Psychostimulants have been used to combat sedation in specialist units

Hallucinations or delirium
- Parenteral rehydration, if appropriate
- Alternative opioid
- Antipsychotic e.g. haloperidol 3–5mg nocte or by CSCI

Myoclonus
Consider renal failure—renal failure alone can cause myoclonus, but also causes opioid metabolites to accumulate, thereby increasing the risk of opioid toxicity. Myoclonus may be more likely in patients also taking anti-depressants , antipsychotics or NSAIDs. Consider the following:
- Parenteral rehydration, if appropriate
- Review other medication which may exacerbate myoclonus
- Alternative opioid
- Clonazepam 2–4mg/24h. Diazepam or midazolam are probably less effective than clonazepam but may be appropriate if sedation is also desirable
- Gabapentin 600–1200mg/24h in divided doses

Constipation
- Constipation can usually be treated acceptably with laxatives
- Fentanyl may cause less constipation than morphine

Increase in generalized pain
Hyperalgesia and allodynia have been reported with high dose opioids. It is usually associated with myoclonus, and an increase in the opioid dose may lead to worsening of the pain. Substitution of an alternative opioid often resolves the symptoms. Alternatively, reduction of dose and the addition of an alternative co-analgesic may be useful.

Nausea and vomiting
Initial nausea may wear off after a week and usually responds to:
- Haloperidol 1.5mg nocte
- Metoclopramide (for opioid-induced gastric stasis)
- Cyclizine or 5-HT$_3$ antagonists
- Alternative opioid

Sweating
- Alternative opioid
- Exclude other causes of sweating
- Antimuscarinic drugs

Pruritus (itching)
More common with spinal than with systemic opioids.
- Alternative opioid
- If unsuccessful, treat opioid induced pruritus with 5-HT$_3$ antagonists such as ondansetron

Respiratory depression/sedation

Reduction of the dose is usually all that is required immediately. Infusion by a syringe driver should be temporarily stopped to allow plasma levels to decrease, before restarting at a lower dose

Naloxone

- Naloxone is only indicated if significant respiratory depression is present; acute opioid withdrawal symptoms and pain can be severe in patients who have been on long-term opioids Naloxone has a half-life of 5–20 minutes. As the half-life of most opioids is longer than this, it is important to continue assessment of the patient and give naloxone at further intervals if necessary

Indications for naloxone:

- respiratory rate <8 breaths/min, or
- <10–12 breaths/min, difficult to rouse and clinically cyanosed, or
- <10–12 breaths/min, difficult to rouse and SaO_2 <90 per cent on pulse oximeter

Method of use of naloxone

- Dilute naloxone 0.4mg vial in 10ml 0.9% sodium chloride
- Use an i/v cannula or butterfly
- Administer 0.5ml i/v every 2 minutes until respiratory status satisfactory
- Repeat further doses as needed

Neuropathic pain

Neuropathic pain: Pain which is transmitted by a damaged nervous system, and which is usually only partially opioid sensitive.

Up to 40 per cent of cancer-related pain may have a neuropathic mechanism involved. Neuropathic pain may be difficult to control. A wide variety of treatments may be needed:

Management

Table 6a.7 Examples of treatments used for patients with neuropathic pain

Opioids	Ketamine
Antidepressants (tricyclic)	Spinal (epidural and intrathecal)
Anticonvulsants	Methadone
NSAID trial	Lidocaine patch/infusion
TENS Accupuncture	Neurolytic procedures e.g. coeliac plexus block, cordotomy
Radiotherapy	Capsaicin
Corticosteroids	

Remember that most cancer pains which seem to be predominantly neuropathic will also probably have a nociceptive *opioid responsive* element. i.e. try WHO analgesic ladder first.

Classes of drugs used in neuropathic pain

Opioid analgesics

Opioids may be effective in both cancer-related and non-malignant neuropathic pain. Opioids other than morphine/diamorphine have been shown to be effective including tramadol, fentanyl, and oxycodone.

Opioids are used in cancer-related neuropathic pain as:
- many patients will have a different, coexisting nociceptive pain
- there may be a nociceptive element to the pain
- opioids alone may control a third of neuropathic pains, and partially control a further third

If the pain seems to be resistant to first-line opioid (or opioid toxicity is a problem):
- an alternative opioid analgesic may be tried for better tolerance
- medication can be given to counteract side-effects (e.g. psychostimulants for drowsiness)
- the pain may be morphine-resistant

Methadone can be considered different from the other opioids with respect to neuropathic pain. It can either be tried as an alternative to a first-line opioid, or introduced later, when other options have failed which is more usual. See p. 196.

Tricyclic Antidepressants

The mechanism of analgesic action is principally by facilitation of descending inhibitory pain pathways.

e.g. amitriptyline 25–100mg

dosulepin 25–100mg

Note that amitriptyline can increase the bioavailability of morphine leading to opioid side-effects.

- Start with amitriptyline 25mg (10mg in the elderly) nocte
- If no response by day five, increase the dose (or, according to clinical circumstances, consider changing to anticonvulsant)
- Some patients do not see benefit until after 4–6 weeks of treatment, and/or doses of up to 50mg/day
  - severity of pain and the patient's prognosis will dictate how long to persevere with antidepressants
  - many patients do not tolerate amitriptyline especially in higher doses, therefore consider changing to dosulepin
- Use lofepramine for frail, elderly, or those already suffering antimuscarinic side-effects from other drugs:
  - start at 70mg nocte
  - may increase to 70mg b.d. on day 5–7

Lower doses of tricyclic antidepressants than those commonly required in depressive illness are reported to be effective in neuropathic pain, and faster responses are to be expected.[9] Other less sedating tricyclic antidepressants (e.g. imipramine) may be more useful for certain patients. Newer antidepressants are being used,[10] but their rôle is as yet unclear and there is growing concern about withdrawal reactions and cardiotoxicity, particularly with venlafaxine. Mirtazapine is a noradrenergic and specific serotonergic antidepressant (NaSSA); there are a few reports of its use in neuropathic pain. Topical tricyclics such as doxepin cream have also been tried.

Amitriptyline

- Tabs. 10mg, 25mg, 50mg
- Syrup 25mg/5ml, 50mg/5ml

Starting dose: 25mg nocte p.o.

Dosulepin

- caps. 25mg
- Tabs. 75mg (Prothiaden)

Starting dose: 25mg nocte p.o.

Lofepramine

- Tabs. 70mg
- Susp. 70mg/5ml

Starting dose: 70mg nocte p.o.

Doxepin

- Cream 5% 30g

Starting dose: Apply t.d.s to q.d.s., maximum 12g daily

9 McQuay H. J. (1996) A systematic review of antidepressants in neuropathic pain. *Pain* **68**: 217–27.

10 Pernia A., Mico J. A., Calderon E., Torres L. M. (2000) Venlafaxine for the treatment of neuropathic pain (letter). *Journal of Pain and Symptom Management*, **19**, **6**: 408–10.

Anticonvulsants[11]

e.g. sodium valproate   100–600mg b.d.
      gabapentin   100–600mg t.d.s.
      carbamazepine   100–400mg b.d.

Anticonvulsants have for a long time been considered better than tri-cyclic antidepressants for lancinating or paroxysmal pain, but evidence from studies does not support this.

There is little to choose overall between antidepressants and anticonvulsants for neuropathic pain in terms of efficacy or adverse effects.

There is little data to compare anticonvulsants in terms of efficacy, although in one trial comparing the efficacy of different anticonvulsants for lancinating pain, the results suggested that clonazepam was superior to phenytoin, sodium valproate and carbamazepine.[12]

- **Carbamazepine** has been used most extensively, but is often tolerated poorly by elderly, frail or ill patients. It has numerous drug interactions and tends to result in more side-effects, particularly when used in combination with other drugs. Doses should be built up slowly to minimize adverse effects
- **Sodium Valproate** has therefore been recommended by many in palliative care, but more data on its efficacy is needed
- **Clonazepam** has been used in cancer-related pain and has the advantage of subcutaneous administration
- **Lamotrigine** has had mixed results
- **Gabapentin** is the only drug licenced for all types of neuropathic pain. Trials have shown it to be effective in non-malignant and cancer-related pain. It appears to be well tolerated in palliative care patients. Doses up to 2.4g/24h have been used successfully
- Pregabalin has recently been introduced and is thought to work in a similar way to Gabapentin. It is unclear if patients who are unresponsive to Gabapentin may gain benefit from Pregabalin apart from its simpler dose regime (Pregabalin—for neuropathic pain November 2004, www.druginfozone.org)

Unlike the antidepressants, anticonvulsants are pharmacologically diverse in their actions, and there is good theoretical reason to try alternative anticonvulsants if one is ineffective.

All anticonvulsants are used in their typical 'anticonvulsant' doses.

- Start with gabapentin: day one—300mg nocte, day two—300mg b.d., day three—300mg t.d.s.
- If no response by day five, either increase dose in 300mg increments every few days (maximum 1800–2400mg/day), use an alternative anticonvulsant, or move on to another method:
- Some patients do not see full benefit from anticonvulsants until after 4–6 weeks of treatment
- The severity of pain and the patient's prognosis will dictate how long to persevere with gabapentin, or with anticonvulsants in general

11 McQuay H. J. (1995) Anticonvulsant drugs for management of pain: a systematic review. *BMJ*, **311**: 1047–52.

12 9. Swerdlow M., Cundill J. G. (1981) Anticonvulsant drugs used in the treatment of lancinating pain. A comparison. *Anaesthesia* **36, 12**: 1129–32.

Gabapentin
- caps. 100mg, 300mg, 400mg
- Tabs. 600mg 800mg

Starting dose; Day 1–300mg nocte, day 2–300mg b.d., day 3–300mg t.d.s. p.o.

Usual maintenance: 0.9–1.2g/24h. Maximum recommended dose 1.8g/24h, but doses up to 2.4g/24h (and even higher) have been used.

Sodium valproate
- Tabs. 200mg, 500mg
- Syrup 200mg/5ml

Starting dose; 200mg t.d.s. p.o. or 500mg nocte p.o.

Increase 200mg/day at 3-day intervals. Usual maintenance 1–2g/24h. Max. 2.5g/24h in divided doses. Supps. are available as special orders.

Carbamazepine
- Tabs. 100mg, 200mg, 400mg
- Liquid 100mg/5ml
- Supps. 125mg, 250mg

Starting dose; 100mg b.d. p.o.

Increase from initial dose by increments of 200mg every week. Usual maintenance dose 0.8–1.2 g/24h in two divided doses. Max. 1.6–2g/24h. Equivalent rectal dosage: 125mg PR $\cong$ 100mg p.o.

Carbamazepine levels are increased (risk of toxicity) by dextro-propoxyphene (co-proxamol), clarithromycin, erythromycin, fluoxetine, fluvoxamine.

Clonazepam
- Tabs. 500mcg, 2mg
- Inj. 1mg/1ml

Starting dose; 1mg nocte for 4 nights

Increase gradually to usual maintenance dose 4–8mg/24h. Oral solutions in various strengths are available from several sources.

Pregabalin
- Caps. 25mg, 50mg, 75mg, 100mg, 150mg, 200mg, 300mg

Starting dose; 75mg b.d.

Increase after three days to 150mg b.d.

Increase after seven days to 300mg b.d.

Corticosteroids

Corticosteroids (usually dexamethasone) may help cancer-related neuropathic pain, either by reducing inflammatory sensitisation of nerves, or by reducing oedema which may cause pressure on nerves. A high initial dose is used to achieve rapid results (dexamethasone 8mg/day will work in 1–3 days); the dose should then be rapidly reduced to the minimum that maintains benefit.

Although long-term corticosteroids may be best avoided, they can sometimes buy useful time whilst allowing other methods (e.g. radiotherapy or antidepressants) time to work.

- Hydrocortisone has a high mineralocorticoid effect
- Dexamethasone has a relatively high equivalent corticosteroid dose per tablet and less mineralocorticoid effects than prednisolone, or methylprednisolone with consequently less problems with fluid retention
- Prednisolone causes less proximal myopathy than dexamethasone.[13]
  If steroids are not helpful for pain within five days, consider stopping

Table 6a.8 Relative anti-inflammatory steroid doses (approximate)

Steroid	Administration	Equivalent dose
Dexamethasone	Oral/SC	2mg
Prednisolone	Oral/Rectal	15mg
Hydrocortisone	Oral/i/m/i/v	60mg
Methylprednisolone	Oral/i/m/i/v	12mg

NSAIDs

NSAIDs are sometimes effective in cancer-related neuropathic pain, either because there is mixed nociceptive pain or because they reduce inflammatory sensitization of nerves. NSAIDs exert an anti-inflammatory action by inhibiting prostaglandin synthesis.

There is considerable variation in individual patient tolerance and response. Pain relief starts soon but an anti-inflammatory effect may take a few weeks. The main differences between NSAIDs are in the incidence and type of side-effect, and efficacy should be weighed against the possible side-effects. NSAIDs vary in their selectivity for inhibiting different types of cyclo-oxygenase; selective inhibition of cyclo-oxygenase-2 (e.g. celecoxib) improves gastrointestinal tolerance but significant cardiac side-effects have created recent concerns and lead to the withdrawal of some preparations, most notably rofecoxib (vioxx). Ibuprofen has fewer side-effects than other non-selective NSAIDs.

e.g. ibuprofen 200–400mg t.d.s. p.o.
diclofenac 50mg t.d.s. (can be used p.o. SC or Supps.)
celecoxib up to 200mg b.d. p.o.
naproxen 250–500mg b.d. (p.o. or PR)
ketorolac 10–30mg SC every 4–6 h p.r.n. Max. 90mg daily (max. 60mg for elderly). Max. duration 2 days
parecoxib 40mg, then 20–40mg every 6–12 h p.r.n. Max. 80mg daily (max. 40mg for elderly).

13 Kingdon R. T. *et al.* (1998) *Handbook for pain management.* London: Saunders.

Elderly patients or those with a past history of peptic ulceration may be more at risk from side-effects. A proton pump inhibitor such as lansoprazole has been shown to reduce this risk.

Aspirin causes long acting inhibition of platelet coagulability and its unique cardiovascular protective effect makes joint prescribing of low dose aspirin and a non selective NSAID appropriate for patients in need of aspirin prophylaxis. However, the reduction in gastrointestinal side-effect risks gained by use of a selective COX2 inhibitor is obviated if given with low dose aspirin.

Risk factors for GI bleed with NSAID

- Age ≥ 75
- Corticosteroids
- Aspirin
- Anticoagulant
- Platelets $< 50 \times 10^9$/t
- Dyspepsia on NSAIDs now or in the past
- Peptic ulceration/ bleed in last year

Other drugs
Topical lidocaine (Lignocaine)
Topical lidocaine may be useful for superficial localized areas of pain such as fungating wounds for short periods of time.[14] A combination of lidocaine gel with diamorphine may also help pain. Prolonged use may lead to skin sensitization. A lidocaine 5 per cent patch has been shown to reduce pain and allodynia from post herpetic neuralgia. Up to three patches for periods of up to 24 h seems to be safe. An adequate trial over several weeks may be required. Mild to moderate skin redness, rash or irritation may occur. While the systemically absorbed dose from topical lidocaine will be small care should be exercised with patients susceptible to cardiac problems.

Oral flecainide and mexiletine
These medications should only be used **under specialist supervision and are rarely used in palliative care**.

Infusions of lidocaine (lignocaine) have been claimed as effective in neuropathic pain, and have been used long-term over many weeks.

As a continuous infusion is not always acceptable, oral drugs with similar sodium-channel blocking properties have been used (flecainide and mexiletine).

A positive response to lidocaine infusion may predict a response to mexiletine, and possibly therefore flecainide.

That neuropathic pain is particularly challenging to treat is illustrated by the very large number of strategies which have been tried to a greater or lesser extent.

- Hypomagnesaemia should be looked for and corrected
- Baclofen may specifically help paroxysmal pain; up to 60mg daily has been used
- Levomepromazine appears to have intrinsic analgesic activity. The sedative/anxiolytic effect may also benefit distressed patients
- Clonidine is used extensively in spinal infusions. Given by mouth, its tolerance is limited by hypotension and sedation. Doses of 25mcg t.d.s. increasing to 100 mcg t.d.s. have been used
- Capsaicin cream has proved useful in neuropathic pain, especially post herpetic neuralgia. The application of the cream can itself cause stinging which can be relieved by the use of Emla cream applied prior to the capsaicin. Capsaicin is a derivative of chilli pepper and must be applied with gloves five times a day. The pain may increase to start with but perseverance may provide relief. Studies suggest its mode of action is mediated by reducing the amount of substance P available for neurotransmission
- Cannabinoids may have a place in neuropathic pain, or pain associated with muscle spasm

Capsaicin
- Cream 0.075% 45g (Axsain)
Starting dose: Apply topically 3–4 times daily
Clonidine
- Tabs. 25mg. Tabs. 100mg, 300mg
- caps. m/r 250mg
Starting dose: Neuropathic pain 25mg t.d.s. p.o. increasing to 100 mg t.d.s.
Baclofen
- Tabs. 10mg; Liquid 5mg/5ml
Starting dose: 5mg t.d.s. p.o.

14 Back I. N., Finlay I. (1995) Analgesic effect of topical opioids on painful skin ulcers. *Journal of Pain and Symptom Management*, **10, 7**: 493.

N-methyl-D-aspartate (NMDA) receptors
The NMDA receptor is thought to be involved in the development of the 'wind-up' phenomenon of neuropathic pain. Ketamine and methadone are NMDA antagonists which may explain their efficacy in neuropathic pain.

The site of action of opioid analgesics is closely related to the NMDA receptor, and anecdotal reports suggest that opioid analgesics may be needed for NMDA receptor antagonists to work.

Wind up is the phenomenon of central sensitization when the experience of unchanged chronic pain stimulation worsens as nerve fibres become 'trained' to deliver pain signals better.

Ketamine
Ketamine is a dissociative anaesthetic with strong analgesic properties. Its analgesic effect may be partly due to NMDA receptor blocking and may be useful clinically in sub-anaesthetic doses for treating neuropathic, inflammatory or ischaemic pain. In higher doses approaching anaesthetic doses, it may be useful for treating terminal uncontrolled overwhelming pain.

It has been used byp.o., CSCI and i/v routes, and in a very wide range of doses.
- CSCI in doses of 50–360mg/24h ± a loading dose of 10mg SC
- p.o. starting doses between 2mg and 25mg t.d.s. have been used, and up to 50mg q.d.s. or 240mg/day
- i/v bolus doses of 0.1–0.5mg/kg (approx. 5–25mg)

Dysphoric effects including hallucinations are reported quite commonly in higher doses. They are more common in anxious patients, and small doses of benzodiazepines may help. Anaesthetic experience suggests pre-treatment may help reduce the incidence.

Neuropathic pain
Use oral route if possible:
- Diazepam 2mg p.o. 2 h before first dose then 2mg nocte for 3 days
- Start ketamine 10mg q.d.s. p.o.
- Increase by 10mg increments once or twice daily, up to 50mg q.d.s. as appropriate

If parenteral route appropriate:
- Ketamine 10mg SC stat. may be given if indicated for severe pain
- Start infusion of ketamine 50–100mg/24h CSCI
- Add midazolam 5mg/24h CSCI to reduce dysphoric effects, or higher dose if patient is very anxious
- Increase ketamine dose by 50–100mg increments as indicated to maximum 500mg/24h CSCI

Oral versus Parenteral doses
Ketamine is effective orally and in view of the wide dose ranges used, it is difficult to assess the potency ratio. It undergoes first-pass hepatic metabolism to an active metabolite, and one study suggests it may be more potent given orally than parenterally. In general, equivalent daily doses should initially be used when changing route.

Ketamine for procedures

Ketamine can be used as an analgesic to allow patients to be positioned for epidural or certain procedures (e.g. dressing changes). It carries a high incidence of dysphoric effects at these doses.

- Ketamine 0.5mg/kg by slow i/v injection (for 50kg man=25mg), or
- Ketamine 1.5mg/kg i/m (for 50kg man=75mg)
- Pre-treatment with a benzodiazepine to reduce the incidence of dysphoric effects:
  - midazolam 2.5mg SC given 30 min before, or
  - midazolam 1-3mg slow i/v immediately before
  (N.B. Anaesthetic dose for 50kg man is 50–150mg i/v over 1 min or 300–600mg i/m)

Terminal overwhelming pain

- Give ketamine 25–50mg slow i/v or SC for immediate effect if needed
- Midazolam 5mg SC stat
- Start ketamine 300–600mg/24h CSCI
- Add midazolam at least 20mg/24h to prevent hallucinations
- Increase ketamine to a maximum of 1,200mg/24h CSCI (up to 3.2g/24h have been given)

Methadone (📖 see p. 220)

Table 6a.9 Efficacy of drugs for neuropathic pain (NNT)[15]

	Diabetic neuropathy	**Postherpetic neuralgia**
Oxycodone	2.7	2.5
Tramadol	3.4	
Tricyclic antidepressants	2.4	2.3
SSRIs	6.7	
All antidepressants	3.4	2.1
Carbamazepine	3.3	
Gabapentin	3.7	3.2
All anticonvulsants	2.7	3.2
Mexiletine	10.0	
Baclofen	1.4	
Capsaicin	5.9	5.3

NNT is the number of patients who have to be treated for one to achieve the specified level of benefit, in this case benefit in terms of pain relief.

15 Sindrup S. H. and Jensen T. S. (1999) Efficacy of pharmacological treatments of neuropathic pain: an update and effect related to mechanism of drug action. *Pain*, **83**: 389–400.

Table 6a.10 Examples of treatments used for patients with neuropathic pain

Opioids	Ketamine
Antidepressants (tricyclic)	Spinal (epidural and intrathecal)
Anticonvulsants	Methadone
NSAID trial	Lidocaine patch/infusion
TENS Accupuncture	Neurolytic procedures e.g. coeliac plexus block, cordotomy
Radiotherapy	Capsaicin
Corticosteroids	

Treatment of other causes of poorly controlled pain

Malignant bone pain

- Radiotherapy—around 50 per cent will experience less pain within two weeks and 85 per cent within four weeks of treatment. In around 5 per cent a 'pain flare' is described with the pain worsening in the first few days after treatment before settling
- NSAID e.g. diclofenac 50mg t.d.s.
- Strong opioids (morphine)
- Corticosteroids
- Bisphosphonates

Bisphosphonates

Bisphosphonates have a rôle in a long-term strategy to reduce skeletal complications, including pain, from bone metastases of any origin (most data available for myeloma, breast and prostate cancer). Bisphosphonates may also have a rôle in the 'acute' management of metastatic bone pain. Patients may experience a 'flu-like reaction post treatment. Doses may need to be altered in renal failure.

Treatment

Bisphosphonates

- Analgesic effect should be expected within 14 days. Disodium pamidronate, sodium clodronate, and ibandronic acid need to be given every three to four weeks, but zoledronic acid has a longer duration of action (four to six weeks)
- It is not clear for how long bisphosphonates should be continued. The rôle of oral bisphosphonates has yet to be clarified in patients with metastatic bone disease

Treat

- Zoledronic acid 4mg i/v over 15 minutes. Calcium levels must be watched closely as hypocalcaemia may need treatment with calcium and vitamin D supplements
- Disodium pamidronate 90mg i/v infusion diluted to 500ml in sodium chloride 0.9 per cent (minimum 375ml), infuse over 2–4h
- Sodium clodronate i/v infusion 1500mg (can exceptionally be given SC)
- Ibandronic acid 6mg i/v every 3–4 weeks. (2–4mg for hypercalcaemia.)

Radiotherapy

- Radionuclides such as strontium are absorbed at areas of high bone turnover. They may take 12 weeks to have full effect and 80 per cent will experience pain relief. External beam hemi-body irradiation is an alternative for multiple-site bone pain

Surgery

- Surgical techniques. The pain of bone metastases may respond to local infiltration or intra-lesional injection with depot corticosteroid ± local anaesthetic. Consideration should be given to prophylactic pinning of osteolytic metastases in long bones. Vertebroplasty, in which injection of acrylic cement is administered percutaneously, into unstable fractures of the vertebrae may be worth considering if the patient is relatively well. Spinal or epidural anaesthetic blocks may also be needed

Bisphosphonates and bone pain

Disodium pamidronate
- Inj. 15mg, 30mg 90mg (dry powder for reconstitution)

Sodium clodronate
- Inj. 300mg/5ml 300mg/10ml

Starting dose: 800mg or 520mg b.d. p.o.

Zoledronic acid
- Inj. 4mg

Ibandronic acid
- Inj. 6mg
- p.o. 50mg daily

Treatment of poorly controlled pain

Pain	Possible co-analgesics
Headache due to cerebral oedema	dexamethasone
Painful wounds	metronidazole
Intestinal colic	hyoscine butylbromide or hydrobromide (Kwells)
Gastric mucosa	lansoprazole
Gastric distension	asilone + domperidone
Skeletal muscle spasm	baclofen/diazepam
Cardiac pain	nitrates/nifedipine
Oesphageal spasm	nitrates/nifedipine

Renal impairment/renal failure[16,17]

Palliative care teams may be involved in the care of patients with different degrees of renal failure. Many drugs and their metabolites accumulate in uraemic patients and cause significant side-effects.

Degree of Renal Impairment

	GFR	Serum Creatinine
Mild	20–50ml/min	150–300 mmol/l
Moderate	10–20ml/min	300–700 mmol/l
Severe	<10ml/min	>700 mmol/l

Drugs in renal failure
- Metabolites of morphine accumulate in renal failure and can cause neurotoxic side-effects such as myoclonus and confusion
- Oxycodone and hydromorphone have active metabolites which are renally excreted, and their value in renal failure is less clear. However, case reports suggest they *may* be better than morphine, at least in individual patients switched from morphine because of problems with metabolite accumulation. In health, there is a large reserve of renal function, urea and creatinine remaining at normal values until there is a reduction of 50–60 per cent in glomerular filtration rate
- Paracetamol is safe in renal failure but should be reduced to 3g every 24 h if the patient has severe renal impairment. Paracetamol is dialysed out by haemodialysis but not by peritoneal dialysis

Factors associated with altered handling of drugs in renal failure

- Loss of plasma protein binding capacity occurs due to uraemia itself, which may be relevant for drugs which are highly protein-bound such as diazepam
- Changes in hydration may affect the distribution of drugs in the body causing overdosage
- Oral absorption of drugs may be reduced because of vomiting, diarrhoea and gastrointestinal oedema
- Increased permeability of the blood brain barrier in uraemia may exaggerate the unwanted central nervous system effects associated with certain drugs

- Codeine and Dihydrocodeine can both cause prolonged narcosis but can be used if necessary in a combined preparation with paracetamol (e.g.co-codamol/co-dydramol) in reduced doses. There is an increase in the CNS side effects of weak opioids in renal failure
- Co-proxamol should be used with caution in patients with severe renal impairment
- Diamorphine is metabolized to morphine which is itself metabolized to morphine-3-glucuronide (M3G) and morphine-6-glucuronide (M6G). Accumulation of M3G may cause clinical excitation or agitation

16 Kirkham S. R., Pugh R. (1995) Opioid analgesia in uraemic patients. *Lancet*, **345**, 8958: 1185.

17 Farrell A., Rich A. (2000) Analgesic use in patients with renal failure. *Eur J Pall Care*, **7, 6**: 201-5.

Accumulation of M6G, the useful analgesic metabolite, may account for symptoms of drowsiness, nausea and vomiting, respiratory depression and even coma. Haemodialysis may produce significant falls in morphine concentration leading to pain during or shortly after dialysis. The complex nature of opioid usage in renal failure requires that, particularly in the opioid naïve, very small doses are used and then only with the ready availability of naloxone. For similar reasons the use of long-acting preparations should be avoided. Opioids which do not have active metabolites may be more suitable for patients in renal failure than morphine or diamorphine. (Alfenanil or fentanyl.)

- Fentanyl is mainly metabolized in the liver to inactive metabolites and it has a short half-life, making it a useful drug in renal impairment
- Alfentanil is a short acting opioid metabolized by the liver to inactive compounds. It is 10 times more potent than diamorphine when given subcutaneously and there are some case studies showing less agitation when changed from diamorphine
- Twenty per cent of methadone is excreted unchanged in urine. With its long half-life the dose should be reduced in renal impairment.
- Hydromorphone has been used in patients with renal failure even though it is metabolized to a metabolite which can potentially accumulate causing neuroexcitatation and cognitive impairment
- Oxycodone is 90 per cent metabolized in the liver. In severe renal impairment, it is contra-indicated because the 10 per cent which is normally excreted unchanged in the urine, may then accumulate. For patients with mild or moderate renal failure, oxycodone can be used with caution, so long as the dose is titrated up slowly
- NSAIDS should be avoided, if possible, in patients with any degree of renal impairment, though this counsel of perfection may not necessarily be appropriate in the palliative care setting. Where appropriate, sulindac is the NSAID of choice as it is reported to have renal sparing effects. These effects are lost with doses above 100mg twice daily. In patients with total renal failure on dialysis NSAIDs should not be forgotten if kidney protection is no longer an issue.

Table 6a.11 Commonly used palliative care medication in different degrees of renal failure

Drug	Mild Creat. 150–300mmol/l GFR 20–50ml/min	Moderate Creat. 300–700mmol/l GFR 20–50ml/min	Severe Creat. >700mmol/l GFR <10ml/min
Analgesics			
Paracetamol	ND	ND	500mg–1g every 8 h
NSAIDs	Avoid if possible	Avoid if possible	Avoid
Weak opioids			
Co-codamol,	ND	6 Tabs. in 24h	4 Tabs. in 24h
Co-dydramol	ND	6 Tabs. in 24h	4 Tabs. in 24h
Co-proxamol	ND		
Tramadol	ND	50–100mg every 12h	50mg every 12h
Strong opioids			
Morphine	75% of ND	2.5–5mg every 6–8 h**	1.25–2.5 every 6–8 h*
Oxycodone	Start at a low dose and titrate slowly	Avoid	
Diamorphine	75% of ND**	2.5mg SC every 6 h**	2.5mg SC every 8 h*
Hydromorphone	ND**	1.3mg every 6–8 h**	1.3mg every 8 h*
Methadone	ND**	ND**	50% of ND
Fentanyl	ND**	75% of ND**	50% of ND
Alfentanil	ND**	ND**	ND**

Antiemetics			
Metoclopramide	ND	75% of ND	50% of ND
Haloperidol	ND but avoid repeated dosing as haloperidol may then accumulate.		
Cyclizine	ND	ND	ND
Levomepromazine	ND	ND	ND
Domperidone	ND	ND	ND
Ondansetron	ND	ND	ND
Anticholinergics			
Hyoscine butylbromide	ND	ND	ND
Hyoscine hydrobromide	ND	ND	ND
Central nervous system			
Baclofen	Max. 5mg o.d.	Max. 5mg o.d.	Max. 5mg o.d.
Benzodiazepines	Start with very small doses. Increased cerebral sensitivity		
Gabapentin	300mg b.d.	300mg o.d.	
Amitriptyline	ND	ND	ND
Fluoxetine	ND	ND	ND on alternate days
Citalopram	ND	ND	No information available
Mirtazepine	ND	15mg o.d.	15mg
Paroxetine	ND	20mg o.d.	20mg o.d.

**Titrate

ND normal dose

From: Bunn R., Ashley C. (1999) *The Renal Drug Handbook*. Oxford: Radcliffe Medical Press

With thanks to the Renal Pharmacists at the Belfast City Hospital Pharmacy Department.

Anaesthetic procedures in palliative care

Presently she cast a drug into the wine of which they drank, to lull all pain and anger and bring forgetfulness of every sorrow

Homer's Odyssey

Introduction

The majority of patients with cancer can have their pain needs met by following the WHO three-step analgesic ladder. For the minority of patients who do not gain satisfactory pain relief, a 'fourth step' (interventional pain management) can be useful in helping to control pain, maintain psychomotor performance and improve quality of life.

As with all interventions, patient selection is vital for success. General selection criteria include:

- Patient competent/consented
- Patient compliant
- Absence of systemic infection
- Absence of specific allergy
- Absence of significant coagulopathy
- Adequate support for post-procedural care and maintenance

Patients with palliative care needs are often debilitated, have limited mobility and have a limited life span. It is therefore imperative that measures to alleviate their pain are minimally disruptive. Many spinal procedures can easily be done at the bedside, while more involved interventions such as chemical neurolysis necessitate radiological guidance, usually in a hospital setting. With this in mind, patients should be selected for procedures acceptable to them and appropriate to their level of disability.

Intrathecal and epidural (neuraxial) techniques

Direct delivery of opioids to the spinal cord via epidural and intrathecal techniques has become increasingly popular in recent decades, and has proven an effective and reversible way to provide profound analgesia with reduced systemic side-effects. Intrathecal opioids bind to the mu and kappa opioid receptors in the substantia gelatinosa of the spinal cord. This is achieved to a lesser extent with epidural opioids, which exert a simultaneous systemic and intrathecal effect (10 per cent and 90 per cent respectively).

Common indications for the use of neuraxial techniques:

- Unacceptable side-effects despite successful analgesia with systemic opioids
- Unsuccessful analgesia despite escalating doses and use of sequential opioids
- Intolerable neuropathic pain which may be amenable to spinal adjuvants
- Sympathetically mediated pain amenable to sympathetic blockade
- Incident pain which may benefit from numbness (local anaesthetic)

Possible contra-indications to neuraxial techniques (risk-benefit decision):
- Platelet count of $<20 \times 10^9/l$ with clinical symptoms of poor clotting
- Full anti-coagulation or INR>1.5
- Active infection with concurrent septicaemia
- Concurrent chemotherapy likely to cause neutropenia
- Occlusion of epidural space by tumour at the site of catheter tip placement (epidural catheters only)
- Allergy or unmanageable side-effects from anticipated treatment
- Psychosocial issues that make technique untenable
- Inadequate professional support to resolve ongoing problems

There is a growing body of evidence favouring intrathecal over epidural administration of opioids in the palliative setting.

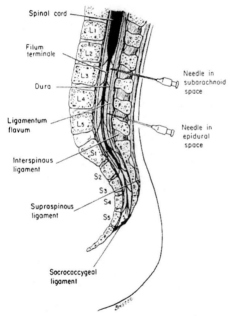

Fig. 6a.5 Schematic diagram of lumbosacral anatomy showing needle placement for lumbar subarachnoid, and epidural spaces.

Table 6a.12 Comparing the two routes of administration

Factors	Intrathecal	Epidural
Infection rate	Same as epidural	Same as intrathecal
Pain relief	Better for long-term	Good only for short-term
Dose	Lower (10–20% of epidural dose)	Higher
Pump refills	Less frequent	More frequent (higher volumes)
Side-effects	Fewer	More
Technical difficulty	Easier to place, less likely to become displaced	Potentially more difficult, and catheter may migrate
Long-term complications	Less (approx. 5%)	More (approx. 55%)
Catheter occlusion and fibrosis	Minimal	Higher frequency (leading to loss of analgesia/pain on injection)
Epidural metastases	Less affected	More affected (may compromise drug delivery)
Overall advantage	Effective analgesia with fewer complications	

Catheters may be externalized through the skin at the puncture site or may be tunnelled subcutaneously away from the spine. Alternatively, a totally implantable pump system may be employed if the patient has a life expectancy of several months.

Table 6a.13 Comparison of continuous versus bolus techniques

Factor	Continuous	Intermittent bolus
Dose escalation	Higher	Lower
Analgesic quality	Better	Fair
Local anaesthetic combinations	Minimal motor or haemodynamic complications	Higher risk of motor or haemodynamic complications (Not recommended for intraspinal administration)

Ideally, the continuous infusion technique should be used, with a familiar delivery system e.g. standard Graseby syringe pump delivering the infusion solution over 24 h.

Technical complications of neuraxial catheters

1 Mechanical problems
2 Skin breakdown at insertion site
3 Infection-local/catheter infection/epidural abscess/meningitis/systemic infection
4 CSF leak, causing headache
5 CSF seroma
6 Haematoma
7 Catheter dislodgement, occlusion or migration
8 Nerve damage (rare but possible).

Adverse effects attributable to spinal opioids

1 Minor sedation (opioid dose excessive)
2 Urinary retention (commonest in males in first 24 h)
3 Persistent nausea
4 Pruritus
5 Respiratory depression (may be severe and insidious if opioid-naïve)
6 Hyperalgesia (at higher doses)
7 Myoclonus (higher doses, indicating toxicity)
8 Constipation.

Management of adverse affects

1 Sedation: reduce dose of opioid
2 Urinary retention: usually requires once-only catheterization
3 Nausea: regular antiemetic
4 Pruritus:
   • consider adding spinal bupivacaine
   • i/v ondansetron 8mg has been shown to be effective
   • i/v nalbuphine may be effective
5 Respiratory depression: (R.R. less than 8/minute or excessive drowsiness)
   • naloxone 100–400mcg
   • stop intrathecal infusion
   • reduce infusion dose
6 Hyperalgesia:
   • reduce opioid dose
   • consider addition of adjuvant agent
7 Myoclonus:
   • reduce opioid dose
   • check renal function
   • encourage rehydration
   • Consider low dose benzodiazepine therapy (myoclonus may not be opioid dose-dependent)
8 Constipation: regular laxatives from the outset of therapy.

Choice of drug: Opioids, local anaesthetics, clonidine

Opioids

Morphine is one of the least lipid soluble opioids available, and when given in the spinal space, it has the slowest rate of uptake into the surrounding vasculature, which gives it a longer and primarily spinal site of action. Intrathecal morphine is regarded as 100 times more potent than a systemically given dose. Data from postoperative pain studies suggest that morphine is twice as potent as diamorphine by the intrathecal route. Intrathecal morphine should be preservative free.

Diamorphine can be administered intrathecally, with a potency ratio of 1:100 (intrathecal:systemic). Diamorphine should be reconstituted in sodium chloride 0.9 per cent. Alternatives to morphine and diamorphine are used less frequently. **Hydromorphone** is an effective and affordable option for the morphine-intolerant patient. The potency of intrathecal hydromorphone is five times that of morphine. Of the lipophilic drugs, both **fentanyl** and **sufentanil** are used. Greater lipid solubility may be an advantage for rapid onset of action, but rapid systemic absorption means shorter duration of action with less dose-sparing effect when compared to systemic administration. There is no published data on dose equivalences.

Typical dosing schedule

- If opioid-naïve, start with intrathecal diamorphine 0.5–1mg/24h or epidural diamorphine 2.5–5mg/24h
- If the patient is established on a systemic opioid, the following regimen may be used to minimize the withdrawal phenomenon during route conversion
  - Give half of the systemic opioid by the established route
  - Convert the remaining half dose to equivalent dose of diamorphine, and then divide by 100 to get the intrathecal dose
- Add 2ml of 0.5 per cent bupivacaine to diamorphine
- Add sodium chloride 0.9% up to total of 10ml
- Infuse solution over 24 h
- After 24 h, reduce the systemic dose by 50 per cent again and titrate upwards the intrathecal dose (usually in increments of 10–30 per cent)
- Attempt to discontinue the systemic opioid by day two (may not always be possible)

Local anaesthetics

Local anaesthetic agents are sodium channel blockers and are unique in their ability to block nerve impulses conducted proximally (pain relief) and impulses conducted distally (motor blockade). The conduction blockade produced is both painless and reversible.

Side-effects of local anaesthetics

- Postural or overt hypotension—sympathetic block
- Numbness—sensory block
- Leg weakness—motor block
- Altered proprioception in low doses, even when motor weakness is not apparent
- Urinary retention
- 'Total spinal'—this potentially catastrophic event can occur if a large dose of local anaesthetic is delivered to the subarachnoid space

erroneously. A profound drop in blood pressure is accompanied by motor paralysis of the lower limbs, spreading to the upper limbs and respiratory muscles and ultimately the brain. Both cardiovascular and ventilatory support are required until the local anaesthetic effects wear off

Table 6a.14 The most frequently used local anaesthetic agents

Agent	Lidocaine	Bupivacaine	Ropivacaine
Onset	Rapid	Slower	Similar to bupivacaine
Duration	Short (h)	2–3 times longer than lidocaine	Slightly longer than bupivacaine
Typical dosage	2ml 2% over 24 h	2ml 0.5% over 24 h	2ml 0.75% over 24 h
Advantages	Rapid onset and offset Synergism with opioids	Synergism with opioids	May preferentially block sensory nerves Two-thirds as potent as bupivacaine Synergism with opioids

Spinal adjuvants
Clonidine
Clonidine is an α-2adrenergic agonist and appears to act at the level of the spinal cord. It acts synergistically with opioids but is also a powerful analgesic when used alone in the management of neuropathic pain. It is a lipophilic compound and its spinal effect may be more pronounced with intrathecal rather than epidural administration. The dose of clonidine is often limited by the appearance of side-effects such as sedation, hypotension and bradycardia. Nausea, pruritus and urinary retention have also been reported. Starting doses range from 10–20mcg/24h and should be titrated for analgesic effect and minimal side-effects. Doses above 150 mcg/24h should not be necessary.

Other analgesics have been tried as intrathecal agents, including midazolam, ketamine, octreotide, calcium channel blockers and neostigmine. As yet, there is no convincing body of evidence to support their use.

Guidelines for percutaneous intrathecal catheter insertion
- Patient consent
- Nurse assistant present
- Adequate space for aseptic trolley
- Patient in sitting or lateral position, with their head and knees curled toward their abdomen
- Skin asepsis (eg. chlorhexidine)
- Local anaesthetic infiltration of skin at chosen level of insertion
- 18G Tuohy needle inserted into spinal space, piercing the dura, until CSF is free-flowing
- Aseptic epidural catheter inserted to 15cm, and free-flow of CSF confirmed
- Catheter secured and dressing applied to insertion site (one which allows daily visual inspection)

- An antibacterial filter should be connected and may remain attached for up to a month
- Connection made to infusion pump or syringe driver

Follow-up care
- All staff involved in aftercare of the patient should be familiar with the possible side-effects and complications listed, and should be vigilant for signs of infection or problems developing
- The catheter insertion site should be inspected on a daily basis
- A pain chart should be kept initially until the analgesia is considered sufficient
- If the patient is being discharged to the community, there should be liaison with the key members of the primary care team (GP, district nurse and community specialist palliative care nurse) prior to discharge and written guidelines should accompany the patient home
- Patients should not be discharged home until dose escalation have been stabilized

Chemical neurolysis for cancer pain

Neurolysis of nerves by chemical means is indicated for patients with limited life expectancy. The use of neurolytic techniques has diminished over recent years due to advancements in spinal analgesia and increased life expectancies in cancer patients. However, neurolysis should be considered in the following circumstances:
- the pain is severe, intractable and has failed to respond to other measures
- the nociceptive pathway is readily identified and related to a peripheral nerve pathway or sympathetic chain
- a trial block of local anaesthetic has been successful
- the effects of the local anaesthetic block are acceptable to the patient

The goals of neurolysis include reduction in pain, and reduction in the need for other pharmacotherapy. Neurolysis is rarely permanent and pain returns as a consequence of regrowth of neural structures or disease progression in the treated area. When used centrally, there is a risk of motor paralysis and sphincter weakness, which are generally unacceptable to most patients. For that reason, patients should be fully consented by the practitioner prior to the procedure.

Neurolytic agents
Alcohol and phenol are the two most commonly used agents.
Effects of alcohol:
- Burning sensation upon injection along the distribution of the nerve, followed by warm numbness
- Pain relief increases over a few days and is maximal by one week
- Alcohol is hypobaric, hence the patient should be able to tolerate a position that allows the alcohol solution to float upwards to the affected nerve root

Effects of phenol:
- Following injection, an initial local anaesthetic effect subsides to neurolysis which may take 3–7 days to become apparent
- Density and duration of block is felt to be less than that of alcohol
- Since phenol is hyperbaric, the patient should be able to tolerate a position that allows the phenol to sink down to the nerve roots

Visceral cancer pain is often produced by a combination of visceral afferent stimulation, as well as somatic and neuropathic elements. The sympathetic chain carries much nociceptive information, and blockade of the sympathetic chain may improve both visceral and sympathetically-mediated pain. Visceral cancer pain can often be alleviated by a combination of oral medication and neurolytic blockade of the sympathetic axis. Since neurolytic techniques have a narrow risk/benefit ratio, they should only be performed by experienced pain clinicians in appropriate surroundings.

Coeliac plexus block

The coeliac plexus is responsible for transmission of nociceptive information from the entire abdominal contents, excluding the descending colon and pelvic structures. It has been successfully used to combat pain from pancreatic cancer and other upper abdominal viscera. For an experienced operator it is a relatively safe and simple technique, performed under CT guidance. Patients referred for this procedure should be able to tolerate lying on an X-ray table, and should have no coagulopathy or local infection.

Possible complications include:
- Orthostatic hypotension (may persist for days)
- Backache at the site of needle insertion (if backache and hypotension persist, observe serial haematocrit measurements to rule out retroperitoneal haemorrhage haematoma)
- Diarrhoea
- Abdominal aortic dissection
- Paraplegia and motor paralysis (rare)

Superior hypogastric block

The superior hypogastric sympathetic ganglion transmits nociceptive information from the pelvis, excluding the distal Fallopian tubes and ovaries. It has been successfully used to manage pain of pelvic origin, other than ovarian pain. Neurological complications have not been reported with this block.

Ganglion of impar block

This ganglion marks the end of the sympathetic chains and is situated at the sacrococcygeal junction. Visceral pain in the perineal area has been successfully treated with neurolytic blockage of this ganglion. These patients often present with a vague, poorly localized perineal pain, accompanied by burning or urgency, and oral medication alone is often inadequate. No complications have been reported with this block.

Other neurolytic blocks
Pleural phenol block

Insertion of an epidural catheter into the pleural space and infusion of local anaesthetic or phenol has been described in the management of visceral pain associated with oesophageal cancer and rib invasion by bony metastases.

It is a relatively simple technique with few complications. These include:
- Pneumothorax (avoid bilateral blocks)
- Phrenic nerve palsy
- Trauma to local structures caused by the needle, catheter or as a consequence of the phenol injection

(a)

(b)

Fig. 6a.6 (a) Positioning for coeliac plexus block; (b) Deep anatomy showing placement of needles for coeliac placement block

Saddle block
This is a modified low spinal technique where phenol is injected into the CSF in the lumbar area, with the intention of causing chemical neurolysis of the low sacral nerve roots that serve the perineum and perianal area. It is useful for patients complaining of pain in the 'saddle' area, but carries the potential risk of sphincter compromise (<10 per cent).

Fig. 6a.7 Technique of intra-pleural block

Further reading

Borgeat A., Stirnemann H. R. (1999) Ondansetron is effective to treat spinal or epidural morphine-induced pruritus. *Anesthesiology*, **90**: 432–6.

Buchheit T., Rauck R. (1999) Subarachnoid techniques for cancer pain therapy: When, Why and How? *Current Pain and Headache Reports*, **3, 3**: 198–205.

Cohen S. E., Ratner E. F., Kreitzman T. R. et al. (1992) Nalbuphine is better than naloxone for treatment of side effects after epidural morphine. *Anesth Analg*, **75**: 747–52.

de Leon-Casasola O. (2000) Critical evaluation of chemical neurolysis of the sympathetic axis for cancer pain. *Cancer Control*, **7, 2**: 142–8.

Hill D. A. (2003) Peripheral nerve blocks: practical aspects. In H. Breivik et al. (eds.) *Clinical Pain Management, Practical Applications and Procedures*, pp. 197–232. London: Arnold.

Lema M. J., Myers D. P., de Leon-Casasola. (1992) Interpleural phenol therapy for the treatment of chronic oesophageal cancer pain. *Rge Anesth*, **17**: 166–70.

Mercadante S. (1999) Neuraxial techniques for cancer pain: an opinion about unresolved therapeutic dilemmas (review). *Regional Anesthesia and Pain Medicine*, **24, 1**: 74–83.

Miguel R. (2000) Interventional Treatment of Cancer Pain: the fourth step in the World Health Organization analgesic ladder? *Cancer Control*, **7, 2**: 149–56.

Schnitzer T. J., Burmester G. R., Mysler E. et al. (2004) Comparison of lumiracoxib with naproxen and ibuprofin in the Therapeutic Arthritis Research and Gastrointestinal Event Trial (TARGET), reduction in ulcer complications. *Lancet*, **364**: 665–74.

Simpson K. H., Russon L. (2000) The use of intrathecal drug delivery systems in pain management. *CME Bulletin Palliative Medicine*, **2**: 17–20.

Twycross R. et al. (2003) Itch. *QJM*, **96**: 7–26.

Zeppetella G. et al. (2004) Topical opioids for painful skin ulcers—do they work? *European Journal of Palliative Care*, **11**: 93–6.

Other non-pharmacological pain interventions

A range of techniques and expertise exists complementing the pharmacological and interventional approaches, which have dominated this module thus far.

These techniques are not just an adjunct to medication but point to the centrality of holistic patient-centred care. Not all approaches will be appropriate for every patient, but for some traditional medicine has little to offer either.

Table 6a.16 Complementary therapies and other non-pharmacological interventions

Complementary therapies	Other non-pharmacological interventions
Acupuncture	Positioning
Reflexology	Catheterization
Aromatherapy	Reassurance
Art therapy	Good communication
Music therapy	Diversional therapy
Touch therapy	TENS
	Splinting of a fractured limb
	Psychological support

📖 See also Chapter 11.

Pain and difficulties in communication

High prevalence of pain in the elderly population is a recognized reality. Almost half of those who die from cancer are over 75 years old. One study showed that 40–80 per cent of elderly in institutions are in pain. There is evidence that many patients suffering from some form of dementia receive no pain relief at all, despite the presence of a concomitant, potentially painful illness.

The reason for this lies in the difficulty in assessing those with communication difficulties. Additionally, the elderly often minimize their pain making it even more difficult to evaluate. The patient's unusual behaviour and its return to normal with adequate analgesia, may be the only indication of pain.

There have been various attempts to evaluate pain in such circumstances. The DOLOPLUS[19] was developed in 1993. It is based on observations of the behaviour of patients in ten different situations that could be associated with pain. The pain is classified into somatic, psychomotor and psychosocial aspects and scores are allocated. A collective score level confirms the presence of pain.

19 (2001) Lefebvre-Chapiro, S. and the DOLOPLUS group. (2001) The DOLOPLUS 2 scale-evaluating pain in the elderly. *European Journal of Palliative Care*, **8**, 5: 191–4

Examples of unusual behaviour indicating pain[20]

Verbal expression e.g.
- crying when touched
- shouting
- becoming very quiet
- swearing
- grunting
- talking without making sense

Facial expression e.g.
- grimacing/wincing
- closing eyes
- worried expression

Behavioural expression e.g.
- jumping on touch
- hand pointing to body area
- increasing confusion
- rocking/shaking
- not eating
- staying in bed/chair
- withdrawn/no expression
- grumpy mood

Physical expression e.g.
- cold
- pale
- clammmy
- change in colour
- change in vital signs if acute pain (e.g. BP, pulse)

Further reading

Back I. N., Finlay I. (1995) Analgesic effect of topical opioids on painful skin ulcers. *J Pain Symptom Manage*,**10, 7**: 493.

Flock P., Gibbs L., Sykes N. (2000) Diamorphine-metronidazole gel effective for treatment of painful infected leg ulcers. *J Pain Symptom Manage*, **20, 6**: 396–7.

Scottish Intercollegiate Guidelines Network (2000). *Control of pain in patients with cancer.* Edinburgh: SIGN.

Ventafridda V., Ripamonti C., De Conno F., Bianchi M., Pazuconi F., Panerai A. E. (1987) Antidepressants increase the bioavailability of morphine in cancer patients (letter). *Lancet* i: 1204.

20 Galloway S. and Turner, L. (1999) Pain assessment in older adults who are cognitively impaired. *Journal of Gerontological Nursing* **25**, 37: 34–9.

Gastrointestinal symptoms

Roast Beef, Medium, is not only a food. It is a philosophy.

Edna Ferber, *Roast Beef, Medium*, 1911

A sizeable proportion of palliative care is concerned with the management of gastrointestinal symptoms. Traditionally such symptoms have received less attention than pain management, yet the same principles apply.

Patients with pain usually show a response or a lack of response to treatment within hours. Patients with gastrointestinal symptoms may take several days to respond to interventions, and the temptation is thus to have a more lax attitude to monitoring gastrointestinal problems. In reality the doctor and nurse need to be much more attentive to these problems which deceptively cause great patient morbidity, yet may not become obvious until major management difficulties arise.

Example

Every time a patient is prescribed a strong opioid for the first time: Waiting to see if the patient will become nauseated or constipated will lead to major problems. The patient may become so sick that they refuse all morphine again. The patient may become severely constipated with serious and unpleasant consequences.

- The patient and family may lose trust in the healthcare professional. Such trust is one of the strongest tools in helping patients and it may be difficult to repair if it is shaken so fundamentally

Therefore

- Every time a strong opioid is prescribed for the first time, or the dose of a strong opioid is markedly increased, always prescribe or increase the dose of a laxative
- Antiemetics should be prescribed for the first five to ten days of a strong opioid being started or a higher dose being initiated, but after five days can, and should be, stopped as nausea due to the opioid side-effects may wear off. In practice, if patients have tolerated analgesics on step two of the analgesic ladder, they will probably not need antiemetics when changing to strong opioids

Anticipation of problems before they occur.
Ongoing assessment of treatments and their effectiveness.
Appropriate prescribing of background medication as well as medication for 'breakthrough' symptoms

Oral problems

Oral problems may affect up to 60 per cent of patients with cancer and can impact greatly on quality of life, both physically and psychologically.

Pathology and physiology

A healthy mouth is moist, clean and pain-free with an intact mucosa. Saliva is a major protector of the tissues of the mouth.

About 1500mL of saliva are produced daily by the parotid, submaxillary, sublingual and several minor salivary glands.

Saliva is composed of a serous part (alpha amylase), which initiates starch digestion, and a mucus component which acts as a lubricant. It also contains calcium, phosphate and bicarbonate which help maintain healthy teeth and other components such as mucin which protects oral tissue from chemical and mechanical trauma and infections.

The majority of oral problems seen in palliative care are related to a reduction in saliva secretion, although poor oral hygiene is also a major factor. Candidiasis and dry mouth (xerostomia) are two of the most common problems. Other problems include pain, stomatitis, mucositis, ulceration, halitosis, altered taste and hypersalivation (drooling).

During cytotoxic therapy the cells of the oral mucosa are vulnerable due to their high proliferation rate. Other treatment complications may arise due to direct stomatotoxicity or indirectly due to myelosuppressive effects. Risk factors for oral problems in patients with advanced cancer:

- Reduced oral intake
- Debility (reduced ability to perform own oral hygiene)
- Dry mouth (often aggravated by medicines, mouth breathing, oxygen therapy)
- Dehydration
- Local irradiation
- Chemotherapy
- Local tumour

General mouth care

The aim of good mouth care is to prevent problems before they arise and to control unpleasant symptoms.

Assessment:

- Assess daily for symptoms or signs of problems such as altered taste, oral pain, dry mouth, halitosis, ulcers, oral or pharyngeal candidiasis or dental problems
- Regular examination of lips, tongue, teeth and oral mucosa
- Involve local dental team if necessary
- Assess patient's ability to carry out mouth care effectively
- Encourage good oral hygiene for general well being

*An oral assessment tool may be useful. Eilers *et al.*'s oral assessment guide has been found to be appropriate for use in patients with advanced cancer.[1]

1 Eilers J., Berger A., Petersen M. (1998) Development, testing and application of the Oral Assessment Guide. *Oncol Nurse Forum*, **15**: 325–30.

Management

Basic oral care—by staff or patient if able.

- Keep mouth moist—encourage regular sips of fluids/oral rinsing
- Brush teeth with toothpaste or clean dentures regularly, especially after meals
- Rinse mouth thoroughly and frequently with sodium chloride 0.9 per cent (helps removal of oral debris and is soothing and non-traumatic[2])
- Gently clean coated tongue with a soft toothbrush or sponge
- Apply moisturizing cream or white soft paraffin (petroleum jelly) to lips
- Soak dentures overnight in cleansing solution

If the patient is unconscious or too unwell to carry out oral hygiene, instruct and involve family in this important area of care.

Management of oral problems[2, 3, 4]

Coated tongue/dirty mouth

In addition to basic oral care, if no candidiasis:

- Use mouthwashes to remove debris e.g. cool water or sodium chloride 0.9 per cent
- Gentle brushing with soft toothbrush or sponge
- Pineapple (fresh or tinned) to chew—contains proteolytic enzyme ananase which cleans the mouth
- Effervescent vitamin C has been used for furred tongue—place ¼ of 1g effervescent tablet on tongue and allow to dissolve; repeat up to q.d.s. for up to one week

Dry mouth (xerostomia)

Xerostomia is the subjective feeling of a dry mouth and is often associated with difficulties with speech, chewing or swallowing, the need to keep drinking and loss of taste. This is a common problem in advanced cancer and appropriate management may involve the use of both saliva stimulants and substitutes.

Causes:

- Drugs e.g. antimuscarinics, antidepressants, opioids, diuretics
- Candidiasis
- Dehydration
- Anxiety
- Mouth breathing
- Radiotherapy
- Oxygen therapy (non-humidified)

2 Miller M., Kearney N. (2001) Oral care for patients with cancer: a review of the literature. *Cancer Nursing*, **24, 4**: 241–54.

3 Twycross R. (2001) *Symptom Management in Advanced Cancer*, 3rd edn. Oxford: Radcliffe Medical Press.

4 Sweeney M. P., Bagg J., Baxter W. P., Aitchison T. C. (1997) Clinical trial of a mucin-containing oral spray for treatment of xerostomia in hospice patients. *Palliative Medicine*, **11**: 225–32.

Management
- Treat underlying cause if possible e.g. infection, dehydration
- Review medication
- Basic oral care regimen (see the previous page)
- General measures (little scientific rationale[2]):
  - sipping semi-frozen drinks
  - sucking ice-chips
  - chewing pineapple pieces
  - sugar-free chewing gum
  - petroleum jelly applied to lips
  - oral sprays may be beneficial[5]

Consider saliva substitutes, especially pre-meals:
- Saliva orthana (NB pork mucin-based spray—may be no more beneficial than placebo)
- OralBalance gel
- Methylcellulose solution e.g. Glandosane spray
- Saliva stimulation
  - Pilocarpine—a parasympathomimetic agent which stimulates salivary gland secretion. (It should be avoided in bowel obstruction, glaucoma, asthma, COPD and cardiac disease)
  - Dose: Pilocarpine 5mg tablets p.o. t.d.s. Sweating is a common side-effect
  - Pilocarpine 4 per cent eye-drop solution has been used in raspberry syrup or peppermint water (2–3 drops taken orally t.d.s.—unlicensed use[6])
  - Bethanechol starting with 10mg t.d.s. with meals and increase if necessary

Painful mouth and stomatitis
Stomatitis refers to painful, inflammatory and ulcerative conditions affecting the mucous membranes lining the mouth and may be caused by:
- Infection
- Ulceration
- Mucositis post radiotherapy or chemotherapy
- Iron deficiency (angular stomatitis and glossitis)
- Vitamin C deficiency (gingivitis and bleeding)
- Dry mouth

Other causes of oral pain include:
- Tumour infiltration
- Dental problems

Management
Non-drug treatment
- Treat underlying cause if possible e.g. infection
- Good oral hygiene
- Avoid foods that trigger pain e.g. acidic foods
- Avoid tobacco and alcohol
- ENT/Oncology review

5 Sweeney M. P., Bagg J., Baxter W. P., Aitchison T. C. (1997) Clinical trial of a mucin-containing oral spray for treatment of xerostomia in hospice patients. *Palliative Medicine*, **11**: 225–32.

6 Back I. N. (2001) *Palliative Medicine Handbook*, 3rd edn. Cardiff: BPM Books.

Drug treatment

Generalized oral pain

- Systemic analgesic:
- Analgesic mouthwash e.g. benzydamine hydrochloride (difflam) 10mL q.d.s. (dilute 1:1 if stings)
- Chlorhexidine 0.2 per cent (Corsodyl)—rinse mouth with 10mL for 1 minute b.d.
- Sucralfate Susp. 10 mL as mouthwash 4-h
- Soluble aspirin 300—600mg q.d.s. (if no contra-indications)
- Cocaine mouthwash 2 per cent is used for mucositis in some centres

Some claim there is no evidence that benzydamine, sucralfate or chlorhexidine ease oral pain.[7]

Localized oral pain

- Topical analgesia e.g.
  - Choline salicylate oral gel (Bonjela/Teegel)—apply q.d.s.
  - Carmellose paste (orabase)—protective oral paste—apply p.r.n.
  - Lidocaine spray, gel or cream (beware pharyngeal anaesthesia and risk of aspiration)
- Systemic analgesics
  - NSAIDs e.g. diclofenac (if no contradictions)
  - Opioids—consider starting or increasing systemic opioids and monitor response
  - Consider ketamine for persistent oral neuropathic pain

Ulceration of oral mucosa

Causes include trauma (chemical or physical), recurrent aphthae, infections, cancer, nutritional deficiencies, haematinic deficiency (iron, folate, B_{12}) and drug therapy.

Management: Identify and treat cause where possible.

- Consider referral for further investigation if mouth ulcer persists
- Pain relief—as for Stomatitis

Aphthous ulcers

- Topical corticosteroids for five days e.g. Adcortyl in Orabase (triamcinolone 0.1 per cent paste) applied twice daily or Corlan lozenges (hydrocortisone) 1 q.d.s. p.o. to ulcerated area
- Tetracycline mouthwash (for resistant ulcers). Caps. 250mg—dissolve contents in water and hold in mouth for 2–3 minutes twice daily for three days. Avoid swallowing. May stain teeth[7]
- Persistent and severe ulcers may respond to thalidomide (seek specialist advice)

Infection

- Fungal—candidiasis is most common in patients with cancer
- Viral—e.g. herpes simplex
- Bacterial—e.g. coliforms or staphylococci

Predisposing factors:

- Reduced salivary flow

7 Regnard C., Hockley J. (2004) *A Guide to Symptom Relief in Palliative Care*. 5th edition. Oxford: Radcliffe Medical Press.

- Immunosuppressants
- Chemotherapy
- Antibiotics
- Poor nutritional state
- Diabetes
- Wearing dentures
- Poor oral hygiene

Candidiasis

Present in up to 80 per cent of patients.[8] (Present in normal oral flora of 50 per cent general population.) May be asymptomatic.

Presenting features may include:
- Dry mouth
- Loss of taste
- Smooth red tongue
- Adherent white plaques on tongue or mucous membranes
- Soreness
- Dysphagia (remember oropharyngeal/oesophageal candidiasis)
- Angular cheilitis

Investigation

In palliative care swabs are not routinely taken, although it may be useful since fungal infections may become resistant to standard treatment.

Treatment

- Specific treatments should be accompanied by good oral hygiene
- There is no clear evidence to suggest superiority of the various antifungal agents in this patient population
- Remember to treat dentures—soak in Nystatin or dilute Milton overnight
- Topical:
  - Nystatin Susp. 100,000 U/mL or Nystatin pastilles 100,000 U
  - Dose: 2–5mL q.d.s. p.o. or 1 pastille q.d.s. p.o. for at least five days (reduced activity if nystatin combined with chlorhexidine mouthwash)
  - Miconazole oral gel 25mg/mL, apply q.d.s. p.o.
  - Amphotericin lozenges 10mg, dose: 1 lozenge q.d.s.
- Systemic:
  - Ketoconazole Tabs./Susp., Dose: 200mg o.d. p.o. (watch liver function)
  - Fluconazole Tabs./Susp., Dose: 50mg o.d. p.o. for seven days

Recurrent candidiasis in patients with AIDS may require prophylactic treatment with fluconazole 50mg daily. Concern is arising that 'azole' (i.e. fluconazole) resistance may become a clinical problem in palliative care.[9]

Herpes simplex infection may require oral Aciclovir 200mg 4-h for one week.

NOTE: Systemic antifungal drugs may interact with several drugs metabolized by the cytochrome P450 enzymes including phenytoin, warfarin, sulphonylureas and midazolam. It is always best to check for possible interactions when co-prescribing.

8 Back I. N. (2001) *Palliative Medicine Handbook*, 3rd edn. Cardiff: BPM books.

9 Davies A., Brailsford S., Broadley K., Beighton D. (2002) Resistance amongst yeasts isolated from the oral cavities of patients with advanced cancer. *Palliat Med*, **16**: 527–31.

Bacterial infection

Malignant ulcers or local tumour may be associated with halitosis due to anaerobic bacteria.

Treatment

- Metronidazole 400mg t.d.s. p.o. or 500mg b.d. PR × 5 days
- May be used as mouthwash if adverse effects. Metronidazole Susp. 400mg (10 mL) t.d.s. and spit out[8]

Drooling

May be due to overproduction of saliva (sialorrhoea) or inability to swallow normal amounts of saliva. Drooling is common in MND (40 per cent) but uncommon in advanced cancer (except head and neck).

Causes

- Neuromuscular:
  - MND
  - CVA
  - Cerebral palsy
  - Carcinoma of pharynx
  - Parkinson's disease
  - Brain tumours
- Oral factors:
  - Ill-fitting dentures
  - Deformity post surgery e.g. oral surgery
  - Dysphagia
- Drugs:
  - Cholinesterase inhibitors
  - Cholinergic agents
  - Lithium

Management

- Non-drug treatment:
  - Head positioning
  - Suctioning
- Drug treatment:
  - Antimuscarinic drugs (if patient is able to swallow) will reduce saliva production
  - Most patients will not be able to swallow tablets or capsules, or large volumes, and a number will have PEG tube feeding
  - Drugs that do not cross the blood-brain barrier minimise the risk of sedation and other central side-effects; however they may also be poorly and unpredictably absorbed when given orally
  - Other drugs with antimuscarinic effects will reduce saliva production, e.g. amitriptyline p.o. 25mg nocte or propantheline 15mg t.d.s., but use is often limited by side-effects
  - Choice will depend on local availability and patient's circumstances

Table 6b.1 Drug treatment

Given by injection	
Glycopyrronium 0.1–0.4mg/24h CSCI	Ideal drug, but requires regular or continuous injection. Most reliable way of establishing effective symptom control rapidly.
Glycopyrronium 25–100mcg b.d. SC increased as needed	
Transdermal patch	
Hyoscine hydrobromide transdermal patch	Central side-effects can occur, especially in the elderly.
Given orally/PEG/sublingual	
Glycopyrronium p.o. 0.6–2mg up to t.d.s.	Solution for injection can be used but may need 3–10mL. Powder for oral solution requires pharmacy to prepare, is not routinely available, and is expensive. Titration to effective dose may take longer.
Atropine eye drops 1% 2 drops p.o./sublingual q.d.s.	Cheapest; least published experience. Central side-effects may occur, but less than hyoscine hydrobromide.

Further reading

Books

Back I. N. (2001) *Palliative Medicine Handbook*, 3rd ed. Cardiff: BPM Books.

Doyle D., Hanks G. W. C., Cherny N. (eds) (2004) *Oxford Textbook of Palliative Medicine*, 3rd edn. Oxford: Oxford University Press.

Regnard C., Hockley J. (2004) *A Guide to Symptom Relief in Palliative Care*. 5th edn. Oxford: Radcliffe Medical Press.

Twycross R. (2001) *Symptom Management in Advanced Cancer*, 3rd edn. Oxford: Radcliffe Medical Press.

Twycross R., et al. (2002) *Palliative Care Formulary*. 2nd edn. Oxford: Radcliffe Medical Press.

Articles

Davies A., Brailsford S., Broadley K., Beighton D. (2002) Resistance amongst yeasts isolated from the oral cavities of patients with advanced cancer. *Palliat Med*, **16**: 527–31.

Eilers J., Berger A., Petersen M. (1988) Development, testing and application of the Oral Assessment Guide. *Oncol. Nursing Forum*, **15**: 325–30.

Regnard C. (1994) Single dose fluconazole versus five-day ketoconazole in oral candidosis. *Palliat Med*, **8**: 72–3.

Sweeney M. P., Bagg J., Baxter W. P., Aitchison T. C. (1997) Clinical trial of a mucin-containing oral spray for treatment of xerostomia in hospice patients. *Palliative Medicine*, **11**: 225–32.

Reviews

Miller M. Kearney N. (2001) Oral care for patients with cancer: a review of the literature. *Cancer Nursing*, **24**, **4**: 241–54.

Nausea and vomiting

Last night we went to a Chinese dinner at six and a French dinner at nine, and I can feel the sharks' fins navigating unhappily in the Burgundy.

Peter Flemming, Letter from Yunnanfu, 20 March 1938

Nausea is an unpleasant feeling of the need to vomit often accompanied by autonomic symptoms.

Vomiting is the forceful expulsion of gastric contents through the mouth.[10]

Nausea and vomiting are symptoms which can cause patients, and their relatives, deep distress. Of the two, nausea causes most misery; many patients can tolerate one or two episodes of vomiting a day while prolonged nausea is profoundly debilitating. Causes of nausea are multiple and it is important to try to analyse the likely cause so that appropriate therapy can be initiated.

Evaluation
- Distinguish between vomiting, expectoration and regurgitation
- Separately assess nausea and vomiting
- Enquire if nausea is absent for prolonged periods after vomiting or is persistent
- Review drug regimen
- If there is a likelihood of cerebral secondaries, check fundi for papilloedema (although its absence does not exclude raised intracranial pressure)
- Examine the abdomen
- Do a rectal examination if faecal impaction is a possibility
- Consider checking plasma concentrations of: creatinine, calcium, albumin, and digoxin
- Consider radiological investigations if major doubt remains about cause
- Note the content of the vomitus e.g. undigested food, bile, faeculent
- Timing of onset of nausea or vomiting
- Associated symptoms (e.g. the headaches of raised intracranial pressure are coincidental with vomiting)

Causes
Common causes of nausea and vomiting in advanced cancer include:
- Gastrointestinal, e.g. gastric stasis, intestinal obstruction
- Drugs, e.g. opioids, antibiotics, NSAIDs, iron, digoxin
- Metabolic, e.g. hypercalcaemia, renal failure
- Toxic, e.g. radiotherapy, chemotherapy, infection, paraneoplastic
- Brain metastases
- Psychosomatic factors, e.g. anxiety, fear
- Pain

Treat reversible causes
- Severe pain
- Infection
- Cough
- Hypercalcaemia
- Tense ascites

- Raised intracranial pressure (using corticosteroids)
- Emetogenic drugs—stop or reduce dose
- Anxiety—pharmacological and psychological management

Opioid-induced nausea and vomiting

Opioids can cause nausea and vomiting through a number of different possible mechanisms. These include stimulation of the chemoreceptor trigger zone, increased vestibular sensitivity, gastric stasis or impaired intestinal motility and constipation.

Haloperidol is usually recommended as first-line for opioid-induced nausea and vomiting, however metoclopramide (for gastric stasis), cyclizine or hyoscine hydrobromide may all be effective in certain patients. 5-HT$_3$ antagonists have also been shown to be useful but are expensive for long term use.

Non-pharmacological management of nausea and vomiting

- Control of malodour from colostomy, fungating tumour or decubitus ulcer
- A calm, reassuring environment away from the sight and smell of food
- Avoid exposure to foods which precipitate nausea which may mean transferring the patient to a single room
- Small snacks, e.g. a few mouthfuls, and not large meals
- If the patient is the household cook, someone else may need to take on this rôle
- Use of acupressure wrist bands, Sea Bands—These devices are helpful to some patients, particularly those who prefer non-pharmacology treatments

Drug management of nausea and vomiting

There are many neurotransmitter receptors involved in nausea and vomiting. These include those for histamine, acetylcholine, 5-hydroxytryptamine and dopamine located in varying concentrations largely in the vomiting centre and the chemoreceptor trigger zone in the mid brain.

In simple terms, neural impulses from a variety of emetic stimuli are relayed to these sites in the brain stem, triggering the vomiting reflex. A single antiemetic may be adequate to suppress symptoms, but if there are different causes for the vomiting in the same patient, it may be necessary to combine drugs. For instance, if the cause of vomiting is thought to be raised intracranial pressure and uraemia, it may be necessary to combine e.g. cyclizine and haloperidol.

Levomepromazine antagonises several receptors and may thus be a useful single alternative at a dose of 6.25mg o.d. or b.d. orally, doses higher than this causing sedation.

It may be possible to control nausea with oral medication, but persistent vomiting requires drug delivery by an alternative route such as per rectum or, more reliably, subcutaneously by means of stat doses or continuously via a syringe driver.

10 Twycross R. (2001) *Symptom Management in Advanced Cancer*, 3rd edn. Oxford: Radcliffe Medical Press.

Side-effects

All antiemetics have side-effects with which it is necessary to be familiar.

It is very easy to overlook minor extrapyramidal effects of the dopamine antagonists which thus adds to a patient's distress. For instance, haloperidol and metoclopramide may cause restlessness and inability to keep still (akathisia). More marked signs include Parkinsonian effects such as stiffness and tremor. The effect can be reversed by stopping the drug. If necessary a small dose of an antimuscarinic drug, such as procyclidine, can be given. Domperidone is an alternative to metoclopramide since extrapyramidal problems are less.

Cyclizine and the phenothiazines (e.g. levomepromazine) are associated with anticholinergic side-effects such as dry mouth, blurring of vision and urinary retention.

5-HT$_3$ antagonists cause constipation.

Table 6b.2

Cause of vomiting	Choice of antiemetic drug
Drug or toxin induced	Haloperidol 1.5mg nocte/b.d. Levomepromazine 6.25mg (a quarter tablet). 6mg Tabs. available soon
Radiotherapy	Granisetron 1mg stat then 1mg b.d. Haloperidol 1.5–3mg nocte/b.d.
Chemotherapy	Granisetron 1mg stat then 1mg b.d. Dexamethasone 4–8mg o.d. (often as part of a chemotherapy regime) Metoclopramide 20mg q.d.s.
Metabolic e.g. hypercalcaemia	Haloperidol 1.5mg nocte/b.d. Levomepromazine 6.25mg nocte
Raised intracranial pressure	Cyclizine 50mg t.d.s./ or 150mg /24h SC. Dexamethasone 4–16mg o.m.
Bowel obstruction[11]	Cyclizine 150mg/24h p.o. or SC Hyoscine butylbromide 40–100mg/24h SC Octreotide 300–1000mcg/24h SC Ondansetron 8–24mg/24h p.o., i/v or SC
Delayed gastric emptying	Metoclopramide 10–20mg q.d.s. Domperidone 10–20mg q.d.s.
Gastric irritation	Treat gastritis e.g. proton pump inhibitor Stop gastric irritants e.g. NSAID Cyclizine 50mg t.d.s. Ondansetron 8mg b.d.

11 Baines M. J. (2000) Symptom control in advanced gastrointestinal cancer. *Eur J Gastroenterol Hepatol*, **12**: 375–9.

Management of nausea and vomiting: practical guide

Identify any causes of nausea and vomiting that can best be treated specifically e.g.

- constipation—remember to do a rectal examination
- gastritis—epigastric discomfort and tenderness
- raised intracranial pressure—neurological signs
- oropharyngeal candida
- hypercalcaemia—dehydration, confusion
- drug induced—recent introduction of morphine?
- intestinal obstruction

Choose an antiemetic based on the most likely cause of nausea and vomiting

- drug or metabolic haloperidol
- gastric stasis metoclopramide
- GI tract involvement or cerebral tumour cyclizine

If first choice drug unsuccessful or only partially successful after 24h, increase dose or use different antiemetic(s)

- nausea and vomiting in cancer is often multifactorial
- if confident that there is a single cause for the nausea and vomiting, consider increasing the dose of antiemetic (especially metoclopramide), or changing to a second-line specific antiemetic (e.g. ondansetron for drug-induced nausea)
- if not confident of cause, empirically try one of the other first-line antiemetics (metoclopramide, haloperidol, cyclizine)
- combinations of antiemetics with different actions (e.g. at different receptor sites) are often needed and can act additively
- if using more than one antiemetic, one from each class of antiemetics should be considered, see Table 6b.3
- cyclizine and haloperidol are a logical combination
- levomepromazine acts at several receptor sites, and alone may replace a previously unsuccessful combination
- levomepromazine may be useful as a non-specific second-line antiemetic for nausea and vomiting of any or unknown aetiology
- cyclizine may antagonise the prokinetic effects of metoclopramide, and they should not usually be mixed

General points

Always give antiemetics *regularly*—not p.r.n.

If vomiting is preventing drug absorption, use an alternative route e.g. CSCI

Dexamethasone 4mg daily often contributes an antiemetic effect for nausea and vomiting of unknown mechanism

Check blood urea and electrolytes, liver function tests and calcium:

- Renal failure—consider lowering the dose of opioids
- Hypercalcaemia—treat with intravenous bisphosphonates

Monitor carefully if giving prokinetic drugs (e.g. metoclopramide) in intestinal obstruction in case intestinal colic and vomiting increase.

Always reassess the patient regularly as the cause of nausea and vomiting can change with time.
- Levomepromazine tends to cause sedation at doses above 6.25mg b.d.
- Octreotide dries up gastrointestinal secretions tending towards constipation
- Granisetron and ondansetron are also associated with constipation

ANTIEMETIC LADDER

	2nd line narrow Spectrum	e.g. ondansetron
	OR combination	e.g. cyclizine + haloperidol
	OR broad spectrum	e.g. levomepromazine

Selected narrow spectrum antiemetic
- metoclopramide
- cyclizine
- haloperidol

Step 1

Step 2

± administer by **CSCI**
± dexamethasone

Antiemetic drugs

Anti-histamines

The *vomiting centre* is rich in histamine and acetylcholine receptors. Most antihistamine drugs are also antimuscarinic.

Cyclizine is a commonly used antihistamine antiemetic. Acting at the vomiting centre, it is useful for vomiting of many causes.

Dose: 25–50mg t.d.s. orally or 100–150mg/24h CSCI.

Side-effects: antimuscarinic effects like dry mouth and drowsiness often abate after a few days.

Antimuscarinics

Hyoscine hydrobromide is a potent antimuscarinic. It is especially useful if there is intestinal obstruction or colic as it reduces peristalsis.

Side-effects of dry mouth, drowsiness or confusion may be more severe than with cyclizine.

It is available as buccal tablets (Kwells), transdermal patch (Scopoderm TTS), and can be used by CSCI. 200–1200 mcg/24h CSCI.

Antipsychotics

Drugs and metabolic disturbances cause vomiting by stimulating the CTZ. Antipsychotics (as potent dopamine antagonists) block this pathway and are very effective against drug or metabolic induced nausea and vomiting (e.g. opioids and renal failure).

Haloperidol. Dose: 1.5mg nocte orally (0.5–1.5mg b.d.) or 2.5–5mg/24h CSCI

Sedation and extrapyramidal effects are rare at these low doses.

Prochlorperazine is relatively more sedative but is available in buccal (Buccastem) and suppository form. Prochlorperazine cannot be given subcutaneously as it is irritant.

Levomepromazine. Dose ranges: 6.25mg–25mg nocte or b.d. orally or 6.25–25mg/24h CSCI. Oral bioavailability of levomepromazine is approx. 40 per cent. Use half the daily oral dose by CSCI.

A sedative, broad spectrum antiemetic which is effective in low doses. Some patients show a narrow therapeutic window.

It also has antimuscarinic, antihistamine and 5-HT$_2$ antagonist effects, as well as an anxiolytic effect.

Phenothiazines and haloperidol should be avoided with amiodarone since there is an increased risk of ventricular arrhythmias. The low, antiemetic doses of haloperidol used in palliative care probably carry a low risk.

Prokinetic drugs/drugs altering gastric motility

Metoclopramide acts peripherally on the gut restoring normal gastric emptying. It also acts at the CTZ and thus helps drug-induced nausea. Dose: 10mg–20mg q.d.s. p.o. or 30–80mg/24h CSCI.

Side-effects: extrapyramidal effects are rare, but most common in young female patients.

Domperidone is very similar to metoclopramide but is less likely to cause extrapyramidal effects because it does not cross the blood brain barrier; it is available as suppositories.

5-HT₃ antagonists

5-HT$_3$ receptors are found in the chemoreceptor trigger zone. They are very effective against acute-phase chemotherapy and radiotherapy induced nausea with little to choose between ondansetron and granisetron, but their place in other situations (e.g. intestinal obstruction) is as yet uncertain.

Ondansetron has been shown to be ineffective in motion sickness, but effective at treating morphine-induced nausea and vomiting. 5-HT$_3$ antagonists may work synergistically with haloperidol in some cases.

In the UK, 5-HT$_3$ antagonists are only licensed for chemotherapy-induced and postoperative emesis.

Other drugs

Corticosteroids often have a non-specific benefit in reducing nausea and vomiting.

Additional drugs

Newer atypical antipsychotics may be expected to show antiemetic effects. Olanzapine has a similar pharmacological profile to levomepromazine and there is weak anecdotal evidence that it may be an effective antiemetic.

Risperidone has potent 5-HT$_2$ antagonist effects as well as being anti-dopaminergic but there is no published evidence to date of any antiemetic effect. It should be avoided in patients with cerebrovascular disease.

Table 6b.3 Receptor affinity of antiemetic drugs

Agonist/Antagonist	ACh$_M$ Ant	H$_1$ Ant	5-HT$_2$ Ant	D$_2$ Ant	5-HT$_3$ Ant	5-HT$_4$ Ag
Hyoscine hydrobromide	+++					
Cyclizine	++	+++				
Haloperidol				+++ (*)		
Ondansetron					+++	
Metoclopramide				++	(+)	++
Domperidone				++		
Levomepromazine	+	+	++	+ (*)		

(*) Prokinetic effect of metoclopramide and domperidone is partly attributed to D$_2$ antagonism—however there is no evidence that haloperidol or other neuroleptics have prokinetic activity.

Avoid dopamine antagonists (particularly haloperidol), in patients with Parkinson's Disease.

Constipation

Constipation is characterised by difficult or painful defaecation, and is associated with infrequent bowel evacuations, and hard, small faeces.

Stool frequency varies considerably in the normal population: 45 per cent of patients are constipated on admission to a hospice. Complications of constipation include pain, bowel obstruction, overflow diarrhoea and urinary retention which cause great distress and every effort must therefore be made to avoid them.

Causes

- Disease-related
  - Immobility
  - Decreased food intake
  - Low residue diet
- Fluid depletion
  - Poor fluid intake
  - Increased fluid loss i.e. vomiting, polyuria, fever
- Weakness
  - Inability to raise intra-abdominal pressure
    - e.g. general debility • paraplegia
  - Inability to reach toilet when urge to defaecate occurs (immobility leads to decreased peristalsis)
- Intestinal obstruction
- Medication
  - Opioids (90 per cent of patients taking opioids need laxatives)
  - Diuretics
  - Antimuscarinics
    - phenothiazines • tricyclic antidepressants • hyoscine derivatives
  - Serotonin inhibitors
    - ondansetron/granisetron/tropisetron
  - Somatostatin analogues
    - octreotide • lanreotide
- Biochemical
  - Hypercalcaemia
  - Hypokalaemia
- Other
  - Embarrassment in public setting
  - Pain on defaecation e.g. fissure in ano

Complications of constipation

- Pain—colic or constant abdominal discomfort
- Intestinal obstruction
- Urinary retention or frequency
- Overflow diarrhoea
- Faecal incontinence
- Confusion or restlessness if severe

Traditionally laxatives are divided into
- Stimulants
- Osmotic agents
- Bulking agents
- Faecal softeners

In reality, these categories are arbitrary as there is much overlap between the agents. For example, an osmotic agent will act as a stimulant by decreasing the GIT transit time by increasing pressure within the bowel.

Management of constipation
- Anticipate this common problem
- Enquire about bowel function regularly
- Start prophylactic laxatives when starting opioid drugs
- Use oral laxatives in preference to rectal measures
- Use a combination of a stimulant laxative with a softener/osmotic laxative if necessary
- Titrate components to achieve optimum stool frequency and consistency

Remember also to:
- Increase fluid intake
- Increase fruit/fibre in diet
- Encourage mobility
- Get patient to toilet, if possible avoiding bed pans
- Provide privacy
- Raise toilet seat for comfort

Laxatives

Choice of laxative
- A number of laxative combinations may be equally effective
- Patient preference may dictate choice
- Mixed preparations of softener/stimulant (e.g. co-danthramer) keep medications to a minimum
- Separate softener and stimulant allows titration of components to give optimum stool frequency and consistency
- Senna has a greater tendency to cause colic than dantron-containing combination laxatives

Stimulants e.g. senna, dantron, bisacodyl
Avoid stimulant drugs if there is the possibility of intestinal obstruction. Dantron is useful with a softener such as docusate (co-danthrusate) or poloxamer (co-danthramer) for opioid-induced constipation, but may colour urine red and cause excoriation around the perineum if in contact with skin. (Dantron is only licensed for use in patients with a terminal illness.)

Osmotic agents e.g. lactulose, magnesium salts, and macrogols
In palliative care, the use of such agents is often inappropriate because of the need to drink 2–3 litres per day for the agents to function well. In addition, lactulose may be unpalatable and cause uncomfortable abdominal bloating and flatus.

Macrogol (polyethylene glycol) in the palliative setting, particularly in intractable constipation and faecal impaction, may have a particular rôle to play.[12]

Lactulose is usually to be avoided in the palliative care setting because:
- It can increase abdominal cramps
- Its sweet taste can be hard for the palliative care patient to tolerate
- It causes flatulence
- It should be consumed with large volumes of liquid which palliative care patients are often unable to take

Faecal softeners e.g. docusate
These are useful in conjunction with a stimulant (e.g. docusate + dantron in co-danthrusate and docusate + poloxamer in co-danthramer). It may be safer to use docusate alone in resolving intestinal obstruction.

12 Culbert P., Gillett H., Ferguson A. (1998) Highly effective new oral therapy for faecal impaction. *British Journal of General Practice*, **48**: 1599–600.

Bulk-forming agents e.g. methylcellulose (Celevac),
ispaghula husk (Fybogel)

Patients are rarely started on these preparations in the palliative care setting because they have been implicated in worsening constipation when used with reduced fluid intake. They are also unpalatable and may aggravate anorexia.

Rectal agents (1 glycerol suppository + 1 bisacodyl suppository)

Bisacodyl is a rectal stimulant and should be placed in direct contact with the rectal mucosa. If appropriately placed, it should stimulate an evacuation within one hour.

Glycerol is a faecal lubricant which facilitates defaecation by softening the stool.

For more severe constipation

Arachis oil enema (130mL) overnight to penetrate hard stool, soften and lubricate. Follow with high phosphate enema in the morning to stimulate bowel clearance.

Do *not* attempt *manual evacuation* of impacted stool without some form of sedation or analgesia.

In circumstances of intractable constipation, close consultation with nursing colleagues is vital if a clear strategy for managing the problem is to be achieved.

Faecal impaction

If the patient has faecal impaction, try:
• Bisacodyl suppositories (must be in contact with rectal mucosa)
• Arachis oil retention enema to soften
• Phosphate enema
• An alternative is polyethylene glycol, *movicol* taken for three days
• Manual removal (with midazolam, diamorphine, or caudal anaesthesia)
• Once successful it is imperative to start regular oral measures to prevent recurrence of the problem

Table 6b.4 Classification of commonly used laxatives

Category	Examples	Description	Comments
Osmotic Laxatives	**Lactulose** **Polyethylene glycol**	Osmotic laxatives are not absorbed from the gut and so retain water in the lumen by osmotic action (this action may be partial). This increase in volume will encourage peristalsis and consequent expulsion of faeces.	Can cause abdominal distension and abdominal cramps. Patients need to drink over a litre a day which may not be practical

Surfactant Laxatives	**Docusate Poloxamer**	Act to reduce surface tension and improve water penetration of the stools.	
Stimulant Laxatives	**Senna Bisacodyl**	Senna and bisacodyl both rely on bacterial transformation in the large bowel to produce active derivatives and so have little small intestinal effect.	Can cause abdominal cramps. Should be avoided in patients with intestinal obstruction.
	Dantron	Absorbed from the small bowel and undergoes first pass hepatic metabolism to glucuronide forms. These may be secreted in the bile and converted to the active drug prolonging its action	Dantron is available only combined with a surfactant softener e.g. Co-danthramer with poloxamer, or Co-danthrusate with docusate. Dantron-containing preps are subject to licence limitations following evidence from animal studies that in high doses it can cause tumours. It is licensed for use in analgesic induced constipation in terminally ill patients. Dantron may colour urine red. It should be avoided in patients who may be incontinent of urine or faeces, as it can cause severe rashes if it comes in contact with the skin.

Table 6b.5 Onset of action

• Bisacodyl tablet	10–12 h	• Laxoberal	10–14 h
• Bisacodyl Supps.	20–60 min	• Microlax enema	20 min
• Dantron	6–12 h	• Phosphate enema	20 min
• Docusate	24–48 h	• Senna	8–12 h
• Glycerin Supps.	1–6 h	• Sodium picosulfate	min
• Lactulose	48 h		

Diarrhoea

Diarrhoea is a less common symptom than constipation amongst patients requiring palliative care and has been defined as the passage of more than three unformed stools within a 24-h period.

As with constipation, patients can understand 'diarrhoea' in different ways and clarification of the term is always required.

Up to 10 per cent of patients admitted to hospice complain of diarrhoea. (In contrast, 27 per cent of HIV infected patients are reported as having diarrhoea).

Treatment of diarrhoea

A **cause** for the diarrhoea should be looked for prior to giving anti-diarrhoeal agents. The presence of fever or blood in the stool should prompt further discussion to ensure the most appropriate treatment.

General measures
• Increase fluid intake, constant sipping
• Reassurance that most diarrhoea is self-limiting

Management
Treat or exclude any specific causes.

Table 6b.6 The most common causes of diarrhoea in the palliative care setting

1 Imbalance of laxative therapy. (Especially when laxatives have been increased to clear severe constipation.)
Diarrhoea should settle within 24 h if laxatives are stopped. Laxatives should be reintroduced at a lower dose.

2 Drugs such as antibiotics and antacids, NSAIDS or iron preparations.

3 Faecal impaction is associated with fluid stool which leaks past a faecal plug or a tumour mass.

4 Radiotherapy involving the abdomen or pelvis is likely to cause diarrhoea especially in the second or third week of therapy.

5 Malabsorption associated with:
Carcinoma of head of pancreas with insufficient pancreatic secretions thus less fat absorption and resultant steatorrhoea.
Gastrectomy resulting in poor mixing of food with pancreatic secretions and consequent resultant steatorrhoea. Vagotomy can cause increased water secretion into the colon.
Ileal resection reduces the ability of the small intestine to reabsorb bile acids. These acids increase fluid in the colon and contribute to explosive diarrhoea.

Table 6b.6 (Continued)

A resection of over 100-cm of terminal ileum will outstretch the liver's capacity to compensate for the bile salt loss, and fat malabsorption will compound the diarrhoea.

Colectomy. Immediately following surgery for a total or a near total colectomy, the water in the gut cannot be adequately absorbed. Although this tends to settle over a week, the bowel seldom returns to its pre-surgical function. The small intestine is unable to adequately compensate for the loss of this colonic water-absorbing capacity. This can lead to an ongoing daily loss of an extra 400–1000mL of gut fluid rectally.

Such patients often require an ileostomy and need an extra litre of fluid and 7g of extra salt a day with vitamin and iron supplements.

6 **Colonic or rectal tumours** can cause diarrhoea through causing partial bowel obstruction or through increased mucus secretion

7 **Rare endocrine tumours** which secrete hormones cause diarrhoea. e.g. carcinoid tumour

8 Concurrent disease such as gastrointestinal infection

9 Odd dietary habits.

Table 6b.7 Diagnostic diarrhoea patterns

Defaecation described as 'diarrhoea' happening only two or three times a day without warning suggests anal incontinence.

Profuse watery stools are characteristic of colonic diarrhoea.

Sudden onset of diarrhoea after a period of constipation raises suspicion of faecal impaction.

Alternating diarrhoea and constipation suggests poorly regulated laxative therapy or impending bowel obstruction.

Pale, fatty offensive stools (steatorrhoea) indicate malabsorption due to either pancreatic or ileal disease.

Table 6b.8 Cause management

Subacute small bowel obstruction	See intestinal obstruction
Laxatives (including self-administered magnesium-containing antacids)	Discontinue and review
Faecal impaction (with anal leakage or incontinence)	Rectal disimpaction /manual evacuation/ macrogol
Antibiotic-associated diarrhoea/ pseudomembranous colitis (recent or broad-spectrum antibiotics)	Check stool for Clostridium difficile (metronidazole 400mg t.d.s. for 7–14 days) vancomycin 125mg q.d.s.
Radiotherapy-induced	Ondansetron, aspirin, colestyramine
NSAID	Try stopping or changing NSAID
Misoprostol	Use a PPI or other alternative
Pre-existing disease e.g. Crohn's or ulcerative colitis	Corticosteroids or sulfasalazine
Ileal resection (causing bile salt diarrhoea)	Colestyramine
Steatorrhoea/fat malabsorption	Pancreatic enzymes ± PPI (reduces gastric acid destruction of enzymes)
Carcinoid syndrome	$5\text{-}HT_3$ antagonists, octreotide
Zollinger –Ellison syndrome	H_2 antagonist e.g. ranitidine
Non-specific profuse secretory diarrhoea	Opioids such as loperamide and codeine and morphine may be necessary. (Loperamide is not absorbed)

Somatostatin has a place in the management of severe, profuse, secretory diarrhoea, such as that associated with HIV infection when other agents have failed to work. It is best given by CSCI.

Intestinal obstruction

This most commonly occurs with carcinoma of the ovary or bowel. The obstruction may be intramural, intraluminal, or extraluminal due to surrounding peritoneal disease, and is often at multiple sites. In addition, there is often a clinical obstruction in the absence of a mechanical lesion (functional obstruction).

A plain abdominal X-ray may be helpful in excluding constipation.

If surgical intervention is inappropriate, symptomatic measures using medication are the mainstay of treatment, avoiding the standard 'drip and suck' approach, which may be distressing and is ineffective in 80% of patients.

- In the presence of advanced peritoneal disease, the most likely cause of obstruction is due to malignant tumour. The cause may also be due, however, to benign factors such as adhesions
- If the patient is fit enough, a surgical opinion should be sought and the advantages and disadvantages of laparotomy assessed
- The potential mortality and morbidity associated with surgery should be weighed against quality of life in a patient whose prognosis may only be predicted to be a few weeks or months
- If the obstruction is incomplete or mainly functional, it may resolve. It may therefore be helpful in the first place to try:

Reducing bowel wall oedema
Using: Dexamethasone 8–16mg SC before midday

The evidence for such an approach is equivocal, but if a three day trial proves beneficial and vomiting subsides it may be useful to consider continuing with reducing doses of oral steroids. Whether improvement is due to steroids or to the passage of time remains the subject of debate.

If dexamethasone is not helpful after three days it should be stopped (unless the patient has been on longer-term steroids (more than a week) in which case it should be tailed off slowly).

Stimulating gut motility
Metoclopramide 30–120mg/24h via subcutaneous infusion. Beware of any increase in gut colic and stop if obstruction is not resolving.

For complete obstruction or obstruction not resolving with the above measures in 24–48 h, focus on treating symptoms rather than the underlying cause:

- **Nausea and vomiting:**
  - cyclizine 100–150mg/24h CSCI
  - ± haloperidol 3–5mg/24h CSCI
  - or levomepromazine 6.25–25mg/24h CSCI
- **Colic:**
  - hyoscine butylbromide 40–100mg/24h CSCI (diamorphine may also be needed for background pain)
- **Diarrhoea:**
  - codeine 30–60mg p.o. every 4 h, or
  - loperamide 2–4mg p.o. every 4 h. *Use with caution if possibility of reversible obstruction*

- **Constipation:**
  - Ensure that reversible constipation is not contributing to the obstruction. Gentle rectal measures or a small dose of a faecal softener such as docusate may be used, particularly if there is no colic and obstruction is thought to be colonic and subacute. More vigorous measures should be avoided for fear of aggravating symptoms

If intestinal obstruction is still not resolving

1 *Reduce* or *encourage reabsorption of gut secretions* and reduce intestinal motility using:
  - hyoscine butylbromide (Buscopan) 40–100mg/24h CSCI
  - octreotide 300–600 mcg/24h CSCI
2 Nasogastric tube
  - *If* vomiting is not subsiding, or *if* very distressing and/or faecal, it may be necessary to use a nasogastric tube after full discussion with patient and carers. Although this is an infrequent practice in a hospice setting, and can be seen as a very undignified approach to patient care, it can bring comfort in exceptional circumstances
3 Venting gastrostomy
  - With occasional, clinically stable patients who are distressed by vomiting but who have a prognosis of at least weeks, and who are keen to resume oral intake, it *may* be an option to discuss venting gastrostomy and subcutaneous fluids.[13] In practice venting gastrostomies are rarely performed

---

13 Roila F. et al. (1996) Comparative studies of various antiemetic regimes. *Supportive Care in Cancer,* **4**: 270–80.

Hiccup

Definition: Spasmodic contraction of the diaphragm that causes a sudden breath in, cut off when the vocal cords snap together, creating the characteristic sound

Hiccups result from diaphragmatic spasms caused by diaphragmatic irritation, which is often associated with liver enlargement or gastric distension.

Causes
- Via vagus nerve
  - gastric distension
  - gastritis/gastro-oesophageal reflux
  - hepatic tumours
  - ascites/abdominal distension/intestinal obstruction
- Via phrenic nerve
  - diaphragmatic tumour involvement
  - mediastinal tumour
  - CNS
  - intracranial tumours, especially brainstem lesions
  - meningeal infiltration by cancer.
- Systemic
  - renal failure
  - corticosteroids
  - Addison's disease
  - hyponatraemia

Management of hiccup

Pharyngeal stimulation is effected in a number of ways. The soft palate can be massaged, the patient can try eating dry granulated sugar or holding the breath or rebreathing into a bag etc. These measures are often effective, at least temporarily. Alternatively:

1 Reduce gastric distension:
- Pro-kinetic drugs e.g.
  - metoclopramide 10mg q.d.s.
  - domperidone 10mg q.d.s.
- Gastric distension may also improve with a change to small frequent meals and using a defoaming antiflatulant with an antacid, such as activated dimeticone and aluminium hydroxide (Asilone) 5–10mL q.d.s.

2 Relax smooth muscle:
- nifedipine 5mg p.r.n. or regularly three times daily, either by mouth or sublingually, may be effective
- baclofen 5mg t.d.s. is an alternative

3 Suppress central hiccup reflex: If symptoms are severe and not responding to other measures including pharyngeal stimulation it may be necessary to give:
- chlorpromazine 25mg p.o. Intravenous administration may cause sedation and hypotension and is only used in intractable cases

4 **Suppress central irritation from intracranial tumour**: This may respond to dexamethasone (starting with high doses e.g. 16mg daily) or to an anticonvulsant e.g. phenytoin 200–300mg given at night. NB Corticosteroids can also cause hiccups—consider stopping if recently started.

Anorexia/cachexia/asthenia

Primary anorexia is the absence or loss of appetite for food.

Cachexia (📖 See Chapter 6c) is a condition of profound weight loss and catabolic loss of muscle and adipose tissue. It is often associated with primary anorexia and fatigue.

Asthenia(📖 See Chapter 6c) is characterized by:

- Fatigue or easy tiring and reduced sustainability of performance
- Generalized weakness resulting in a reduced ability to initiate movement
- Mental fatigue characterized by poor concentration, impaired memory, and emotional lability[14]

Secondary anorexia is often due to several conditions and may be reversible and should be actively sought.

- Dyspepsia
- Altered taste
- Malodour
- Nausea and vomiting
- Sore mouth
- Pain
- Biochemical
  - Hypercalcaemia
  - Uraemia
- Gastric stasis
- Constipation
- Secondary to treatment
  - Drugs
  - RT
  - CT

Early satiety (patient hungry but then feels full) occurs with small stomach, hepatomegaly and gross ascites. Anxiety and depression will contribute to loss of appetite. Patients are 'put off' by too much food and food which is unappetizing.

These symptoms which are closely interrelated occur in about 70 per cent of patients with advanced cancer particularly gastric and pancreatic cancer.

Management

1 Assess and treat any reversible causes as outlined above.
2 Involve the dietician and multidisciplinary team to maximize treatment goals.
3 Non-drug treatment:
  - Explore the patients' and carers' fears of anorexia
  - Reassure patients that it is normal to feel satisfied with less food
  - Consider if advice on food fortification/supplementation would be appropriate for this patient at this point of their illness
  - Suggest smaller helpings to allow patients to eat frequently small amounts of what they enjoy
4 Evidence-based drug treatments:
  - **Corticosteroids** e.g. dexamethasone 2–4mg o.d.
    - Appetite stimulant and may help nausea
    - May improve subjective feeling of anorexia and weakness

- Non-specific central euphoric effects
- Effects generally short lasting (weeks)
- Onset of side-effects rapid
- **Progestogens** e.g. megestrol acetate 160–800mg o.d.
  - Improves appetite, nutritional status and calorie intake
  - Take two—three weeks to produce effect
  - Associated with modest weight gain, (though not gain in lean body mass)
  - Effects may last for months
  - Increased incidence of thrombotic episodes
  - Expensive
- **Prokinetic drugs** e.g. metoclopramide 10mg q.d.s.
  - Try if early satiety, gastric stasis (many patients with malignancy have associated autonomic dysfunction)

Total parenteral nutrition (📖 See Chapter 10c)

In case of total parenteral nutrition (TPN) in the palliative care setting, some studies have shown an association with survival shortened with the introduction of TPN.

Universal benefit and efficacy have not been clearly proven with TPN and its routine use is not recommended in view of this, the practical disadvantage, and the risk of side-effects and complications.

Aggressive nutritional therapy could perhaps be justified in particular situations such as when patients are recovering from surgery or awaiting chemotherapy.

Hydration (📖 See Chapter 1)

There is often an overwhelming need for relatives and staff to give dying patients food and water but this must not be allowed to override the patients need for comfort.

Avoiding overhydration in a dying patient may improve comfort, by minimizing urinary output (and therefore the need for catheterisation) and the volume of distressing bronchial secretions. In bowel obstruction gastric secretions will be minimised, thereby reducing the frequency of vomiting and the need for a nasogastric tube. A dry mouth can be treated with local measures.

In contrast, those patients who may survive for many months but who are unable to swallow adequately may find life easier with, for instance, a percutaneous gastrostomy tube. However, when these patients are dying it is necessary to explain to the relatives why it may be helpful to reduce fluid input.

14 Woof R. (1998) Asthenia, cachexia and anorexia. In C. Faull *et al.* (eds) *Handbook of Palliative Care.* Oxford: Blackwell.

Ascites (📖 See Chapter 16)

The healthy adult has about 50mL transudate in the peritoneal cavity. This has a protein level of about 25 per cent of that found in plasma. Peritoneal fluid turnover is 4–5mL/h in health.

Malignant ascites
- Malignant ascites accounts for about 10 per cent of all cases of ascites and occurs in up to 50 per cent of all patients with cancer
- Malignant ascitic fluid is an exudate with a protein content of about 85 per cent of that found in plasma. This protein-rich fluid is an excellent culture medium for malignant cells and bacteria. It may also have high levels of certain enzymes
- In malignant ascites, the ascitic fluid turnover can be twenty-fold of that found in healthy individuals
- Ascites may be the presenting feature of the malignancy or be indicative of recurrence or metastatic spread. It is often indicative of end-stage disease
- It is caused by malignant peritoneal deposits, blockage of sub-diaphragmatic lymphatics and secondary sodium retention

Causes of malignant ascites
- Ovarian primary (50 per cent of cases)
- Unknown primary (20 per cent of cases)
- Stomach, colon, pancreatic primary (most of the remainder)

Non-malignant ascites
- Cardiac failure, liver failure and renal failure are common causes of non-malignant ascites, accounting for 90 per cent of cases
- The significance of this for patients with palliative care needs is that ascites should not automatically be attributed to underlying malignancy
- Management options, however, are similar for both malignant and non-malignant disease

Management

Treatment of the primary cancer, usually with chemotherapy, may be the most effective measure to reduce ascites. Analgesics and good symptom control may be all that is necessary, particularly for a patient who is bed-bound and has a short prognosis.

Diuretics may alleviate symptoms over several days. Doses must be adequate and include a combination of spironolactone (100mg b.d. and possibly higher) and a loop diuretic e.g. furosemide (40–80mg o.d.).

Patients with liver metastases are more likely to respond to diuretics; paracentesis will provide more immediate relief (see below).

A peritoneo-venous shunt could be considered and inserted under general or local anaesthesia.

Shunts comprise a multi-perforated catheter in the peritoneal cavity which joins to a one-way valve positioned subcutaneously just above the costal margin. From here ascitic fluid is drained into the superior vena cava via a tunnelled catheter which enters the external or internal jugular vein. Fluid flows through the shunt on inspiration. Patients are encouraged to pump the reservoir to keep fluid flowing through the shunt. The two commonest shunts in use (Denver and LeVeen) have similar performance profiles. Results from use of such shunts have been mixed as they are prone to blockage.

Paracentesis

General

Paracentesis is a simple procedure, which can be performed as a day case (usually only removing 2–4 litres maximum), or as an inpatient.
- In tense, symptomatic ascites there may be up to 12 litres of ascites present
- Removal of 4–6 litres is usually enough to give symptomatic relief
- Removal of more than 4–6 litres increases the risk of hypovolaemia and adverse effects, but may give symptom relief for longer until ascites re-accumulates
- For an ill, elderly patient, small volume paracentesis repeated as needed may be preferable

Indications
- Pain, discomfort, or tightness due to stretching of the abdominal wall
- Dyspnoea, usually exacerbated by exertion, due to upward pressure on the diaphragm
- Nausea, vomiting and dyspepsia due to the 'squashed stomach' syndrome
- Patients are usually symptomatic only when the abdominal wall is tensely distended. Patients who are also bothered by ankle (or generalized) oedema, may fare better with diuretic therapy

Complications of paracentesis
- After a large volume paracentesis, the compensatory large fluid shifts from circulating volume into extracellular fluid can decompensate the patient's cardiovascular system leading to hypovolaemia, and in severe cases, collapse and renal failure
- A low albumin or sodium level will exacerbate this effect
- The cannula site may continue to leak ascites after removal
- If a limited, partial paracentesis has been performed, this may rarely become a continuing leak over days to weeks. (Use colostomy bag to collect leakage)
- The patient needs to be warned about possible leaking which may otherwise cause distress
- Bowel perforation is a risk, especially if intestinal obstruction is present
- Infection is a rare complication, providing an aseptic technique is used

Investigations prior to paracentesis
- An ultrasound scan will confirm the presence of ascites, and may determine if it is 'pocketed' by tumour adhesions
- A scan should be performed if:
  - ascites is not easily clinically identified
  - there is a chance of bowel obstruction
- A serum albumin and urea and electrolytes should be taken if:
  - more than 4–6 litres is to be removed and the patient has oedema, or
  - the patient is clinically dehydrated, or
  - the patient has reacted badly to a previous paracentesis
- A platelet count and clotting screen should be measured in at risk patients

Contra-indications to paracentesis
- Local or systemic infection
- Coagulopathy—platelets $<40 \times 10^9$ /l or INR >1.4
- Limit paracentesis to 4–6 litres maximum if:
  - Hepatic or renal failure (creatinine >250mmol/L)
  - Albumin <30g/L or sodium <125mmol/L

Follow-up care to paracentesis
- Ascites will usually re-form after a paracentesis; this can vary between one and many weeks
- Diuretics may reduce the rate of re-accumulation, or prevent it becoming as tense again
- Repeated paracentesis on an as-needed basis is appropriate management for patients with advanced cancer

The procedure of paracentesis
- The patient should be asked to pass urine before the procedure
- Blood pressure should be measured and recorded
- The patient should lie in a semi-recumbent position
- It may be helpful if the patient tilts 30 degrees towards the side of the paracentesis
- Use left iliac fossa unless local disease is present, avoiding scars and inferior epigastric artery (see Fig. 6b. 1)
- Confirm that site is dull to percussion
- Using aseptic technique, anaesthetize skin locally
- A large bore intravenous cannula or 'Bonanno' catheter can be used
- Avoid clamping the catheter if possible, since malignant ascites can be very proteinaceous and is likely to block it

Large volume paracentesis (>6 litres)
If it is intended to drain to dryness, or >6 litres:
- Stop diuretics (if used solely for ascites) 48h before procedure
- Check blood pressure and pulse every 30 minutes during paracentesis, then hourly for 6h
- Some units give plasma substitutes such as intravenous dextran 70 or gelatin infusion (e.g. Gelofusine), 150mL for every litre of ascites drained, during the paracentesis or shortly afterwards to reduce hypovolaemia

Tenesmus and tenesmoid pain

Tenesmus is the painful sensation of rectal fullness, usually caused by local rectal tumour. There may be associated spasm of smooth muscle, or neuropathic pain from lumbosacral plexus infiltration causing stabbing or more continuous pain. It may be difficult to distinguish from pudendal neuralgia.

Management
- Prevent and treat constipation
- Opioid analgesia may be helpful but not reliably
- NSAID e.g. diclofenac 50mg t.d.s.
- Radiotherapy
- Nifedipine m/r 10–20mg b.d.
- Co-analgesics as for neuropathic pain
- Amitriptyline
- Anticonvulsants
- Corticosteroids
- Lumbar sympathectomy: >80 per cent success rate
- Spinal infusion of local anaesthetic ± opioids

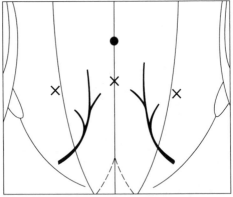

Figure 6b.1 Usual sites for paracentesis, avoiding the inferior epigastric arteries

Dyspepsia

Gastro-oesophageal reflux/oesophagitis (GORD)

Assessment
- Exclude or treat oesophageal candida
- Consider oesophageal spasm
- Avoid drugs which cause oesophagitis—potassium, NSAIDs
- Consider pain of cardiac origin

Treatment
- Raise head of bed to reduce acid reflux
- Consider paracentesis for tense ascites
- Metoclopramide 10mg t.d.s. if signs of gastric stasis or distension
- Antacid e.g. Gaviscon 10mL q.d.s. for mild symptoms
- Proton pump inhibitor (PPI) e.g. lansoprazole 30mg daily for moderate or severe symptoms; start with treatment dose then step-down after a few weeks

NSAID and steroid-related dyspepsia

Treatment of drug-related dyspepsia
- Consider stopping or reducing dose of NSAID/steroids
- PPI e.g. lansoprazole 30mg o.d. for severe symptoms or proven pathology. Start with treatment dose and reduce after four weeks. For milder symptoms start with maintenance dose (15mg) and increase later if needed
- If symptoms persist on treatment dose of PPI, and NSAID needed by the patient to control pain, consider changing to a selective COX-2 inhibitor (e.g. Celecoxib)

Indications for prophylaxis
- Prescribing NSAID with recent history of dyspepsia
- Prescribing steroids with recent history of dyspepsia
- Co-prescribing NSAID with steroids, anticoagulants, or aspirin
- Prescribing NSAID in elderly patient >70 years (less clear evidence—use judgement)

Drugs for dyspepsia
Proton pump inhibitors (PPIs)
- There is little difference in efficacy between the current PPIs available
- A single daily dose is appropriate for PPIs rather than divided doses
- Lansoprazole and omeprazole can be taken before or after food with equal efficacy

Despite the variations in dose recommendations in the product literature, omeprazole, lansoprazole and pantoprazole display similar dose-response relationships with similar potency at the same milligram doses. Daily doses of 15–20mg PPI are appropriate for maintenance therapy, prophylaxis, or less severe gastro-oesophageal reflux disease. Doses of 30–40mg daily are appropriate for treatment.

Antacids

Aluminium-containing antacids cause constipation whereas magnesium-containing antacids are laxative. Dimeticone in asilone is a defoamer, useful for gastric distension/hiccups.

Prostaglandin analogues

Misoprostol is effective at preventing NSAID-induced ulcers, but is less well tolerated than PPIs, and diarrhoea is a common side-effect. Misoprostol is available in combination with diclofenac.

H2 antagonists

H2 antagonists are less effective at acid suppression than PPIs, and are less effective clinically at healing ulcers. Ranitidine has significantly fewer drug interactions and adverse affects than cimetidine.

Gastrointestinal bleeding

Gastric bleeding and melaena

Assessment

Consider the commonest causes:
- Tumour bleeding
- Clotting disorders
- Peptic ulcer ±NSAIDs

Management considerations for gastrointestinal bleeding

- Review or stop NSAIDs, aspirin, corticosteroids, warfarin
- Commence PPI in treatment dose, e.g. lansoprazole 30mg o.d. when able to take orally
- Blood tests for clotting screen and platelets and treat if appropriate
- Consider radiotherapy referral if bleeding due to tumour
- Tranexamic acid 1–2g t.d.s. p.o. (or by slow i/v until able to take p.o.)
  - Stop if no effect after one week
  - Continue for one week after bleeding has stopped, then discontinue
  - Only continue long term (500mg t.d.s.) if bleeding recurs
  - Avoid tranexamic acid with history of thromboembolism/CVA etc.
- Small bleeds can herald a larger haemorrhage;
  - consider siting an i/v cannula to administer emergency drugs
- Intravenous high-dose PPI e.g. omeprazole 80mg i/v stat., then 8mg/h i/v infusion
- Arterial embolization
- Oral sucralfate
- Octreotide which is an accepted medical management for bleeding from oesophageal or colonic varices. Circumstantial evidence indicates that the actions of octreotide are mainly mediated by a splanchnic vasoconstrictive effect, possibly with gastric acid suppression and enhancement of platelet aggregation. It is uncertain whether it has a rôle in gastrointestinal bleeding of other aetiology
- Etamsylate

Rectal bleeding

Assessment

Consider the commonest causes:
- tumour bleeding
- clotting disorders
- pelvic infection
- haemorrhoids

NSAIDs can cause lower gastrointestinal bleeding as well as the better-documented upper GI bleeding.

Treatment
- Review or stop NSAIDs
- Treat any evidence or signs suggestive of pelvic infection
- Consider radiotherapy referral
- Blood tests for clotting screen and platelets and treat as appropriate
- Tranexamic acid 1–2g t.d.s. p.o. (or by slow i/v until able to take p.o.)
  - Stop if no effect after one week
  - Continue for one week after bleeding has stopped, then discontinue
  - Only continue long term (500mg t.d.s.) If bleeding recurs
  - Avoid tranexamic acid with history of thromboembolism/CVA etc.
- Small bleeds can herald a larger haemorrhage;
- Consider siting an i/v cannula to administer emergency drugs
- Arterial embolization
- Etamsylate
- Oral sucralfate for post-radiation proctitis applied topically

Major gastrointestinal or rectal bleeding

If patient's condition is not stable, with history of major haemorrhage or ongoing bleeding:
- Consider if the patient should be transferred to an acute medical/endoscopy unit
- Site an i/v cannula to anticipate need for emergency drugs

Treat anxiety or distress as needed:
- Midazolam 2–5mg initially by slow i/v titration (diluted 10mg in 10mL with saline)
- If no i/v access, midazolam 5–10mg SC (or i/m if shocked/vasoconstricted)

The case for proton pump inhibitors in gastrointestinal bleeding

- Acid suppression in early studies did not help in the management of acute bleeding
- It has more recently been shown that intensive therapy aimed at achieving complete acid suppression does substantially reduce the risk of recurrent bleeding after initial endoscopic treatment
- Pharmacokinetic studies have shown that a bolus of 80mg pantoprazole or omeprazole followed by immediate continuous infusion of 8mg/h will result in an intragastric pH of 7 within 20 minutes This has been continued for 72h in studies[15]

Support for patient and family

Bleeding is very frightening. Ensure that the patient and family are well supported. Ensure that drugs are readily available for sedation if necessary and that dark bed linen (to disguise the amount of blood loss) is accessible.

15 Lau JY et al. (2000). Effect of intravenous omeprazole on recurrent bleeding after endoscopic treatment of bleeding peptic ulcers. *N Eng J Med*, **343**: 310–16.

Bowel stoma care

A bowel stoma is an artificial opening, created surgically, for patients to allow faeces to leave the body by a new route through a spout or outlet on the abdomen.

The majority of stomas encountered in patients with palliative care needs have been fashioned following surgical resection for cancer or as a bypass for inoperable or recurrent cancers of the bowel or ovary causing obstruction.

Any patient with a stoma (whether newly created or created many years ago, for example in Crohn's disease) and malignant intra-abdominal disease is at risk of a number of different symptoms which need appropriate management. These include abdominal pain (constant or intermittent colic), nausea, vomiting, abdominal distension, constipation, diarrhoea and depression all of which may impact on the holistic management of the patient.

Bowel stomas are generally created from the colon (colostomy) or ileum (ileostomy). The bowel proximal to the stoma continues to function in the normal way whereas function distal to this is normally lost.

Temporary (de-functioning) stomas

These include loop ileostomies or colostomies which are usually created to protect an anastomosis or to facilitate decompression or healing in the distal bowel. The bowel loop is usually brought out onto the abdominal wall (right and left iliac fossa respectively for ileostomy and colostomy) and may be supported by a temporary rod or bridge so that it does not retract. The proximal opening allows the passage of stool which is collected in a stoma bag and the distal opening leads to the redundant section of bowel. Mucus and old faeces may be expelled through the rectum. A temporary transverse colostomy may be created at an emergency operation for bowel obstruction since it is a relatively easy procedure in a sick patient.

Permanent stomas

These are end sections of bowel which are brought to the skin surface. The potential stoma site along the path of the bowel is planned preoperatively, if possible, to allow optimal positioning of a stoma bag for the individual.

- Panproctocolectomy—a permanent ileostomy is created from the terminal ileum. The rectum and anus are removed
- Total colectomy—an ileostomy is formed and the rectal stump is retained which may be brought out onto the abdominal wall as a mucus fistula
- Abdominoperineal (A–P) excision—the rectum and anus are removed leaving a colostomy in the left iliac fossa
- Hartmann's procedure—procedure for excision of sigmoid colon or upper rectum. An end colostomy is formed and the rectal stump is closed and left in the pelvis
- Pelvic exenteration—a radical operation removing pelvic organs. A colostomy and urostomy are formed. Men are likely to become impotent. An artificial vagina can be created for a woman

Issues in stoma management

The stool consistency of a sigmoid colostomy is no different from that passed naturally in health through the anus. The stool is less formed the further proximal in the colon the colostomy is. The formation of an ileostomy or colostomy should not in itself interfere with sexual function unless the definitive surgery interfered with the pelvic nerve supply.

Stoma appliances and problems

Stoma appliances are disposable, self-adhesive and skin-friendly. The type of appliance used is determined by several factors which include the shape and position of the stoma itself, including body contours, the type of effluent, skin type and the needs of the individual such as lifestyle and ability to self care. Adequate adherence, comfort and skin protection are paramount.

Ileostomy appliances are drainable for ease of emptying semi-formed/ liquid stool. Modern appliances have integral velcro-type closures. The bags are emptied several times a day and changed every 1–3 days.

- Colostomy appliances may be in one piece such that the whole appliance needs removing every time the bag needs changing. Alternatively, a two-piece appliance is used which allows the flange to remain in position for for several days, allowing the non-drainable bag to be changed as necessary, protecting the skin from the trauma of frequent changes
- The flange size should be cut to fit accurately around the base of the stoma. The peristomal skin must be kept healthy and intact
- A stoma usually shrinks in size during the first few months but should always retain the bright red colour, indicating a good blood supply
- Checks for colour, odour, consistency and volume should be made routinely

Psychological care

Enjoyment, comfort and satisfaction with life for the patient and his/her family needs support from healthcare professionals, giving adequate time for answering questions and responding to needs. Frequently patients have a short prognosis and the stoma is a visible daily reminder of this. In addition, they may be distressed by a feeling of no longer being in control. They have to learn new skills at a time when it is important to be concentrating on other more important issues, and they may be having to adapt reluctantly to relying on others for care. Relationships with family, friends and particularly spouses may be affected.

Overactive stoma

A cause may need to be identified and treated. Diet may need to be altered until overactivity settles. Foods such as cooked white rice and stewed apple may help. Marshmallows and 'jelly babies' may help in thickening the output from an ileostomy. Extra fluids orally should be encouraged to maintain hydration, especially in hot weather. A drainable bag may be necessary temporarily for a colostomy if the output is liquid. Some medication, particularly longer-acting modified release preparations e.g. MST, enteric coated drugs and capsules, may not be absorbed adequately and are not recommended with ileostomies.

Loperamide (taken three-quarters of an hour before meals) with an ileostomy in the form of 'melts' or tablets but not capsules may be helpful. If all else fails, systemic opioids and antisecretory agents may be needed. 📖 See the section on diarrhoea, p. 258.

Constipation

A cause should be sought where possible and may include medication, particularly opioids, partial/complete bowel obstruction and dehydration. It may be necessary to instil warm arachis oil through a Foley catheter with the balloon inflated (only 5mL for a short time) to aid enema retention. The patient will usually be turned on the right side if the stoma is in the left iliac fossa to allow oil to flow across the transverse colon. The oil may cause difficulties with flange adhesion and the possibility of nut allergy should always be considered. Suppositories, phosphate and microlax micro-enemas may also be useful. As a general rule, bulking aperients such as ispaghula husk (Fybogel) are not used in palliative care.

Odour

This is rarely a problem with modern appliances which contain charcoal filters. Proprietary stoma deodorizing agents are available. A few drops of vanilla essence placed in a bowel stoma bag may help. Topical metronidazole may be helpful for offensive fungating tumours in the region of the stoma.

Bleeding

The stoma may bleed due to clotting deficiencies and fungating tumour. Wafers of kaltostat soaked in tranexamic acid or epinephrine may help with local pressure. Silver nitrate may be used for oozing granulation tissue. Bleeding from local cancer growth may abate with radiotherapy or cryotherapy.

Skin excoriation

Skin excoriation is a rare occurrence with modern appliances and good skin care. Various preparations are available to aid skin protection, including pastes to make a level surface onto which an appliance can be fitted. This is particularly important with an ileostomy, when damage to the skin from digestive enzymes must be avoided.

Flatulence

Flatulence can usually be minimized by avoiding various foods and medication such as lactulose.

A diet with fibre such as porridge, root vegetables and brown bread is advised although the terminally ill may not find these foods palatable. In relatively good health, most people with stomas can eat most foods, although certain food such as vegetables and fruit may cause an increase in stoma activity with embarrassing flatulence and odour. Camomile tea and peppermint tea or capsules may be helpful.

Enterocutaneous fistulae

Enterocutaneous fistulae may occur in 3 per cent of patients with advanced malignant disease. Patients with gastrointestinal tumours and those who have had abdominal radiotherapy are most at risk. A dehisced wound may also need management with a stoma appliance. If the effluent is greater than 100mL per 24 h a stoma appliance will probably be needed.

Meticulous preparation of the skin will be needed prior to applying an appliance. Suction may be needed while cleansing and preparing the fistula if there is excessive exudate, or it may need to be spigotted with a balloon catheter for a while. Various pastes, fillers and skin barriers may be needed to protect the skin and ensure a good fit to the edges of the wound. The stoma appliance may need to be adapted with time to take account of the change in size of the tumour and the weight loss of the patient.

Gastrostomy

A gastrostomy is used for the purpose of feeding when the patient is unable to swallow adequately or safely such as in motor neurone disease, or with head and neck cancers. A venting gastrostomy is occasionally used in a relatively fit patient with intestinal obstruction who wants to be able to eat. In this situation, the patient is able to take nutrients by mouth but food contents are expelled through the gastrostomy.

In patients with advanced disease, the decision to insert a gastrostomy has to be judged carefully.[16] It is important to distinguish starvation, which responds to feeding, from cachexia, which does not respond to feeding alone. The latter is more likely in the presence of large tumour masses, certain tumour types or ongoing sepsis.

Types of gastrostomy

Percutaneous endoscopic gastrostomy (PEG): Inserted under sedation and local anaesthetic using a 'pull' technique. Throughout its lifetime, the PEG tube should be rotated through 360° at least twice a week to prevent adhesion formation.

Radiologically inserted gastrostomy (RIG): Inserted in the radiology department without sedation by a 'push' technique under fluoroscopic control. The tube is thinner than a PEG tube, and is held in place by its pigtail shape. It should NOT therefore be rotated, or it will dislodge.

Surgical gastrostomy: Carried out under general anaesthetic, usually when it is impossible to insert a PEG or RIG.

Care of the gastrostomy tube: The fixation plate should be maintained at 1 to 1.5cm from the abdominal exit stoma. A 50mL flush of sterile water should be used before and after every feed or administration of medication and regularly three times a day. Soda water, but not other fizzy drinks (they are too acidic) can be used to unblock stubborn blockages.

Feeding: Patients should be maintained at an angle of 30–45° during feeding and for two h after to reduce the risk of aspiration. Many centres are less keen for feeding to occur during sleep because of the aspiration risk.

Problems with gastrostomies

- Dislodgement
- Leakage: chemical digestion of surrounding skin
- Overgranulation
- Infection

16 Rabeneck L., Wray P., Petersen N. J. (1996) Long-term outcomes of patients receiving percutaneous endoscopic gastrostomy tubes. *Journal of General Internal Medicine*, **11**, 5: 287–93.

A major concern with the use of PEG and RIG tubes in the UK involves ensuring that the best possible decision about when to insert a tube is taken.

Often the clinical team which asks for a tube to be inserted is different from the team which carries out the procedure which in turn is different from the team who manage the tube once it has been inserted.

While tube insertion can play a crucial rôle for certain patients, especially where clear objectives for the intervention have been discussed and documented with the patient and family, figures show that a large percentage of patients die within weeks of tube insertion, perhaps before they have had time to gain benefit from the procedure and its management.

Further reading

Books

Doyle D., Hanks G., Cherny N. (2004) *Oxford Textbook of Palliative Medicine*. 3rd edn. Oxford: Oxford University Press.

Twycross R. (2001) *Symptom Management in Advanced Cancer*. 3rd edn. Oxford: Radcliffe Medical Press.

Watson M., Lucas C. (2003) *Adult Palliative Care Guidelines*. London: The South West London and the Surrey, West Sussex and Hampshire Cancer Networks.

Articles

Coco C., Cogliandolo S., Riccioni M. *et al.* (2000) Use of a self-expanding stent in the palliation of rectal cancer recurrences. A report of three cases. *Surgical Endoscopy*, **14, 8**: 708–11.

Potter K. (2000) Surgical oncology of the pelvis: ostomy planning and management. *Journal of Surgical Oncology*, **73, 4**: 237–42.

Baines M. J. (2000) Symptom control in advanced gastrointestinal cancer. *Eur J Gastroenterol Hepatol*, **12**: 375–9.

Culbert P., Gillett H. and Ferguson A. (1998) Highly effective new oral therapy for faecal impaction. *British Journal of General Practice*, **48**: 1599–600.

Cachexia, anorexia, and fatigue

Background

Cachexia and fatigue are common symptoms affecting patients with advanced or chronic disease. They are closely related in 70 per cent of patients with advanced cancer, particularly gastric and pancreatic cancer. Apart from marked weight loss and lethargy, there is also an association with physical, emotional and mental symptoms and loss of motivation and social contact.

'Listless, sluggish, faint, despondent, apathetic, tired, slack, indifferent, paralysed', are some of the adjectives used by patients and some describe the fatigue of advanced disease as 'pain'.

Cachexia and fatigue are multifactorial. They are seldom seen in isolation from other symptoms experienced by patients with advanced disease, thus adding to the disease burden.

Cancer has become more of a chronic rather than an acute illness, due to improvements in its management. There is an increased awareness of the suffering caused by cachexia and fatigue but they still remain poorly recognized by clinicians. Advances in management have not kept pace with that for other common symptoms in advanced disease.

Definitions

Cancer-related fatigue is defined by the National Comprehensive Cancer Network as 'a persistent, subjective sense of tiredness related to cancer or cancer treatment that interferes with usual functioning'.[1] It has further been described in terms of

Perceived energy, mental capacity, and psychological status. It rises over a continuum, ranging from tiredness to exhaustion. In contrast with the tiredness sometimes felt by the healthy individual, cancer-related fatigue is perceived as being of greater magnitude, disproportionate to activity or exertion, and not relieved by rest.[2]

Patients may describe fatigue **subjectively** in 3 dimensions:-
Physical sensations—unusual tiredness, and decreased capacity for work
Affective sensations—decreased motivation, mood and energy
Cognitive sensations—decreased concentration and mental agility

Patients may describe fatigue **objectively** as a quantifiable decrease in physical or mental performance

These two experiences of fatigue may not be related, and patients may feel fatigued without any loss of objective performance and vice versa[1]

1 Mock V. *et al.* (2000) NCCN Practice Guidelines for cancer-related fatigue. *Oncology (Huntington)*, **14**: 151–61.

2 Ahlberg K. *et al.* (2003) Assessment and management of cancer-related fatigue in adults. *Lancet*; **362**: 640–50.

Cancer cachexia involves involuntary loss of weight that is not caused simply by anorexia. The syndrome includes anaemia and immunosuppression along with a number of biochemical changes indicating some systemic effects of malignancy. Cachexia is a term derived from the Greek word *kakos*, meaning bad, and *hexis*, meaning condition.

Cancer Cachexia:-

- Weight loss (usually defined as more than five percent of premorbid weight in the previous six months)
- Cancer tumours produce cytokines e.g. cachectin—tumour necrosis factor, interleukin I and VI, lipolytic hormones and proteolysis inducing factor (PIF) which cause metabolic abnormalities such as lipolysis and protein loss
- Progressive loss of lean and adipose tissue that is unrelated to anorexia
- Cannot be reversed by feeding
- Is commonly associated with **anorexia** (the absence or loss of appetite for food) and **asthenia** (a syndrome of physical fatigue, generalised weakness and mental fatigue)
- Affects over eighty percent of patients with advanced cancer and is a major contributor to cancer morbidity and mortality
- Occurs more commonly in solid tumours such as pancreas, lung, stomach, colorectal and oesophagus, but less frequently in carcinoma of the breast and prostate and haematological malignancies
- Creates a major source of distress to patients and families who often seek to reverse it by pressurising the patient to eat more
- Has a negative psychological impact due to body image changes
- Is a constant reminder to patients of underlying disease
- Decreases social interaction and support
- Decreases ability to tolerate and respond to oncological treatments

Prevalence

Fatigue

- Approaching one hundred per cent of patients treated for cancer are affected by fatigue
- Patients report fatigue more commonly when undergoing chemotherapy or radiotherapy, or in the presence of advanced malignancy

Cachexia

- More than 80 per cent of patients with advanced cancer are cachexic

Aetiology

Non-malignant causes of cachexia and fatigue all of which can also contribute to symptoms in advanced cancer.

Infection	Metabolic and electrolyte	Pharmacological toxicity
Anaemia	disorders	Cachexia due to HIV/AIDS or
Chronic hypoxia	Insomnia	progressive illness
Neurological disorders	Malnutrition	Chronic pain
Psychogenic causes	Over-exertion	Dehydration

Reversible causes of 'secondary' anorexia should be actively sought and corrected as appropriate. They include:
- Dyspepsia
- Altered taste
- Malodour
- Nausea and vomiting
- Sore mouth
- Pain
- Biochemical
  - Hypercalcaemia
  - Hyponatraemia
  - Uraemia
  - Gastric stasis
- Constipation
- Secondary to treatment
  - Drugs
  - Radiotherapy
  - Chemotherapy
- Anxiety
- Depression

Psychological and CNS
Learned food aversion
Alterations in taste perception
Psychological stress

Treatment-related effects
Chemotherapy
Nausea, stomatitis,
mucositis
Radiation therapy
Xerostomia, fatigue
Surgery
Pain, ileus

Tumour effects
Mechanical obstruction
Substrate consumption
Cytokine production by tumour
Lipid mobilizing factors

Host-related effects
Increased resting energy expenditure
Alterations in intermediary metabolism
Cytokine production by host macrophages
Autonormic dysfunction
↓ Gastric emptying

Fig. 6c.1 Multifactorial causes of cancer fatigue and cachexia. From Bruera and Higginson, *Cachexia-anorexia in cancer patients* (1996), Oxford University Press.

Metabolic effects

The metabolic changes seen in cachexia differ from those seen in starvation. In starvation, protein is conserved, energy expenditure reduced and fatty acids and ketones become a major source of energy. This contrasts with cancer cachexia where the resting energy expenditure is *increased* and both protein and fat are inefficiently utilized, in association with increased gluconeogenesis.

The reasons behind these metabolic changes are unknown, but postulated mechanisms may include the following:

A non-specific response to the tumour or factors released by the tumour. The presence of a tumour may cause chronic stimulation of the body's inflammatory system leading to classic cachexic metabolic changes, including an increase in carbohydrate, fat and protein catabolism.

- Solid tumours metabolize glucose anaerobically and thus inefficiently, increasing the resting energy expenditure of the body
- The neuroendocrine axis appears to be important in the regulation of appetite
- There is evidence of increased insulin resistance in patients with cancer, and reduced glucose tolerance, perhaps caused by an imbalance of cortisol, insulin and glucagons
- An increase in protein turnover, particularly in skeletal muscle, is associated with the striking loss of lean muscle mass occurring in malignancy associated cachexia
- The acute phase response is the systemic response to inflammation or tissue damage occurring in trauma and sepsis, as well as cancer cachexia. This response appears to be mediated by cytokines. The activity of this response has been shown to correlate with the development of cachexia in patients with malignancy

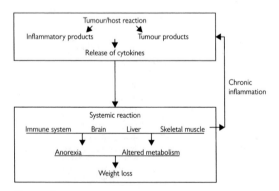

Fig. 6c.2 The systemic inflammatory response and cancer

Management

Cachexia and fatigue can often be anticipated and potentially correctable causes **actively** sought. A multidisciplinary approach maximizes the potential to improve symptoms.

National Comprehensive Cancer Network cancer related fatigue guidelines propose the following:[1]

1 Regular screening of patients using an instrument to evaluate degree of fatigue
2 For those who describe mild fatigue, the subject is discussed and education provided. For those who describe moderate or severe fatigue a fuller, *primary* assessment is required, looking in particular for the presence of:
   • Pain
   • Emotional distress
   • Sleep disturbance
   • Anaemia
   • Hypothyroidism

If such primary factors are detected, they should be treated according to practice guidelines.

If primary factors are not detected a *secondary* comprehensive assessment is advocated, with referral to other healthcare professionals as appropriate, including:
   • Review of medications
   • Assessment of co-morbidities e.g.
      • Nutritional/metabolic evaluation
      • Assessment of activity level

3 If specific causes (and therefore treatment) of fatigue and weakness cannot be found, symptomatic interventions should be considered.

Non-drug interventions

● There is a large body of evidence to suggest that a moderate exercise programme can improve functional capacity, reduce fatigue and improve mood
● Nutritional advice—to eat when hungry, what is enjoyed, in frequent small amounts
● Pacing activity so that important activities can be carried out. Pacing allows gradual adaptation to lower levels of energy
● Promotion of good sleep hygiene
● Help the family: listen to their concerns and explain cachexia. They may need to find other ways of expressing love than being obsessional about quantities of food that can no longer be eaten and that will not alter prognosis

Drug interventions

Corticosteroids (i.e. dexamethasone 4mg o.d.)
● Rapid onset of benefits within 2–3 days
● Rôle is limited by the rapid onset of side-effects (proximal myopathy, fluid retention and insulin resistance) and loss of effectiveness after only a few weeks
● They do not increase lean body mass
● They may be useful to improve appetite and well-being, particularly when prognosis is limited and a fast response is needed

Progestogens (i.e. megestrol acetate 160–320mg/day; medroxyprogesterone acetate 200mg t.d.s.)
- Onset of benefit may take up to two weeks
- Clear evidence of appetite improvement but less clear evidence of anything other than minimal weight gain. Fluid retention may be a problem
- Does not increase lean body mass
- Higher doses of progestogens above 800mg/day not noted to be more effective than lower doses
- Comparisons between corticosteroids and progestogens show no survival advantage, but more side-effects are noted with corticosteroids

Metoclopramide
- Useful in situations where there is gastric stasis
- Prokinetic action counteracts autonomic dysfunction which is common in malignancy
- Reduces nausea

Erythropoietin
- For patients with anaemia, erythropoietin on a weekly basis has been shown to reduce fatigue
- It is unclear if the beneficial effect is due to anaemia correction or a direct erythropoietin effect on its receptors, which have been isolated in several different tissues including the brain
- Expensive treatment
- Most efficient dosage schedules still to be worked out

Future treatment possibilities

There is growing understanding as to the complex nature of the pathophysiological basis of cachexia. Cytokine activity has been strongly implicated in much of the recent research.

However, the processes involved remain complex, with both procatabolic and anticatabolic cytokine involvement, altered inflammatory responses, neuroendocrine effects and the interactions of both tumour and host. Drugs which interrupt the harmful catabolic effects of cytokines are being developed, though it is unlikely that any single agent will be able to benefit every patient with cachexia or fatigue.

The causes of cachexia and fatigue are so multifactorial that it is essential to develop individualized treatment approaches for each particular patient. Such a strategy requires a careful clinical history and examination in order to decide which interventions are appropriate.

As yet the therapeutic tools for such intervention are limited, but if the current research activity bears fruit, the management of patients with anorexia/cachexia syndrome will be transformed.

Table 6c.1 Possible mechanisms of action of established and emerging pharmacological agents in the management of cachexia

Possible mechanism	Agent
Central nervous system effects	Metoclopramide
	Corticosteroids
	Progestational agents
	Cannabinoids
	Thalidomide
Modulate immune response/reduce inflammation	Corticosteroids
	Progestational agents
	Polyunsaturated fatty acids
	Thalidomide
	Melatonin
	NSAIDs
Anabolic effect	Growth hormone/insulin growth factors
	Anabolic agents
	Beta 2 adrenergic agents
Stimulate gastrointestinal motility/ increased gastric emptying	Metoclopramide

Further reading

Books

Doyle D., Hanks G., Cherny N. (2004) *Oxford Textbook of Palliative Medicine*. 3rd edn. Oxford: Oxford University Press.

Bruera E., Higginson I. (1996) *Cachexia-anorexia in cancer patients*. Oxford: Oxford University Press.

Neuenschwander H., Bruera E. (1996) *Cachexia-Anorexia in Cancer Patients*. Oxford: Oxford University Press.

Articles

Ardies C. M. (2002) Exercise, cachexia, and cancer therapy: a molecular rationale. *Nutr Cancer*, **42, 2**: 143–57.

Bruera E., Macmillan K. *et al.* (1990) A controlled trial of megestrol acetate on appetite, caloric intake, nutritional status, and other symptoms in patients with advanced cancer. *Cancer*, **66, 6**: 1279–82.

Bruera E., Neumann C. M. *et al.* (1999) Thalidomide in patients with cachexia due to terminal cancer: preliminary report. *Ann Oncol*, **10, 7**: 857–9.

Curt G. A. (2000) The impact of fatigue on patients with cancer: overview of FATIGUE 1 and 2. *Oncologist*, **5, (Suppl. 2)**: 9–12.

Inui A. (2002) Cancer anorexia-cachexia syndrome: current issues in research and management. *CA Cancer J Clin*, **52, 2**: 72–91.

MacDonald N., Easson A. M. *et al.* (2003) Understanding and managing cancer cachexia. *J Am Coll Surg*, **197, 1**: 143–61.

McMillan D. C., Watson W. S. *et al.* (2001) Albumin concentrations are primarily determined by the body cell mass and the systemic inflammatory response in cancer patients with weight loss. *Nutr Cancer*, **39, 2**: 210–3.

McMillan D. C., Wigmore S. J. *et al.* (1999) A prospective randomized study of megestrol acetate and ibuprofen in gastrointestinal cancer patients with weight loss. *Br J Cancer*, **79, 3–4**: 495–500.

Nelson K. A., Walsh D. (2002) The cancer anorexia-cachexia syndrome: a survey of the Prognostic Inflammatory and Nutritional Index (PINI) in advanced disease. *J Pain Symptom Manage*, **24, 4**: 424–8.

Stone P., Richardson A. *et al.* (2000) Cancer-related fatigue: inevitable, unimportant and untreatable? Results of a multi-centre patient survey. Cancer Fatigue Forum. *Ann Oncol*, **11, 8**: 971–5.

Tchekmedyian N. S., Hickman M. *et al.* (1992) Megestrol acetate in cancer anorexia and weight loss. *Cancer*, **69**: 1268–74.

Toomey D., Redmond H. P. *et al.* (1995) Mechanisms mediating cancer cachexia. *Cancer*, **76, 12**: 2418–26.

Willox J. C., Corr J. *et al.* (1984) Prednisolone as an appetite stimulant in patients with cancer. *Br Med J (Clin Res Ed)*, **288, 6410**: 27.

Wolfe G. (2000) Fatigue: the most important consideration for the patient with cancer. *Caring*, **19, 4**: 46–7.

Sweating and fever

Definition
- Sweating (diaphoresis) is the secretion of fluid onto the skin surface to aid cooling
- Hyperhydrosis is the production of large volumes of sweat
- Sweating is a normal phenomenon in the regulation of body temperature, but in illness can be a troublesome and distressing symptom
- Severity of sweating can change with climate, and perception of the symptom may differ with varying cultural norms

Measurement tools include:
- Symptom diary
- Three grade
- Severity scale (Quigley and Baines 1997[1])
- Six point rating scale (Deaner 2000[2])

To date, none of these tools have been validated nor have their reliabilities been tested.

Causes (common):
- Tumour burden (Chang 1988[3])
- Sepsis
- Lymphoma (neoplastic fever)
- Disseminated malignancy esp. hepatic and renal metastases (neoplastic fever)
- Sex hormone insufficiency due to cancer treatment, especially breast cancer (tamoxifen, induction of menopause by chemotherapy or radiotherapy) and prostate cancer (gonadorelin analogues)

Causes (less common)
- Endocrine disturbance e.g. hypoglycaemia, hyperthyroidism
- Thermoregulation in response to increase in temperature, exertion or nutrition
- Weakness
- Hypoxia
- Severe pain (infarction, fracture)
- Fear and anxiety
- Medication e.g. opioids (rare), antidepressants, ethanol
- Drug reactions; blood products (transfusion reaction)
- Neuropathy (diabetic, autonomic); autoimmune disease, idiopathic

1 Quigley C. S., Baines M. (1997) Descriptive epidemiology of sweating in a hospice population. *Journal of Palliative Care*. **13**: 22–6.

2 Deaner P.B. (2000) The use of thalidomide in the management of severe sweating in patients with advanced malignancy: trial report. *Palliative Medicine*. **14**: 429–31.

3 Chang J. C. (1988) Antipyretic effect of naproxen and corticosteroids on neoplastic fever. *J Pain and Symptom Management*, **3**: 141–4.

Management

- Exclude reversible cause(s) and treat if appropriate
- Supportive measures:
  - decreasing ambient temperature
  - lowering humidity
  - increasing airflow around patient (fan)
  - clothing (modern synthetic materials, e.g. Gore-Tex, allow evaporation)

Pharmacological measures

- Sepsis:
  - Antibiotics if appropriate
  - Paracetamol 1gram p.o./PR qds (effective in palliating sepsis induced sweating)
- Neoplastic fever:
  - Naproxen 250–500mg p.o. b.d. can relieve neoplastic fever for 10–14 days; once stopped, fever recurs in 66 per cent of patients[3]
  - Patients may benefit from switching to an alternative NSAID[4]
  - Corticosteroid therapy with dexamethasone has been shown to reduce symptoms, independently of NSAIDs. However, there is no agreement on starting dose. Suggestion:
    - Start dexamethasone at 1–2mg o.d. and titrate to effect (or to corticosteroid side-effects)
- Sex hormone insufficiency:
  - Venlafaxine 37.5mg p.o. o.d. is effective as is clonidine 0.3–0.4mg p.o. nocte
  - Higher doses of venlafaxine may be required, though this drug can also *cause* sweating[5]
  - Diethylstilboestrol 1–3mg p.o. o.d. improves symptoms in men but risk of thromboembolic events is increased
  - Progestogen therapy is effective in women but has a high side-effect profile
- Non specific treatments:
  - antimuscarinic therapy can block parasympathetic mediated sweating e.g. propantheline p.o. 15mg nocte
  - drugs used for other antimuscarinic effects such as glycopyrronium may also help
  - thalidomide 100mg p.o. nocte[2] has been used in the hospice setting with some effect, though controlled studies are still required
  - Other drugs of reported benefit include:
    - Cimetidine (for opioid induced sweats)
    - Beta-blockers
    - Calcium channel blockers (e.g. diltiazem)
    - Benzodiazepines
    - Olanzapine

4 Tsavaris N., Zinelis A. *et al.* (1990) A randomised trial of the effect of three non-steroid anti-inflammatory agents in ameliorating cancer induced fever. *J of Int Med,* **228**: 451–5.

5 Loprinzi C. L., Barton D. L. *et al.* (2001) Management of hot flashes in breast cancer survivors. *Lancet Oncol,* **2, 4**: 199–204.

Further reading

Books

Back I. (2001) *Palliative Medicine Handbook*. BPM Books: Cardiff.

Doyle D., Hanks G., Cherny N., Calman K. (2004) *Oxford Textbook of Palliative Medicine*. Oxford: Oxford University Press.

Watson M., Lucas C. (2003) *Adult Palliative Care Guidelines*. London: The South West London and the Surrey, West Sussex and Hampshire Cancer Networks.

Articles

Chang J. C. (1988) Antipyretic effect of naproxen and corticosteroids on neoplastic fever. *J Pain and Symptom Management*, **3**: 141–4.

Chang J. C. (1989) Neoplastic fever: a proposal for diagnosis. *Arch Int Med*, **149**: 1728–30.

Loprinzi C. L., Barton D. L. *et al.* (2001) Management of hot flashes in breast cancer survivors. *Lancet Oncol*, **2, 4**: 199–204.

Miller J. I., Ahmann R. D. (1992) Treatment of castration induced menopausal symptoms with low dose diethylstilboestrol in men with advanced prostate cancer. *Urology*, **40, 6**: 499–502.

Quigley C. S., Baines M. (1997) Descriptive epidemiology of sweating in a hospice population. *J Pall Care*, **13, 1**: 22–6.

Further reading

Respiratory symptoms

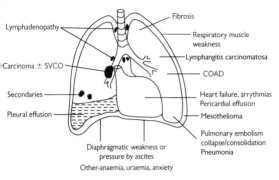

Fig. 6e.1 Causes of breathlessness

Breathlessness[1]

- Breathlessness is common in palliative care (the prevalence is 40–80 per cent in some series)
- Breathlessness is common in patients with cancer
- The pathophysiology of breathlessness is complicated and not fully understood
- Normal breathing is maintained by regular rhythmical activity in the respiratory centre in the brain stem. This is stimulated by *mechanical receptors* (stretch receptors in the airways, lung parenchyma, intercostal muscles and diaphragm) and by hypoxia and high levels of CO_2 (detected by *chemoreceptors* in the aortic and carotid bodies and in the medulla)
- In malignant lung disease, breathlessness is usually due to distortion and stimulation of the mechanical receptors, and blood gases are often normal
- Fatigue, muscle weakness (often due to cachexia or steroid myopathy), phrenic nerve palsy and restrictive chest wall tumours are common problems in cancer that can cause or exacerbate breathlessness
- Muscle weakness, fatigue and anxiety are the predominant factors correlating with breathlessness in cancer

1 Bruera E. (2000) The frequency and correlates of dyspnoea in patients with advanced cancer. *J Pain Symptom Manage*, **19**: 357–62.

Management

Look for reversible causes of breathlessness

- Do not assume that breathlessness is directly caused by cancer
- Reversible causes of breathlessness, such as congestive heart failure, an exacerbation of chronic obstructive airways disease, cardiac arrhythmias, anaemia, pleural/pericardial effusions, bronchial infection and pulmonary emboli, should be treated appropriately
- Breathlessness due to lung cancer per se, can be alleviated in a high proportion of patients with radiotherapy or chemotherapy

Consider causes that may best be treated specifically:	
Lung tumour	Radiotherapy (**RT**) or Chemotherapy
Bronchospasm	Bronchodilators Corticosteroids
Infection	Antibiotics
Pleural effusion	Pleural tap Pleurodesis
Anaemia	Blood transfusion Iron Erythropoetin
Lymphangitis carcinomatosa	Can only be diagnosed on X-ray, and even this may not be diagnostic; suspect when consistent severe breathlessness at rest or on exertion, and widespread fine crepitations in lungs Corticosteroids Diuretics?? Bronchodilators
Large airway obstruction	Diagnosed clinically by difficulty on breathing in, and inspiratory stridor **RT** Stent Laser treatment Brachytherapy Corticosteroids
SVC obstruction	Dilated veins over upper chest and neck, swollen face, neck and arms **RT**

Symptomatic treatment of breathlessness

General management

Relaxation techniques, physiotherapy in the form of percussion, postural drainage or breathing exercises may all be very helpful. Directing a stream of air over the face can reduce the sensation of breathlessness. Explanation and patient confidence that the awareness of breathing will be reduced by the drugs, and that he or she can feel more in control, is essential. Breathlessness clinics, where a multidisciplinary team approach is used to

help breathless patients using a full range of routine and alternative therapies, are available
- Breathlessness tends to cause at least as much (if not more) concern
  among healthcare professionals than other common distressing
  symptoms such as pain
- A calm, positive, logical approach can do much to alleviate the
  distress of the patient and their family as well as other members
  of the healthcare team
- Occasionally breathlessness is very difficult to control despite general
  measures and medication, especially in the terminal situation
- Sedation may then be necessary to alleviate patient and family distress

Medication

Bronchodilators
Even in the absence of obvious 'wheeze', there may be an element of
reversible bronchoconstriction.
- Try:
  - Salbutamol 2.5–5mg 6 h via nebuliser, or 2 puffs q.d.s. via spacer
    device. (Beware of increased anxiety, tremor and tachycardia if used
    regularly)
  - Ipratropium bromide 250–500 mcg 6 h via nebuliser, or 2 puffs q.d.s.
    via spacer device
  - Sodium chloride 0.9 per cent via a nebuliser. (May help liquidize
    tenacious secretions)

Corticosteroids
Steroids are thought to reduce the oedema associated with tumour.
Breathlessness may improve if due to multiple lung metastases, stridor due
to tracheal obstruction, SVCO and lymphangitis carcinomatosa. Benefit
should be apparent within seven days.
- Try:
  - Dexamethasone 4–8mg p.o. daily, for a one week trial. If there
    is no improvement, **stop**

Theophyllines
These can significantly reduce the sensation of breathlessness in the absence
of any bronchodilator effect.
- Try:
  - Theophylline m/r 200mg b.d. (uniphyllin continus)
  - Aminophylline m/r 225–450mg b.d. (phyllocontin continus)
  - Aminophylline can also be given by i/v infusion. (see the *BNF*)
- The half-life of theophylline may be *increased* in hepatic impairment,
  heart failure and with certain drugs including cimetidine, ciprofloxacin,
  and erythromycin
- The half-life is *decreased* in smokers, heavy drinkers and by phenytoin,
  carbamazepine and barbiturates

Opioids
Morphine reduces inappropriate and excessive respiratory drive
and substantially reduces the ventilatory response to hypoxia and
hypercapnia. By slowing respiration, breathing may be made more
efficient, and the sensation of breathlessness reduced.

Morphine does not cause CO_2 retention if used appropriately, and is useful in patients with cancer and with terminal respiratory failure due to chronic obstructive airways disease.
- Try:
  - oral morphine 2.5mg p.o. p.r.n. or regularly 4-h if dyspnoea is continuous

The dose may be escalated if well tolerated but doses above 10–20mg 4-h are unlikely to produce further benefit. Morphine modified release (MST) seems to be less effective for breathlessness than immediate release morphine preparations given 4-h. Nebulised morphine is probably no more useful than nebulised saline, which has some benefit.

Benzodiazepines
Panic with hyperventilation and the fear of suffocation may worsen breathlessness.
- Try:
  - diazepam 2–5mg b.d. and p.r.n.
- Benzodiazepines with shorter half-lives (such as lorazepam or midazolam) can be useful in crisis situations, but there is then a risk of reactive agitation and anxiety as the effect wears off quickly
  - lorazepam 1–2mg p.r.n. (works fast and is well absorbed sublingually)
  - midazolam 5–10mg SC or buccal stat

Oxygen
Oxygen may help breathlessness (or confusion) in patients who are hypoxic either at rest or on exertion. It may help other breathless patients (with a normal PaO_2) because of the effect of facial or nasal cooling, or as a placebo.

Hypoxic respiratory drive usually only starts with $PaO_2 < 8kPa$ (roughly equivalent to an oxygen saturation (SaO_2) of 90%); hypoxic drive is often not significant until $PaO_2 < 5.3kPa$ (approx. SaO_2 75%). Most breathless cancer patients are not hypoxic to this degree and will not benefit from oxygen physiologically. It is difficult to predict those patients who will perceive benefit from oxygen purely from their oxygen saturation.

It is best to avoid *unnecessary* dependency on oxygen, which can limit mobility, may become a barrier between patient and family, and is expensive and inconvenient in the community. Much dependency is caused by injudicious use, leading to habit.

Assessment
If available, a pulse oximeter should be used, and patients with an $SaO_2 \leq 90\%$ (after exertion if appropriate) *should* be offered a trial of oxygen. Those with an $SaO_2 > 90\%$ (or if pulse oximeter not available) *may* be offered a trial if desired.

Trial of oxygen
A trial of oxygen for a fixed period e.g. 15–30 minutes is recommended. After this time the patient should be reassessed, and a decision made as to its benefit. (If it is agreed that it has not helped, the oxygen cylinder/mask may be discontinued). Explanation of the rationale for lack of benefit from oxygen, and offer of alternative strategies, such as a fan, open windows etc. will help.

Domiciliary oxygen

Intermittent or continuous domiciliary oxygen can be prescribed for palliation of breathlessness in patients with cancer. An oxygen concentrator is generally more cost-effective for patients requiring oxygen more than 8 h/day, unless it is only very short term. The 1,360l size of cylinder is the one usually dispensed in the community and at 2l/min this gives about 11 h of use. Warn families about smoking! (Less of a problem with a concentrator.)

Oxygen concentration

Method	Flow rate	% O₂delivered
Nasal cannulae	1l/min	24%
	2l/min	28%
Ventimask	2l/min	24%
	6l/min	35%

Patients with severe COPD who are chronically hypoxic should not be given more than 28% oxygen unless properly monitored for respiratory depression. Many patients with carcinoma of the bronchus also have COPD.

Flow rates of <4l/min via nasal cannulae do not require humidification.

The costs of initiating oxygen therapy are considerable in financial, social, psychological, logistical and safety terms. It should not be undertaken lightly and only after a full discussion of the cost benefits have been explored.

Cannabinoids

Nabilone 0.1–0.2mg orally four times a day may be given for patients who are continually breathlessness, anxious and who do not tolerate other conventional respiratory sedatives. Sedation and dysphoria may occur with higher doses. It is unsuitable for patients with atrial fibrillation or heart failure.

Breathlessness symptomatic treatments summary

Trial of oxygen if patient is hypoxic SaO₂ <90%

Massage, aromatherapy or other relaxation methods

Advise patient on non-drug measures:

    position—sitting upright rather than lying

    cool air from fan or open window

Consider a trial of bronchodilators e.g. nebulised salbutamol 2.5mg q.d.s. Bronchospasm is not always associated with wheeze, and bronchodilators can improve breathlessness without measurable changes in lung function; a therapeutic trial is appropriate for any patient with advanced cancer. Other drug measures include steroids, opioids, and benzodiazepines.

Non-pharmacological management of breathlessness

A non-pharmacological approach to breathlessness in lung cancer works well alongside existing medical treatment. This approach may also be helpful to patients suffering from breathlessness due to end-stage non-malignant disease.

Exploring the patient's experience of breathlessness

An essential prerequisite to managing breathlessness involves understanding what it means to be that person in that particular situation.

- The patient is asked to describe his/her breathlessness experience
- Open acknowledgement of the feelings of 'terror' associated with breathlessness is encouraged
- The patient is helped gently to confront fears of suffocation, choking, not being able to get another breath, or dying during an episode of acute breathlessness. Reassurance is offered that these fears are unlikely to be realized
- The patient's exercise tolerance is ascertained and he/she is asked to identify things which either trigger or alleviate breathlessness
- The impact of breathlessness on the patient's daily life is explored and he/she is assisted in coping with and adjusting to the loss of rôles and activities. It is important to be aware of the extent to which depression may be a component of breathlessness
- Time is given to talk sensitively and at the patient's pace about the disease and associated feelings

Teaching skills to assist the patient in managing breathlessness

The patient is offered an educational programme, consisting of a number of skills and strategies, to manage breathlessness. The programme is dependent on a partnership and therapeutic working relationship between the patient and professional, and has three main aims:

1 **To enable efficient and effective breathing, where possible**. Breathing re-training is a core part of this approach. This involves teaching the patient to use diaphragmatic breathing exercises as a controlled breathing technique when they feel breathless (as opposed to the tendency to breathe rapidly using the upper respiratory, accessory muscles, which tire easily leading to inefficient lung aeration). Diaphragmatic breathing exercises involve a combination of:
   - pursed lip breathing which promotes control, slows the respiratory rate, increases tidal volume and decreases the possibility of airway collapse
   - controlled breathing with the diaphragm, or lower chest which helps to improve function and breaks the pattern of upper chest breathing
2 **To enable the patient to feel in control by reducing anxiety and panic**. The effect of tension and anxiety versus the effect of relaxation on breathlessness, and the concept of the mind–body link are fully discussed with the patient. Relaxation and distraction techniques are taught with the purpose of reducing residual tension, and for use when anxiety and panic are exacerbating breathlessness.
3 **To enable the patient to adjust and conserve energy for activities which are important to them**. Pacing, prioritizing and problem-solving in relation to activity are explored with the patient. Advice is offered on managing activities of daily living such as:
   - washing/showering/bathing
   - dressing and undressing
   - bending
   - climbing stairs
   - talking on the telephone
   - making love
   - carrying shopping/heavy objects
   - gardening

Goal-setting for learning breathing techniques, in relation to activity, is encouraged. It is important that this is realistic and achievable. The patient is given both verbal and written information focusing on the skills taught.

Other non-pharmacological measures

- A draught of air from a fan, or open window may be helpful to some patients
- Massaging the patient's back during an episode of respiratory panic can encourage muscular relaxation and may be comforting to someone experiencing an attack of breathlessness
- Positioning of the patient in bed is important. The upright position uses gravity to assist in lung expansion and to reduce pressure from the abdomen on the diaphragm. Lying high on one side can be helpful to the patient with copious secretions by preventing aspiration. Getting the patient to sit in a good position assists relaxation of the upper chest muscles and encourages freer use of the diaphragm. The patient can achieve this by sitting forward and resting the arms on the thighs. The wrists should be relaxed

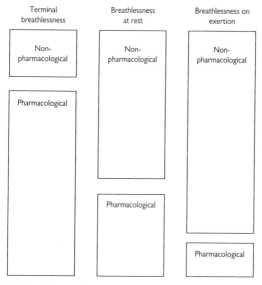

Fig. 6e.2 The relative contributions of pharmacological and non-pharmacoligical approches for the management of breathlessness in patients with cancer according to the severity of the breathlessness and the patient's prognosis. From J. Corner et al. (1997) *The Palliative Management of Breathlessness*. London: European Congress for Palliative Care

Pleural aspiration (thoracocentesis)

General

Aspiration of a pleural effusion can give symptomatic relief from dyspnoea. A pleural effusion large enough to cause dyspnoea will be detectable clinically. Aspiration of 300–500mL fluid will usually give some symptomatic improvement, but up to 1.5 litres may be aspirated in some cases.

Complications

Haemothorax can occur, either from damage to the lung or from vascular pleural tumour. Pneumothorax can occur due to puncture of the lung. A significant pneumothorax is unlikely after an uncomplicated aspiration if simple precautions are taken. A routine check X-ray after aspiration is not essential in a palliative care setting.

If a small i/v cannula is used for aspiration as opposed to a large-bore chest drain, very little air can enter through the cannula if reasonable care is taken. Aspiration of a very large effusion that is causing the heart and mediastinum to be displaced may cause cardiovascular embarrassment.

Infection is a rare complication, providing an aseptic technique is used.

Investigations

A chest X-ray will show a pleural effusion, but it can be difficult to differentiate an effusion from collapse/consolidation or a mixture of the two. An ultrasound scan will confirm the presence of a pleural effusion, and many radiologists will mark a site for aspiration if requested.

Chest X-ray or ultrasound scan should be performed if:
- A clinically-diagnosed pleural effusion has not been confirmed radiologically
- The clinical signs are not straightforward

Platelet count and a clotting screen should be checked if the patient has any symptoms of bleeding or unexplained bruising.

Contra-indications
- local skin infection
- coagulopathy—platelets <40 or INR >1.4
- the presence of local pleural tumour is a relative contra-indication, as tumour cells may be 'seeded' in the chest wall

The procedure
- The patient should sit on a chair, leaning forward, resting the head on folded arms on a pillow on a bedside table
- Use the site marked by ultrasound scan, OR
- Choose a point in the posterior chest wall, medial to the angle of the scapula, one intercostal space below the upper limit of dullness to percussion. The mid-axillary line can also be used
- Confirm that the site is dull to percussion
- Avoid the inferior border of the rib above since the neurovascular bundle runs in a groove inferior to the rib
- Inject local anaesthetic into the skin over the area. When the area is anaesthetized, it is helpful to advance the needle until pleural fluid is obtained which will confirm the depth of the pleural fluid beneath the skin surface and confirm a suitable site for aspiration, thereby minimizing the risk of complications

- Introduce a large-bore i/v cannula with syringe attached until fluid is just obtained, then advance a further 0.5–1cm to ensure that the cannula is in the pleural space
- Asking the patient to exhale against pursed lips (to increase intrathoracic pressure), remove the metal trochar or needle and immediately attach a 50/60mL syringe via a three-way tap
- Aspirate fluid 50mL at a time, until:
  - 1 litre has drained (1500mL maximum),
  - or the patient starts to cough,
  - or giddiness, light-headedness or chest discomfort occur
- Remove the cannula, having asked the patient to take a breath, and immediately seal with flexible collodion BP, and cover with a dressing

Further reading

Books

Ahmedzai S. (1998) Palliation of respiratory symptoms. In D. H. Doyle et al. (eds) Textbook of Palliative Medicine, 2nd edn, pp. 583–616. Oxford: Oxford University Press.

Davis C. L. (1998) Breathlessness, cough and other respiratory problems. In M. Fallon, B. O'Neill (eds) ABC of Palliative Care, pp. 8–11. London: BMJ Books.

Wilcock A. (1997) Dyspnoea. In P. Kaye (ed.) Tutorials in Palliative Medicine, pp. 227–49. Northampton: EPL Publications.

Articles

Booth S., Kelly M. J., Cox N. P., Adams L., Guz A. (1996) Does oxygen help dyspnoea in patients with cancer? American Journal of Respiratory and Critical Care Medicine **153, 5**: 1515–18.

Bredin M., Corner J., Krishnasamy M., Plant H., Bailey C., A'Hern, R. (1999) Multicentre randomised controlled trial of nursing intervention for breathlessness in patients with lung cancer. British Medical Journal, **318**: 901–4.

Bruera E. et al. (1990) Effects of morphine on the dyspnoea of terminal cancer patients. Journal of Pain and Symptom Management, **5**: 341–4.

Connolly M., O'Neill, J, (1999) Teaching a research-based approach to the management of breathlessness in patients with lung cancer. European Journal of Cancer Care, **8**: 30–6.

Reuben D. B., Mor V. M. (1986) Dyspnoea in terminally ill cancer patients. Chest, **89, 2**: 234–6.

Ripamonti C. (1999) Management of dyspnea (sic) in advanced cancer patients. Supportive Care in Cancer, **7, 4**: 233–43.

Van der Molen B. (1995) Dyspnoea: a study of measurement instruments for the assessment of dyspnoea and their application for patients with advanced cancer. Journal of Advanced Nursing, **22, 5**: 948–56.

Cough

Cough may be present in up to 50 per cent of patients with terminal cancer and in up to 80 per cent of patients with lung cancer. It occurs as a result of mechanical and chemical irritation of receptors in the respiratory tracts. The cough reflex involves afferent nerve input to the medulla and efferents to the respiratory muscles. The causes are similar to those causing shortness of breath.

Prolonged bouts of coughing are exhausting and frightening, especially if associated with dyspnoea and haemoptysis, and can also lead to vomiting.

Management

This will depend on the cause of the coughing, which may or may not be reversible, and the clinical status of the patient. The glottis has to close briefly in order to generate sufficient intrathoracic pressure to expel sputum, which may not be possible if there is paralysis of one vocal cord, as can occur in carcinoma of the left upper lung. Coughing in this situation becomes less effficient and may become physically tiring. Active intervention, such as drainage of a pleural effusion, may be appropriate for patients with a relatively long prognosis, whereas comfort and relief of symptoms would be the therapeutic aim for patients in the terminal phase.

The palliation of distressing cough should follow the same general principles as for dyspnoea, remembering that reversible underlying causes should be sought and treated where possible and appropriate.

Symptomatic management of cough

The main distinction to be made is between a productive, wet cough and a dry cough.

Productive/wet cough

Promotion of an easy, effective cough to clear the mucus should be the aim, unless the patient is dying, and too weak to expectorate. Antibiotics may be appropriate, even in very ill patients, as symptomatic treatment for cough.

For patients still able to cough effectively with help:
• Nebulised sodium chloride 0.9 per cent 2.5mL q.d.s. and p.r.n.
  • May help to loosen tenacious mucus and aid expectoration, but patients must be capable of swallowing the large amounts of sputum/liquid that may collect. The evidence for using drugs which aim to reduce the viscosity of mucus, such as carbocysteine (500–750 t.d.s. p.o.) is weak, but they do have some effect on reducing the number of exacerbations of COPD and the length of the episode. Again, patients must be able to swallow well, as the production of copious amounts of secretions may be triggered

Bronchospasm should be treated with nebulised salbutamol.

Patients who are not imminently terminal may benefit from standard vibration, percussion and postural drainage, to help clear sputum, from the physiotherapist. Weaker patients are helped by explanations and being shown breathing techniques.

For chronic persistent infection causing cough, nebulised gentamicin can be considered.

Antitussives should ideally be avoided, but may be helpful at night to aid sleep (📖 see below for choice).

For patients who are dying and too weak to cough:

Antimuscarinics and cough suppressants should be used. Occasionally bronchorrhoea (voluminous amounts of clear frothy sputum which occurs in 6 per cent of cases of alveolar cell cancer of lung and 9 per cent of other lung cancers), may be very debilitating. Radiotherapy should be considered, but other suggested symptomatic treatments are largely **anecdotal**;

- Antimuscarinic drugs (e.g. ipratropium (nebulised) or glycopyrronium (SC) or hyoscine (SC))
- Cough suppressants (see below—usually diamorphine CSCI if patient is dying)
- Corticosteroids p.o.
- Macrolide antibiotics (erythromycin, clarithromycin)
- Nebulised furosemide 20mg q.d.s.

Dry cough

A dry cough should be suppressed, once measures have been taken to exclude or treat an underlying reversible cause.

- Nebulised sodium chloride 0.9 per cent 2.5mL q.d.s. may be helpful, by reducing the irritation of dry airways (breathing oxygen or mouth-breathing) and helping loosen the normal bronchial secretions

Cough suppressants

If it is not possible to reverse the cause of the cough or appropriate to continue to encourage expectoration, cough suppressants will be needed.

1 Peripheral suppressants:

- As an alternative to relieving the cause of the cough or to aiding expectoration, it may be more appropriate to aim for cough suppression, particularly in a patient who is terminally ill. Local anaesthetics block cough receptors in the carina and bronchioles and may therefore be useful in endobronchial malignancy. Bupivacaine (5mL of 0.25 per cent t.d.s.) and lidocaine (5mL of 0.2 per cent t.d.s.) have been used via ultrasonic nebulisers with effect. Pharyngeal anaesthesia occurs and food and drink should be avoided for an hour or so after treatment to avoid aspiration. The first dose should be given as an inpatient in case of reflex bronchospasm

Cause	Treatment
Pharyngeal irritation	Simple linctus
Bronchial irritation	Nebulised bupivacaine

2 Central suppressants:

- Pholcodine 10mL t.d.s. is non-analgesic, causes less sedation and constipation than analgesic opioids and should be tried first for patients not already on opioids
- Codeine 30mg q.d.s. and increased if needed to 60mg q.d.s. may be useful or alternatively morphine 5mg 4-h p.o., or diamorphine 5–10mg/24h CSCI, as appropriate. The dose should be titrated as for pain until either it is successful or side-effects intervene. If a patient is already taking opioids, a dose increment or two should be tried, but there is little evidence supporting the use of high

doses of opioids for cough. Nebulised morphine has been tried but may not be much more effective than nebulised sodium chloride 0.9 per cent
- The efficacy of hydromorphone, oxycodone and fentanyl is not well described
- Methadone is a little more potent than morphine and may be more useful. The long duration of action means that a single dose may be given. A trial should be considered if the patient cannot tolerate morphine in low doses (e.g. <10mg 4-h). The usual starting dose is methadone 2mg (2mL of 1mg/mL solution)
- Inhaled sodium cromoglycate 10mg q.d.s. has been used for cough in lung cancer, usually acting within 48 h

Diazepam may also be needed to relieve anxiety and distress and as a central cough depressant.

	Comparable antitussive dose
Pholcodine	10mg
Dextromethorphan	10–15mg
Dextropropoxyphene	10–12.5mg
Codeine	15mg
Dihydrocodeine	15mg
Morphine	2.5–5mg
Methadone	2mg
Benzonatate	100mg

Haloperidol and antitussives
Studies on experimental models have shown that pre-treatment with haloperidol markedly reduces the antitussive effect of pentazocine and dextromethorphan. Haloperidol is a potent sigma-ligand and it is suggested that the antitussive effect is mediated by sigma-sites. Clinical relevance is unknown, but a trial of an antiemetic other than haloperidol may be worth trying if a patient has intractable cough resistant to antitussives.

Oncological measures
As a generalization, palliative radiotherapy (for non-small cell lung tumours) and chemotherapy (for small cell lung tumours and metastatic lung disease) is good palliative treatment. Cough may be relieved in up to 80 per cent of patients.

Antibiotics
Chest infections commonly occur in the last few days of life. It may be inappropriate to treat relatively asymptomatic bronchopneumonia. However, infected chest secretions may be copious and more effectively treated with antibiotics than with symptomatic measures alone. Frequently patients have had several prior courses of antibiotics, in which case a short course of a broad spectrum antibiotic may be justified. Offensive sputum suggestive of anaerobic infection may respond to metronidazole.

Nebulised gentamicin is used quite frequently in cystic fibrosis. Purulent secretions colonized with gram negative organisms can be treated with nebulised gentamicin 80mg b.d.–t.d.s. with a significant reduction in the volume of secretions. Negligible systemic absorption has been shown.

Anecdotally, massive terminal haemoptysis is associated with anaerobic smelling foetor.

Further reading

Doyle D. H., Hanks G. W. C., McDonald N. (1998) *Oxford Textbook of Palliative Medicine*. 3rd edn. Oxford: Oxford University Press.

Zylicz Z., Krajnik M. (2004) The use of antitussive drugs in terminally ill patients. *Europ J Pall Care*. **11**: 225–9.

Skin problems in palliative care

A man's illness is his private territory and, no matter how much he loves you and how close you are, you stay an outsider. You are healthy.

Lauren Bacall, *By Myself*, 1978

Wound care in cancer

Skin infiltration with subsequent ulceration or fungating wounds can be distressing. A small metastatic skin nodule is a visual reminder of disease progression and a fungating carcinoma with malodour, discharge and bleeding add to the misery of advanced and uncontrolled metastatic disease.

Loco-regional skin involvement (e.g. breast fungation) should be distinguished from generalized skin metastases which imply very late disease. Local extension of malignant tumour leads to embolization of blood and lymphatic vessels, compromising tissue viability. Infarction of the tumour leads to necrosis with subsequent infection, particularly anaerobic.

The ideal aim is complete healing through either local or systemic treatment, which may involve surgery, radiotherapy, hormonal manipulation or chemotherapy. If such treatment is inappropriate, then care is directed to the minimisation of:

- pain
- infection
- bleeding
- odour
- psychological trauma

Treatment should be realistic and acceptable to the patient and carers. The primary aim is the promotion of comfort (as opposed to healing) and the enhancement of quality of life, which may hitherto have been severely impaired.

Following assessment of the problems, choose a dressing regime to meet the needs of the patient. Be prepared to change and experiment since there are no rights or wrongs. The aim is to contain problems and improve quality of life.

Continually re-evaluate

There are numerous commercially available products: alginates, hydrocolloids, hydrogels, semi-permeable films, cavity foams, desloughing agents and charcoals. All may have a place in the management of chronic wounds. The health professional must keep abreast of the merits of established and newer products. The simplest products may be the best and the most cost-effective.

The criteria are comfort, acceptability, and availability.

Choosing a wound care regime
Consider:-
- Pain
- Exudate
- Necrotic tissue
- Bleeding
- Comfort
- Odour
- Infection
- Cosmesis
- Patient Lifestyle
- Psychological Effects

Pain
Ensure that pain is caused neither by infection nor the dressing itself. Try to stick to simple regimes, limiting the frequency of dressing changes. Non-stick and sealed dressings may be useful. Prior to applying the dressing, use short-acting analgesia, or relaxation techniques after discussing the options with the patient.

Exudate
Use dressings with high absorbency and further packing on top in addition to plastic pads to protect clothing. Change the top layer as often as necessary, avoiding frequent changes of dressings placed directly over the wound. Protect the surrounding good skin with Cavilon TM barrier cream or, if skin is broken, use Cavilon TM no-sting barrier film spray.

Necrotic tissue
Surgical debridement may be necessary to remove dead tissue and larvae therapy may also be appropriate.

Bleeding
Gauze soaked in adrenaline 1:1000 or sucralfate liquid or alternatively kaltostat may be used over bleeding points. Gentle removal of dressing with normal saline spray, Steripods or irrigation using a syringe containing warm sodium chloride 0.9 per cent prevents trauma at dressing changes. Kaltostat becomes a jelly-like substance and can be easily lifted off using forceps or gloved fingers. Sorbsan dressings become liquefied and can be washed off with sodium chloride 0.9 per cent. It is preferable to use dressings that can be left in place for a few days to prevent frequent dressing changes—these include the alginates kaltostat, sorbsan and sorbsan plus.

Odour
Use systemic or topical metronidazole but consider limiting to seven days use, as aerobes may increase in numbers on removal of natural competition of anaerobic bacteria. Charcoal dressings are useful and the wound should be sealed. Disguise the smell with deodorizers used sparingly on top of the dressing.

Infection
This is usually chronic and localized. The wound should be cleaned with sodium chloride 0.9 per cent or preferably under running water in the shower or the bath. If the surrounding areas are inflamed, especially if there is spreading inflammation, not just a red rim, antibiotic(s) should be used.

The commonest organisms grown in fungating, cancerous wounds and in pressure sore areas include coliforms, anaerobes, staphylococcus aureus and group G beta-haemolytic streptococcus. Staphylococcus aureus is probably the commonest pathogen.

Antibiotics such as flucloxacillin or, failing this, trimethoprim or erythromycin should cover most common infections, but metronidazole may be needed for anaerobic infections and topical metronidazole gel is particularly useful for eradicating the associated noxious smell. Methicillin-resistant Staphylococcus aureus (MRSA) is difficult to eradicate. It may not necessarily result in morbidity to the patient, but there is clearly a transmission risk to other immunocompromised individuals. Present guidelines for inpatients suggest isolation of patients who are MRSA infected or colonized and the observance of strict 'standard' isolation precautions.

Remember that agents such as cephalosporins, which cover a wider spectrum of bacterial infections, increase the risk of Clostridium difficile diarrhoea.

Comfort
By trial and error, a combination of dressings and top packing that is most comfortable for the individual patient will be needed.

Cosmesis
The best cosmetic effect possible should be achieved, in order to boost confidence.

Lifestyle
Patients may need different regimes for different occasions. For social occasions, avoid bulky unsightly dressings. Large sheet hydrocolloids may be more appropriate. Daily relaxing baths, perfumes and cosmetics should be encouraged to promote well-being and confidence. Use minimal skin strapping by fixing dressings with vests, cling film, netelast or incontinence pads (which may be more comfortable).

Psychological effects
Attention to detail and, in particular, ensuring leakproof/odourproof appliances and giving information and explanation will lessen the sense of isolation and enhance confidence and morale.

Further reading

Books

Grocott P., Dealey C. (2004) In D. H. Doyle et al. (eds) Textbook of Palliative Medicine, pp. 628–40. 3rd edn. Oxford: Oxford University Press.

Mill C. (1998) Skin problems in palliative care: nursing aspects.

Pruritus (itch)

Pruritus may be defined as 'an unpleasant sensation that provokes the desire to scratch'. The prevalence is 27 per cent with the common cancers and 80 per cent in the presence of cholestasis.

Pathogenesis of pruritus

This is complex and not fully elucidated, but it is known that both central and peripheral mechanisms are involved. A number of mediators including serotonin, neuropeptides, cytokines, prostaglandins and growth factors are being studied to generate future treatment options.

Complications of pruritus

- Excoriation +/– secondary infection
- Lack of sleep, social unacceptability, interference with daily functioning
- Depressive symptoms in up to one third of patients with generalized pruritus

Medical history assessment of the pruritic patient

- Generalised or localised itch
- Drug history
- Exacerbating factors
- Previous medical history

Causes of pruritus in patients with cancer

These can be divided into general causes of pruritus (which occur in the healthy population as well as those with cancer) and those specifically related to malignancy. In either case pruritus may be localized or generalized.

Senile itch

This is experienced by 50–70 per cent of those over the age of 70 years. The majority have xerosis and skin atrophy, in others the cause is unknown. It is best treated with general measures (see below) and the application of emollient cream.

Iatrogenic itch

The following drugs are common causes: opioids, aspirin, amfetamines and drugs that can cause cholestasis such as erythromycin, hormonal treatment and phenothiazines.

Iron deficiency

This can cause pruritus with or without anaemia, and responds to iron replacement.

Hormonal itch

Pruritus occurs in up to 11 per cent of patients with thyrotoxicosis, particularly long-term untreated Graves' disease, and less commonly in hypothyroidism. The link between diabetes mellitus and pruritus is controversial.

Management of pruritus

Removal of causative agents (e.g. drugs) and the appropriate investigation and treatment of underlying disease are essential first-line measures. Management can be divided into general and cause-specific.

Evidence for the use of different systemic agents in the treatment of pruritus is limited, but specific drugs may be useful for specific situations as outlined below.

General management

For intact skin

- Ensure that the skin is not dry
- Discontinue using soap
- Use emulsifying ointment or aqueous cream as a soap substitute, or add oilatum to bath water
- Avoid hot baths
- Dry skin gently by patting with soft towel (not rubbing)
- Apply aqueous cream or alternative emollient ('moisturizer') to the skin after a bath or shower each evening
- Avoid overheating (wear light clothes) and sweating day and night (may need an antimuscarinic agent)
- Use sedatives, such as benzodiazepines, to help improve associated anxiety and insomnia
- Discourage scratching; keep nails short; allow gentle rubbing; wear cotton gloves at night
- Avoid exacerbating factors such as heat, dehydration, anxiety and boredom
- Avoid alcohol and spicy foods which may worsen itch
- Consider behavioural treatments and hypnotherapy, which may help ease associated psychological issues and break the cycle of itching and scratching
- Consider TENS and acupuncture

For macerated skin

- Dry the skin and protect from excessive moisture
- Use a hair dryer on cool setting
- Apply surgical spirit to assist evaporation
- Apply a wet compress t.d.s. and allow it to dry out completely
- If infected, use an antifungal solution e.g. clotrimazole
- If very inflamed, use 1 per cent hydrocortisone solution for 2–3 days
- Avoid adsorbent powders e.g. starch, talc, zinc oxide which may form a hard abrasive coating on the skin and be abrasive

Cause-specific management

Itchy skin rashes and insect bites

One–two per cent menthol in aqueous cream or oily calamine lotion with 0.5 per cent phenol (which can be enhanced up to 1 per cent) may be useful. Antihistamine creams should be used when the cause of itch is thought to be histamine-related, e.g. acute drug rash. Prolonged topical use, however, may lead to contact dermatitis, which is best treated with 1 per cent hydrocortisone until it has settled.

Paraneoplastic itch

Cancer per se is an infrequent, but important, cause of generalized pruritus (paraneoplastic itch), the mechanism for which is unknown. Pruritus is particularly associated with haematological malignancies such as Hodgkin's lymphoma and polycythaemia rubra vera.

Treatment of an underlying lymphoma with steroids (dexamethasone 4–8mg o.d. or prednisolone 30–60 o.d.) may be helpful. There is some evidence that paroxetine 5–20mg o.d. (see below), mirtazepine 7.5–15mg o.n. or cimetidine 800mg a day (or other H_2 receptor antagonists) may be effective (see below). Thalidomide may also be useful but its association with teratogenicity and peripheral nerve damage may be difficult to manage.

Cimetidine, an H_2 receptor antagonist, has been shown to be helpful in itch associated with lymphoma and polycythaemia rubra vera. This is not thought to be a direct antihistaminic effect as it has little effect on itching caused by histamine, but is thought to be related to its inhibitory action on liver enzymes which are involved in the synthesis of endogenous opioids, and possibly other agents, causing pruritus.

Paroxetine, a selective serotonin reuptake inhibitor (SSRI) antidepressant, has been shown to relieve itch in a case series of patients with advanced cancer with paraneoplastic and opioid-induced itch probably due to downregulation of $5\text{-}HT_3$ receptors, but side-effects (nausea, vomiting and sedation) may limit its use.

Opioid-induced pruritus

Itch is a well recognized side-effect of opioids and a switch to an alternative opioid (or stopping if possible) may be helpful.

Ondansetron has been shown to be useful in opioid-induced itch at traditional antiemetic doses, although most studies pertain to its success in treating the pruritus associated with opioids given by infusion into the epidural/spinal area. Opioid antagonists are theoretically useful in reducing pruritus but may reverse the essential analgesic effects.

Cholestasis

In palliative care, cholestasis (causing itch) occurs most commonly due to obstruction of the common bile duct from primary or secondary tumours involving the pancreas and biliary tree. (It may also occur as a result of gallstones, drugs or intrahepatic disease.) Stenting of the common bile duct and relief of jaundice should relieve the itch and dexamethasone may be of some help. Drug treatment may include an opioid antagonist (e.g. naltrexone 12.5–25.0mg o.d.) which may be helpful if the patient is not taking opioids for pain relief or an androgen (e.g. methyltestosterone 25mg SL o.d., or danazol 200mg o.d.–t.d.s.). Alternatively, rifampicin 75mg o.d.–150mg b.d. may be used or colestyramine (unpalatable and not effective in complete biliary obstruction) or charcoal which is equally unpalatable.

Renal failure

The pathogenesis of pruritus in renal failure has not been fully defined, but is thought to be multifactorial. Pruritus may be localized (in 70 per cent) or generalized, and is more common in patients receiving dialysis than in those who are not. Ultraviolet light/phototherapy may be helpful. Opioid antagonists such as naltrexone may be effective but cannot be used in patients already receiving opioids because of the risk of reversing analgesia. Ondansetron, mirtazepine and thalidomide have been shown to be effective for generalized itch, whereas topical capsaicin cream can be effective for localized itch.

Further reading

Books

Doyle D. H., Hanks G. W. C., McDonald N. (2004) *Oxford Textbook of Palliative Medicine*. 3rd edn. Oxford: Oxford University Press.

Articles

Borgeat A., Stirnemann H. R. (1999) Ondansetron is effective to treat spinal or epidural morphine-induced pruritus. *Anesthesiology*, **90**: 432–6.

Breneman D. L., Cardone J. S., Blumsack R. F. *et al.* (1992) Topical capsaicin for treatment of hemodialysis-related pruritus. *J Am Acad Dermatol*, **26**: 91–4.

Connolly C. S., Kantor G. R., Menduke H. (1995) Hepatobiliary pruritus: What are effective treatments? *J Am Acad Dermatol*, **33**: 801–5.

Daly B. M., Shuster S. (2000) Antipruritic action of thalidomide. *Acta Dermato-vener*, **80, 1**: 24–5.

Ebata T., Izumi H., Aizawa H. *et al.* (1998) Effects of nitrazepam on nocturnal scratching in adults with atopic dermatitis: a double blind placebo-controlled crossover study. *Br J Dermatol*, **138, 4**: 631–4.

Krajnik M., Zylicz Z. (2001) Understanding pruritus in systemic disease. *J Pain Symptom Manage*, **21, 2**: 151–68.

Sheehan-Dare R. A., Henderson M. J., Cotterill J. A. (1990) Anxiety and depression in patients with chronic urticaria and generalized pruritus. *Br J Dermatol*, **123, 6**: 769–74.

Zylicz Z., Smits C., Krajnik M. (1998) Paroxetine for pruritus in advanced cancer. *J Pain Symptom Manage*, **16**: 121–4.

Lymphoedema

Lymphoedema is a collection of excessive interstitial fluid with a high protein content and is associated with chronic inflammation and fibrosis. It may occur in any part of the body, generally in a limb. It is progressive and may become a grossly debilitating condition. Acute inflammation and trauma cause a rapid increase in swelling. In patients with cancer, lymphoedema is usually due to blockage of lymphatic vessels and glands by malignancy or by fibrosis as a result of previous radiotherapy or surgery.

The aim of treatment is to prevent complications developing, and to achieve maximum improvement and long-term control. Success requires full patient cooperation and treatment strategies devised by the physiotherapist or lymphoedema nurse may include the following:

- Explanation, information and encouragement
- Scrupulous skin care
- Avoidance of trauma, such as sunburn, or venepuncture to minimize infection risks

Massage

- *Manual lymphatic drainage* is a very gentle form of massage used to encourage lymph flow from areas of congestion to areas of normal lymphatic drainage
- *Simple lymphatic drainage* is taught to patients and their carers and, paradoxically, involves very gentle, slow massage beginning from areas of healthy lymphatic drainage towards areas of lymphatic obstruction, 'opening up' the drainage channels

Additional management

- Compression stockings and sleeves can give support and help to prevent fluid accumulating. These may be extremely effective within 24–48 h in patients suffering from lymphorrhoea
- Exercises which should be gentle but performed regularly within compression hosiery
- Compression pumps and intensive low compression bandaging may also be needed for slowly resolving oedema

Contra-indications to compression include local extensive cutaneous metastases, truncal oedema (since fluid from a limb may be diverted to an already congested area), infection or venous thrombosis. Various drugs which influence capillary protein flux and filtration and reduce protein viscosity in interstitial spaces are currently under evaluation but are not in regular use.

Chronic lymphoedema leads to changes in both subcutaneous tissue and skin which make them vulnerable to infection

- Careful hygiene reduces the risk of infection and moisturizing skin creams should be liberally applied to prevent drying and cracking. Any suggestion of impending infection requires prompt treatment with antibiotics
- Diuretics are of limited value in the treatment of lymphoedema, unless the swelling has deteriorated since the prescription of a NSAID or systemic corticosteroid or there is a cardiac or venous component

Further reading

Doyle D. H., Hanks G. W. C., Cherny N. (2004) *Oxford Textbook of Palliative Medicine*. 3rd edn. Oxford: Oxford University Press.

Portenoy R. K., Thaler H. T., Kornblith A. B. *et al.* (1994) Symptom prevalence, characteristics and distress in a cancer population. *Quality of Life Research*, **3**: 183–9.

Twycross, R., Jenns K., Todds J. (2000) *Lymphoedema*. Oxford: Radcliffe Medical Press.

Genito-urinary problems

Anatomy and physiology of the bladder and micturition

Patients with palliative care needs may suffer a variety of symptoms attributable to dysfunction of the urinary system. In order to focus treatment appropriately, it is helpful to understand the basic anatomy and physiology.

Bladder wall

- Made up of detrusor muscle, which is a smooth muscle with an adventitial outer covering together with a supporting inner submucosa for a specialized transitional cell epithelium
- Detrusor muscle forms a functional syncitium with relatively indistinct muscle layers. The outer and inner layers of muscle bundles tend to be longitudinal in orientation with a middle layer circularly orientated
- Bladder emptying is accompanied by detrusor contraction
- The trigone is a smooth, sensitive triangular area at the base of the bladder with apices formed by the ureteric orifices and the internal urinary meatus or bladder neck

Sphincter active urethra

- The distal sphincter mechanism is situated just beneath the prostate in males and in the distal half of the urethra in females. There is a smooth muscle component and a striated muscle component within the wall of the urethra
- The striated muscle component, the intrinsic rhabdosphincter, is the most important component for maintaining continence
- The striated sphincter contains fatigue-resistant, slow-twitch fibres that are responsible for passive urinary control. Voluntary contraction of the levator ani musculature is responsible for active continence

Nerve supply of bladder and urethra

- Micturition is partly a reflex and partly a voluntary act
- Parasympathetic nerve fibres in the anterior sacral roots of S2 to S4 are the principle motor supply to the detrusor muscle. Parasympathetic (cholinergic) nerve stimulation results in bladder contraction and bladder neck sphincter relaxation, allowing micturition
- Smooth muscle in the region of the bladder neck and prostate is regulated by sympathetic fibres from the hypogastric plexus arising from T11 to L2. Sympathetic stimulation relaxes the detrusor muscle (beta-adrenoceptors) and contracts the bladder neck sphincter, preventing micturition. The rôle of the sympathetic nervous system in the female is less exact
- The functional innervation of urethral smooth muscle is adrenergic

- Somatic innervation comes from S2 to S4 as the pudendal nerve to the striated muscle of the sphincter
- The neurovascular bundles running alongside the prostate carry the autonomic innervation of the sphincter active urethra as well as the cavernous nerves responsible for erections. It is these nerves which may be damaged during radical prostatectomy with resulting erectile dysfunction

Clinical relevance of nerve supply

Anticholinergic drugs, including hyoscine and tricyclic antidepressants, cause urinary retention by causing relaxation of the detrusor muscle and contraction of the bladder neck mechanism. Alpha blockers (including doxazosin and tamsulosin) increase urinary flow in bladder outflow obstruction by relaxing the smooth muscle of the bladder neck and prostate.

Pain

Bladder pain is referred to the hypogastric (suprapubic) region of the abdomen.

Blood supply of the bladder

The bladder has a considerable blood supply from the vesical arteries and from branches of the anterior division of the internal iliac arteries. This facilitates reconstructive surgery of the bladder but makes the management of haemorrhagic cystitis difficult.

Bladder pain

Bladder discomfort or pain presents in the hypogastric (suprapubic) area and may be associated with other symptoms such as dysuria, frequency, nocturia and urgency as well as urine retention and/or incontinence. If the trigone is affected the pain may radiate to the tip of the penis. Pain may be constant (e.g. urinary tract infection) or intermittent (e.g. bladder spasm). It may vary in intensity from a dull ache (e.g. urinary tract infection) to acute disabling pain (e.g. acute obstructive pathology causing retention of urine).

Commonest causes of bladder pain in palliative care

- Urinary tract infection (UTI)
  - Bacterial (see later) including tuberculous cystitis
  - Fungal (immunocompromised patients)
  - Urethritis
  - Genital herpes
  - Vaginitis
- Anatomical
  - Pelvic mass
  - Urethral obstruction
  - Cystocoele
- Neoplastic
  - Bladder cancer
  - Urethral cancer
- Foreign body
  - Urethral or suprapubic catheter (usually comfortable unless infected or blocked)
  - Bladder calculus

- Bladder instability
  - Bladder spasm may be idiopathic or more commonly due to contraction around the balloon of an indwelling catheter, blood clots, tumour and infection
- Inflammatory
  - Radiotherapy
  - Chemotherapy—cyclophosphamide
  - Intravesical chemotherapy or immunotherapy for bladder cancer
  - Interstitial and eosinophilic cystitis
  - Amyloid

Treatment of bladder pain/irritability
Treat reversible causes.

Non-drug management
Regular toileting, good fluid intake (which may be difficult for the terminally ill), avoiding caffeine and alcohol, drinking real cranberry juice (although evidence is limited).

Drug management
- Antimuscarinic drugs may be helpful but should be avoided in significant bladder outflow obstruction or urinary retention
- Antispasmodics
  - Oxybutinin 2.5–5mg b.d.–q.d.s. (also has a topical anaesthetic effect on the bladder mucosa and can be given intravesically as 5mg in 30mL o.d. to t.d.s.). Modified preparations available
  - Tolterodine 2mg b.d. (better tolerated than oxybutinin, use lower dose if hepatic impairment). Modified release preparations available
  - Propiverine hydrochloride 15mg o.d.–t.d.s.
  - Trospium chloride 20mg b.d.
- Tricyclic antidepressants
  - Amitriptyline 25–50mg o.n.
  - Imipramine 25–50mg
- NSAIDs may be useful
- Corticosteroids may reduce tumour-related inflammation of the bladder and thereby improve bladder comfort
- Local anaesthetic and opioids can be used intravesically. Lidocaine 2 per cent (diluted in sodium chloride 0.9 per cent) can be instilled through an indwelling catheter, which should then be clamped for 20 minutes to 1 hour. Bupivacaine 0.5 per cent can be combined with morphine 10–20mg and instilled t.d.s. through an indwelling catheter which should be clamped for 30 minutes[1]

Terminal situation
- Antimuscarinics can be given CSCI: hyoscine butylbromide 60–120mg over 24h glycopyrronium 0.2–0.4mg over 24h

1 McCoubrie R., Jeffrey D. (2003) Intravesical diamorphine for bladder spasm. *Journal of Pain and Symptom Management*, **25**: 1–2.

Urinary tract infection (UTI)

UTI is common in palliative care patients and presentation may be non-specific. The clinical picture may vary from asymptomatic to severe symptoms to septicaemia.

Presentation: Dysuria, incontinence, urinary retention, haematuria, supra-pubic pain, loin pain, pyrexia of unknown origin, confusion.

Risk factors: Low urinary output (dehydration), bladder dysfunction (outlet obstruction, neuropathic bladder), catheterization, atrophic vaginitis, renal calculi, diabetes mellitus, immune impairment, vesical fistulae.

Pathogens: *E. coli* commonest, also *Strep. faecalis, Proteus, Klebsiella, Pseudomonas.*

Management: Bedside testing for protein, blood, leucocytes and nitrates (any or all may be positive). UTI unlikely if all bedside tests negative. MSU for culture: clinical diagnosis and positive bedside testing sufficient to start treatment in most patients. Catheter *in situ*—do not treat unless symptomatic or undergoing re-catheterization/instrumentation. Encourage increased fluid intake.

- Antibiotic regime:
  - Trimethoprim 200mg b.d. for three days effective in most uncomplicated infections
  - Other regimes:
  - Ciprofloxacin 250–500mg b.d. p.o./i/v, co-amoxiclav 375mg t.d.s. p.o./i/v, cephalexin, 250mg q.d.s. p.o., cefuroxime 125–250mg b.d. p.o./i/v.
  - Recurrent symptomatic UTI (proven on MSU):
  - Prophylaxis with trimethoprim 200mg o.d. or nitrofurantoin 50–100mg nocte

Renal pain

Renal pain is characteristically a dull ache in the loin caused by capsule distension, irritation or obstruction.

Causes

- Infection—pyelonephritis, abscess
- Haematoma (trauma)
- Infarct
- Tumour—renal cell carcinoma, transitional cell carcinoma, oncocytoma, bleed into angiomyolipoma
- Hydronephrosis

Diagnosis

Urine culture, ultrasound scan, CT scan (MRI may be useful if contrast contra-indicated).

Management

Treat underlying cause if possible, consider dexamethasone 8–16mg for enlarging tumour, analgesics (WHO ladder).

Ureteric colic

Ureteric colic is a severe constant pain, usually located to the loin and may radiate to the ipsilateral groin and testicle. Its onset is typically over 15 to 20 minutes building to an intense plateau of pain with fluctuations in intensity but never disappearing, as for example in small bowel colic.

It relates to acute ureteric obstruction, and depending on the cause may abate with a similar time course to its onset. The patient will become agitated, unable to settle and roll around in agony, unlike the patient with peritonitis who lies still.

Causes
Calculus, tumour, clot, renal papillae, fungal infection.

Treatment
NSAIDs will inhibit the renal response to acute urinary obstruction (*avoid with impaired renal function*) and opioid analgesia may also help. Treating tumour-related oedema with dexamethasone 8–16mg may be useful. Anticholinergics (e.g. hyoscine butylbromide) play no rôle in the management of acute ureteric colic.

Pelvic pain
Can be highly problematic and multifactorial. Assessment needs a logical and thorough approach.

1 Consider which structures may be the site of pain:
   - GU tract:
     - Males: Ureters, bladder, prostate, urethra, penis, testes
     - Females: Ureters, bladder, urethra, ovaries, uterus and fallopian tubes, vagina
   - Perineum
   - GI tract: Distal colon, rectum, anus
   - Bones: Sacrum, pelvis
2 Consider pathological process leading to pain:
   - Cancer—can be nociceptive (visceral or somatic), musculoskeletal or neuropathic and due to the tumour itself/local invasion/ metastases/extrinsic compression of nearby structures
   - Concurrent non-cancer disease (e.g. UTI)
   - Iatrogenic (caused by cancer treatment or non-cancer treatment, e.g. radiotherapy, surgery, constipation)
3 Treat underlying cause—but also consider:
   - Medical treatment
     - Specific to the cause (e.g. antibiotics for infection)
     - Symptomatic: Follow WHO ladder, adjuvant analgesia as appropriate to type of pain
     - Consider dexamethasone 8–16mg daily for extrinsic compression from tumour as a 3 day trial
   - Surgery: e.g. stabilization of fractures such as neck of femur
   - Oncological treatment: Palliative chemotherapy or radiotherapy, hormone therapy (hormone sensitive tumours)
   - Anaesthetic analgesic interventions: Interruption of the pre-sacral sympathetic nerve supply may help pelvic pain. A caudal or lumbar epidural may be useful. Neurolytic techniques may result in lower limb paralysis and double incontinence[2]
   - Non-physical treatments: Complementary therapies, psychological support, spiritual input, social support

2 Wilsey N., Ashford N., Dolin S., (2002) Presacral neurolytic block for relief of pain from pelvic cancer. *Palliative Medicine*, **16**: 441–4.

Urinary retention

Urinary retention is common in palliative care patients and should always be considered in those showing non-specific symptoms such as confusion, restlessness and agitation. Patients presenting with retention often have a previous history of urological difficulties. Risk factors for retention include drugs (such as opioids, anticholinergics), constipation, poor mobility and inadequate toileting facilities and should be avoided as far as possible.

Causes
Local
- Urinary tract infection
- Benign prostatic hypertrophy (BPH)
- Pelvic tumours (any)—primary or secondary
- Constipation
- Urethral stricture—rare, since usually presents with bad lower urinary tract symptoms first
- Haematuria with clot retention

Drugs
- Tricyclic antidepressants
- Phenothiazines
- Opioids
- Anti-cholinergics e.g. oxybutinin, hyoscine, glycopyrronium
- Alpha agonists (contained in some proprietary cough medicines)

Neurological
- Spinal cord compression
- Pre-sacral plexopathy
- Intrathecal/epidural anaesthesia

Debility
- Immobility/weakness
- Decreased conscious level

Acute obstruction
Symptoms: hesitancy and poor urinary stream, post micturition dribbling, early morning frequency and nocturia. Subacute symptoms may have been present previously but may be of sudden onset.

Diagnosis
- Severe lower abdominal pain
- Intense desire to urinate
- Anxiety/irritability—may be the only symptom in terminal or unconscious patient
- Distended, tense bladder: Tender to palpation, increases desire to urinate, dull to percussion
- >500mL on catheterization in presence of symptoms

Chronic obstruction
Symptoms: classic and cardinal symptom is nocturnal enuresis. The onset is often slow and insidious, and is often missed or misdiagnosed as incontinence.

Diagnosis
- Dribbling incontinence
- Large, non-tender bladder (low pressure chronic retention)
- Percussion dull (may extend to above umbilicus)
- High residual volume (>300mL) post micturition. (May be otherwise symptomless). Acute on chronic volumes may be >800mL on catheterization

Complications
- Urinary infection (📖 see also infection as cause in acute obstruction, p. 324) and bladder stones
- Hydronephrosis and post renal failure (high pressure chronic retention)
- Constipation refractory to laxatives
- Agitation, confusion
- Post-catheterization diuresis: due to released pressure on renal cortex and osmotic effects of high urinary urea. A record should be kept of urine output and if excessive, intravenous fluid should be replaced accordingly, with measurement of serum biochemistry. It is no longer good practice to clamp catheters to allow slow drainage

Treatment
Acute retention
- Immediate catheterization with 16–18Fr gauge urethra catheter
- Antibiotic cover e.g. gentamicin 120mg stat (well tolerated and safe as single dose even in renal failure). Ciprofloxacin is a possible alternative
- Catheter should be left in if the patient is in agreement. There are risks of bacteraemia when catheters are both inserted and removed. In the terminally ill, this will prevent risk of further retention and aid in nursing management
- Measure residual volume
- Rectal examination in male and vaginal examination in female as appropriate

If it is not possible to pass a urethral catheter, a suprapubic catheter will be needed. In a hospice setting in the terminally ill, a Bonanno catheter can be used. It should be inserted in the midline away from scars, two finger breadths above the symphysis pubis. This is a short term measure and the catheter should be changed by a urologist to a more appropriate tube if appropriate for the patient. A suprapubic catheter is contra-indicated with clot retention.

Chronic retention
- catheterization—as above
- fluid balance and monitor electrolytes Na^+ and K^+
- consider IVI.

Clot retention
- This should ideally be managed by the urologists who will use a stiff 22 Fr catheter and may need to use an introducer. In a hospice setting with a terminally ill patient a 22 Fr catheter should be tried.

Treat underlying cause as appropriate for the patient

- Laxatives for constipation
- Treat UTI
- Review medication and reduce or stop drugs causing retention (if possible)
- Clot retention—stop anticoagulants and correct bleeding diathesis if possible. NB Tranexamic acid should be used with caution since it might exacerbate the situation
- Consider and treat spinal cord compression. Investigate/treat pelvic tumour (surgery, radiotherapy or chemotherapy according to type)
- Urethral stent e.g. in patients too unwell for surgery
- Debilitated patient—regular toileting, use commode rather than bedpan (women), sit/stand at edge of bed (men), privacy—anxiety will inhibit micturition

Further investigations (unnecessary if patient is in terminal decline)

- CSU for culture and sensitivity
- Urea and electrolytes, creatinine—uraemia not improving after catheterisation may indicate other cause e.g. NSAID nephropathy or a high obstruction not corrected by catheterization
- Consider urinary imaging: IVU, USS, cystoscopy if patient is well and corrective treatment is contemplated

Choice of catheter

Size 16Fr is the smallest useful size in adults, smaller sizes tending to curl in the urethra. A 22Fr gauge will be needed for clot retention. The French (Fr) gauge is the circumference of the catheter in mm. Silastic catheters are most appropriate.

Ureteric obstruction

This may be unilateral or bilateral and is caused, in palliative care, largely by pelvic tumours, e.g. carcinoma of the cervix in women and carcinoma of the prostate in men. A reduction in urine volume, abdominal pain and/or serial blood tests of deteriorating renal function alert the team to the possibility of bilateral obstruction and impending renal failure. Renal ultrasound will confirm the diagnosis of ureteric obstruction due to tumour and rule out other contributing factors.

Obstructing stones are best diagnosed on plain abdominal X-ray. In the presence of ureteric obstruction, cystoscopy and retrograde pyelograms can be carried out which should outline the level/s and cause of obstruction. An indwelling ureteric stent can then be passed under cystoscopic control if there appears to be reasonable potential for regaining function. If this is not possible a percutaneous nephrostomy could be considered under ultrasound guidance. This can sometimes be replaced by antegrade insertion of ureteric stents. In some circumstances, antegrade ureteric insertion into an ileal conduit may be appropriate. With modern equipment and techniques, long-term nephrostomies are a possible option but this needs very careful discussion with patients who may already be suffering from pelvic pain, fistulae or other tumour related problems. They may not want artificial prolongation of life at the expense of relentlessly distressing symptoms.

In palliative care this discussion with the patient and family is crucial in guiding the patient to the correct management for them. Clearly if restoration of renal function with reasonable quality of life and minimal symptoms and disruption to life is a possibility, interventional management will be in the patient's best interests. On the other hand, if the patient is in the terminal phase of cancer with a known large pelvic mass that is already causing pain and debility, the patient might not wish to undergo procedures that might not be successful and that, if technically successful, might prolong life for a short time but with the added burden of further discomfort. This is the choice of the patient and should be discussed adequately with him/her.

Urinary incontinence

This is a distressing symptom for patients, affecting their lives physically, psychologically, socially and sexually. Patients may become isolated from family and friends as they try to maintain their own personal hygiene, fearing to lose their dignity in public. A good history is essential and may indicate that the cause is simply an inability to mobilize and reach the toilet in time. Pelvic disease in a female patient may result in a vesicovaginal fistula leading to constant urinary drainage through the vagina.

Total urethral incontinence

This type of incontinence is relatively common for patients with advanced malignant disease. Uncontrollable loss of urine occurs secondary to local incompetence of the urethral sphincter (due to direct tumour invasion or previous surgical intervention) or central loss of sphincter control (due to confusion or dementia).

Treatment includes regular toileting for central loss of control to allow continence to be regained. Females will need a urethral catheter. A male sheath catheter can be tried first but these are often problematic since they may be difficult to fit securely and twist easily.

Neurological incontinence

Loss of neurological bladder control may be due to damage to the sacral plexus or spinal cord/cauda equina compression. A hypotonic neuropathic bladder may result in overflow incontinence and a reflex/automatic bladder empties automatically. Patients who are well, willing and dextrous enough may be taught intermittent self-catheterization. Other patients will require long-term catheters. Anticholinergics may help.

Overflow incontinence

This is associated with obstruction of the bladder outlet or a poorly contractile floppy bladder. Small volumes of 'overflow' urine may be passed without control. A palpable, distended bladder alerts the clinician to overflow incontinence, although a large distended but floppy bladder, particularly in a patient with other abdominal pathology, may be difficult to diagnose. Permanent catheterization will probably be necessary. Definitive treatment may be possible if the patient is well enough and if the obstruction is amenable to surgery or other intervention such as an intraurethral stent.

Urge incontinence

A sudden urge to urinate and subsequent urinary loss may be particularly distressing for patients with poor mobility who are unable to reach the toilet in time. The causes include all factors that contribute to an irritable bladder. The underlying cause should be treated and anticholinergic agents may help. Patients may be able to manage timed voiding.

Stress incontinence

Involuntary urethral loss of urine with increased intra-abdominal pressure from coughing, sneezing, laughing, jumping or even walking in severe cases in the absence of bladder contraction may occur. It is more common in multiparous women and is associated with poor urethral support and reduced pelvic floor tone. Support prostheses (e.g. ring pessary) and urethral inserts may be a possibility in the absence of local tumour.

Haematuria

A normal urinary tract does not usually bleed, even if the patient is on warfarin. Haematuria is a frequent presentation of urological disease. It ranges from microscopic haematuria discovered incidentally on urinalysis to frank haematuria with the passage of clots and clot retention of urine. The extent of the bleeding does not always correlate with the severity of the underlying aetiology. The bladder is a very vascular organ and will not have a chance to stop bleeding unless it is collapsed. Dantron may tint the urine pink or orange which may be confusing.

Causes:

- Tumour: Renal, ureteric, bladder, prostate (post radiotherapy or locally advanced)
- UTI
- Drug-induced—aspirin or NSAIDs do not usually cause gross haematuria in a normal urinary tract, but any bleeding associated with surgical interventions may be exacerbated. Cyclophosphamide and ifosfamide may cause haemorrhagic cystitis (see below)
- Systemic coagulation disorder—usually evidence of bruising or bleeding elsewhere. Platelets may be low due to leucoerythroblastic anaemia and marrow infiltration
- Urinary calculus

Investigations:

- Urinalysis, microscopy and urine culture
- Intravenous urography
- Ultrasound scan
- Cystourethroscopy (visualizes the bladder and urethra)

Treatment

Treat any reversible causes i.e. treat UTI and systemic coagulation disorder and stop precipitating drug.

General measures:

- Encourage oral fluids to promote a good urine output (to avoid clot retention)
- Transfusion may improve symptoms due to anaemia

- Etamsylate: (reduces bleeding by enhancing platelet adhesion). The use of tranexamic acid (prevents fibrinolysis by inhibiting plasminogen activation) is controversial. It may result in the formation of hard clots which then need to be irrigated cystoscopically; urological surgeons describe bladders lined with clot which can be difficult to manage. As ever, however, the decision must be made on an individual basis. Terminally ill patients may prefer to risk clot retention than to continue with gross haematuria and significant blood loss
- Palliative radiotherapy often reduces haematuria from a bleeding urinary tract cancer
- Instilling 1 per cent alum, formalin, 0.5–1.0 per cent silver nitrate or epsilon aminocaproic acid solutions may be tried. (Discuss with urologists)
- Internal iliac artery embolization may provide effective relief from severe bladder haemorrhage[3]
- Bleeding from the prostate may respond to finasteride 5mg o.d. (a specific inhibitor of 5 alpha-reductase which metabolizes testosterone to the more potent androgen, dihydrotestosterone) even if patients are on other drugs
- Cystectomy may be the final option in a patient able to undergo the procedure which would be most unusual in the palliative care situation

Clot retention

The principle in the management of clot retention is to evacuate bladder clots. A non-distended bladder bleeds far less than a distended bladder. A large bore 22 Fr catheter will be needed. Patients may need referral to a urologist for insertion of a 3-lumen catheter (to permit irrigation with sodium chloride 0.9 per cent and allow removal of clots) which is stiff and may need to be inserted with an introducer. Cystoscopic bladder washouts may be necessary. Percutaneous insertion of a suprapubic catheter is contra-indicated in the presence of clot retention since the catheter is of insufficient diameter to allow satisfactory irrigation; there is also the potential for seeding of bladder tumour through the percutaneous tract.

Haemorrhagic cystitis

This may require clot evacuation and irrigation, and instillation of alum. Intravesical prostaglandin E2 may be helpful. In selected fit patients, urinary diversion, cystectomy or selective embolization of the internal iliac artery may be appropriate, but this would be very rare in the palliative care population.

---

3 Gujral S., Bell R., Kabala J., Persad R. (1999) Internal iliac artery embolisation for intractable bladder haemorrhage in the perioperative phase. *Postgraduate Medical Journal*, **75**: 167–9.

Catheterization

Indications: Urinary retention (acute and chronic), incontinence, patients in whom toileting is problematic e.g. pathological fracture femur.

Indwelling urethral catheterization

The French scale of catheter size is measured in mm. A 16Fr silicone catheter is most commonly used in adults since smaller diameters tend to coil in the urethra. A larger size may be needed (e.g. 18Fr) if debris and infection is suspected. A size 22Fr will be needed for clot retention (see above). Long term catheters should be changed every 6 weeks to avoid blockage, encrustation and formation of stones in the catheter.

For male urethral catheterization:
- Retract foreskin to view urethral meatus
- Clean glans with sodium chloride 0.9 per cent or aqueous chlorhexidine
- Anaesthetize and lubricate with 10mL lignocaine 2 per cent gel via syringe
- Wait for a few minutes and gently pass catheter using aseptic technique. Resistance may be encountered at the level of the distal sphincter complex or bladder neck. Sphincter spasm will diminish in a few minutes. Asking the patient to cough, may facilitate passage of catheter
- A catheter introducer should only be used by experienced urological surgeons
- The female meatus may be difficult to identify and is often situated in the vaginal introitus or along the anterior vaginal wall
- Inflate catheter with required volume of water to prevent catheter dislodging

Urethral catheter problems[4]
- Trauma and false passages—refer to urological team
- Haematuria
- Infection is extremely common with long term catheterization. The incidence of UTIs is related to the duration of catheterization, bacteriuria developing at a rate of about 5 per cent per day of catheterization. Antibiotic treatment should be given if the patient is symptomatic (fever, urinary symptoms, delirium etc). Antibiotic prophylaxis should be used for catheter insertion and removal (gentamicin or ciprofloxacin) but this should be judged in relation to the individual clinical circumstances
- Bladder spasm—Caused by irritation of trigone of bladder by balloon. Often this is relieved by removing water from the balloon, although most long-term silicone catheters have only a 10mL balloon and there is the risk that the problem will not be solved and the catheter will fall out. Antispasmodics (e.g. oxybutynin) may be helpful
- Blockage may occur from debris or clots. Flushing the catheter with antiseptic (0.02 per cent chlorhexidine) or sodium chloride 0.9 per cent may relieve the situation but at the risk of encouraging further infection. This decision will depend on the particular clinical circumstances
- Bypassing is due to a blocked catheter or bladder spasm

- Paraphimosis—failure to reposition foreskin may lead to constriction causing swelling and pain of glans penis. Reduction with gentle squeezing pressure over 1/2 hour using swab soaked in 50 per cent dextrose may allow foreskin repositioning
- Undeflated balloon—if the balloon will not deflate to allow removal of the catheter, it will need deflating with a wire, usually under ultrasound control

Suprapubic catheter

A suprapubic catheter is indicated if passing a urethral catheter has failed. This may be due to a stricture, obstruction due to intrinsic or extrinsic compression or distorted anatomy of the urethral meatus due to tumour or lymphoedema. It may also be used as an alternative to a urethral catheter in a patient with an unstable bladder in whom the balloon is constantly irritating the trigone. A suprapubic catheter is contra-indicated in clot retention.

For suprapubic catheterization:
- The distended bladder is palpated suprapubically
- Patient placed with foot of bed raised
- The skin is infiltrated with lignocaine 1 per cent about two finger breadths above the pubis in the midline and urine aspirated with a 21G needle
- A suprapubic catheter is inserted using an aseptic technique. A pigtail (e.g. Bonanno) catheter may be needed as a short term measure if the patient is not well enough for transfer for the more appropriate insertion of a 16Fr silicone catheter, which should be sited by a urologist
- Caution: Midline scar, previous pelvic surgery, unsuccessful urine aspiration with needle. In these situations, the insertion should be under ultrasound control

Intermittent self catheterization[5] is unusual in patients with palliative care needs. It may be used in patients with a neuropathic bladder e.g. after spinal cord compression. Clean catheter insertion at least four times daily frees patients from indwelling catheterization, gives them control, and prevents renal damage from urinary retention. Patients need to be highly motivated, have manual dexterity and be well enough to perform the task. Refer to incontinence advisor for counselling/instruction.

General management of catheters

Catheters (especially suprapubic) need skin protective agents around the base of the catheter to stop leakage spilling directly onto the skin. Secretions around the catheter site should be removed with soap and water. Over-granulated areas can be removed with silver nitrate. Meatal cleaning around urethral catheters is necessary since secretions are increased due to urothelial irritation. The secretions form crusts which, when removed, form areas of exposed damage which are prone to bacterial colonization and can then ascend into the bladder.

4 Zylicz Z., Krajnik M. (1999) Improvement of transurethral catheterization in male patients. *Palliative Medicine*, **13**: 261–2.

5 Hunt G., Oakeshott P., Whitaker R. (1996) Intermittent catheterisation: simple, safe, and effective but underused. *BMJ*, **312**: 103–7.

Genito-urinary fistulae

Fistulae (abnormal communications between two hollow viscera or viscera and body surface) are common in patients with advanced cancer, causing considerable morbidity and distress. They may be associated with previous radiotherapy and are managed where possible, and appropriate for the clinical circumstances, with bypass surgery.

General management includes:

- Meticulous skin protection—barrier creams, e.g. zinc and castor oil, sudocrem or cavilon (applied as a spray or stick protector and dries to form a protective membrane). Lutrol gel (solidifies when warmed in contact with skin, forming a protective layer) is not commercially manufactured but some hospital pharmacies may be able to prepare it
- Water absorbent pads or tampons
- Treatment of odour: Metronidazole 400mg t.d.s. may reduce odour from anaerobic infection. Charcoal dressings and charcoal placed in the room may have some effect. Masking the smell with lavender oil etc. has been tried but is often ineffective

Vesicoenteric fistulae

A fistula may develop between the bladder and any segment of bowel. The cause in palliative care is usually colonic malignancy, although diverticulitis or small bowel inflammatory disease may also be responsible. Vesicoenteric fistulae rarely occur secondary to bladder pathology. A characteristic symptom is pneumaturia (passage of gas or froth in the urine) and there may also be a foul odour to the urine, persistent urinary tract infections and the presence of faecal matter in the urine (especially with large fistulae). Cystoscopy, contrast cystography or intestinal barium-studies will normally demonstrate the fistula. Ideally, the management is surgical removal of the segments of bowel and bladder, together with repair of the bowel and bladder. Otherwise a bypass procedure may be performed, a colostomy or ileostomy may provide complete relief. Some patients may be too unwell for surgery or prefer not to have a stoma.

Vesicovaginal fistulae

These are characterized by a continuous leakage of urine from the bladder into the vagina and needs to be distinguished from total urethral incontinence. Intravenous urography will identify a ureterovaginal fistula and a cystogram will identify a vesicovaginal fistula. Cystoscopy and retrograde ureterography may be helpful. Surgical excision provides the most effective solution but is often not feasible. Urinary diversion, e.g. ileal conduit, may be necessary if the patient is well enough, but this a formidable undertaking in patients who have had radiotherapy. Bilateral nephrostomy is a potential but radical alternative. As ever the advantages and disadvantages of procedures need discussing with the patient.

Sexual health in advanced disease

Patients with palliative care needs who are very ill and symptomatic may not be interested in sexual intercourse, although they may want to maintain intimacy with their partner. Discussions of sexuality issues may be very helpful for patients and their partners.

Background

- Individuals with advanced cancer may remain sexually active
- Problems may be physical, psychological or relational and are frequently multifactorial and complex
- Many sexual problems are solvable
- Patients with cancer often fear transmission of cancer (especially genito-urinary) to their partner or partners fear contracting cancer themselves
- Patients often find it difficult to ask for help and are embarrassed, fearing that professionals might see sexual difficulties as frivolous in the context of serious disease. They also assume that nothing can be done
- Healthcare professionals without specialist knowledge find it difficult to address this area since they too may be embarrassed

General Issues

- Lack of libido in both sexes can be caused by: Change in body image (surgery to /disfigurement of face, presence of stoma etc.), depression, relationship problems, hormone deficiency, drug related side-effects (see below)
- Physical problems such as breathlessness, weakness and pain may lead to difficulties, some of which may be addressed. Catheterization does not preclude sexual intercourse, a male catheter may be folded inside a condom

Issues for males:

- Impotence:
  - Drug causes (see below)
  - Disease/treatment effects: Spinal cord compression, pelvic malignancy, pelvic surgery/radiotherapy, orchidectomy, brain neoplasm
  - Concurrent disease: Diabetes, peripheral vascular disease, age-related
  - Psychological: Fear of failure to acquire or maintain erection for fear of experiencing or causing pain
- Treatment:
  - Stop or change medication
  - Discuss trial of sildenafil with urologist. Patients with psychogenic ejaculatory dysfunction, spinal cord injury, nerve-sparing prostatectomy and hypertension may get a response of approximately 80 per cent. Absolute contra-indications include the use of nitrates, liver impairment, hypotension and recent stroke or myocardial infarction (MI). Relative contra-indications include poor libido, history of priapism (may be associated with myeloma, sickle cell disease and leukaemia), bleeding disorders and active peptic ulceration

- Intercavernosal drugs (prostaglandin E), vacuum devices and prosthetic implants may very rarely be appropriate for selected patients in palliative care

Issues for females:
- Lack of libido:
  - Change in body image: disease/surgery of breast, genitals, reproductive organs. Associating gynaecological cancer with 'punishment' for previous lifestyle. Fear of pain on intercourse
- Dyspareunia:
  - Vaginal dryness: Lack of oestrogen, infection e.g. candidiasis, vaginal stenosis following radiotherapy or surgery
  - Post-pelvic surgery, pelvic tumour, pelvic infection
- Treatment:
  - Local oestrogen creams, HRT, treat infections, lubrication using KY jelly, use of vaginal dilators post-surgery/radiotherapy (needs to be started early and used persistently), encouragement of regular intercourse to maintain vaginal passage

Approach to management:
- Pre-treatment counselling, regarding sexual issues, may help to avoid problems
- Exploration of issues with open questions: e.g. 'has your disease affected the way you view yourself?'…'has it affected your relationships?'…while allowing the patient to guide the consultation into more specific areas
- General patient information literature available
- PLISSIT model framework for exploring/managing sexual problems
- Referral for further counselling with specialists who will have information/skills addressing this area. Psychosexual counsellors are available for complex situations

Drugs associated with sexual dysfunction
- Antihypertensives
  - Thiazide diuretics
  - Beta-blockers
- Psychotropic drugs
  - Phenothiazines e.g. levomepromazine
  - Butyrophenones
  - Anxiolytics and hypnotics
  - Antidepressants
- Endocrine drugs
  - Antiandrogens
  - Oestrogens
  - Gonadorelin analogues
- Other
  - Recreational drugs
  - Digoxin
  - Spironolactone
  - Ranitidine
  - Metoclopramide
  - Carbamazepine

Further reading

Books

Back I. N. (2001) *Palliative Medicine Handbook*. 3rd edition. Cardiff: BPM Books.

Norman R. W., Bailly G. (2004) Genitourinary problems in palliative medicine. In D. Doyle, G. W.C. Hanks, N. MacDonald (eds) *Oxford Textbook of Palliative* Medicine, 3rd edn, pp. 647–58. Oxford: Oxford University Press.

Tomlinson J. (ed.) (1999) *ABC of Sexual Health*. London: BMJ Books.

Twycross R., Wilcock A. (2001) *Symptom Management in Advanced Cancer*. 3rd edn. Oxford: Radcliffe Medical Press.

Articles

Gujral S., Bell R., Kabala J., Persad R. (1999) Internal iliac artery embolisation for intractable bladder haemorrhage in the perioperative phase. *Postgraduate Medical Journal*, **75**: 167–9.

Hunt G., Oakeshott P., Whitaker R. (1996) Intermittent catheterisation: simple, safe, and effective but underused. *British Medical Journal*, **312**: 103–7.

Law C. (2001) Sexual health and the respiratory patient. *Nursing Times*, **97**: NT Plus XI–XII.

Mercadante S. (1992) Treatment of diarrhoea due to enterocolic fistula with octeotide in a terminal cancer patient. *Palliative Medicine*, **6**: 257–9.

McCoubrie R., Jeffrey D. (2003) Intravesical diamorphine for bladder spasm. *Journal of Pain and Symptom Management*, **25**: 1–2.

Penson R., Gallagher J., Gioiella M., Wallace M., Borden K., *et al.* (2000) Sexuality and cancer: conversation comfort zone. *Oncologist*, **5**: 336–44.

Wilsey N., Ashford N., Dolin S. (2002) Presacral neurolytic block for the relief of pain from pelvic cancer. *Palliative Medicine*, **16**: 441–4.

Zylicz Z., Krajnik M. (1999) Improvement of transurethral catheterization in male patients. *Palliative Medicine*, **13**: 261–2.

Palliation of head and neck cancer

Basic epidemiology and pathology

General background

Head and neck cancer makes up about 3 per cent of all cancer deaths in the UK. It is more common in men and occurs more commonly in France, Italy, Poland, Thailand, and the Indian subcontinent than in the UK. Common primary sites include the oral cavity, pharynx, larynx, paranasal sinuses and salivary glands. Presentation is commonly with pain, hoarseness, recurrent sinusitis and a 'lump' in the neck.

Prognosis

About 50 per cent of patients overall are cured while 50 per cent die of their disease, though the mortality varies widely according to site, histology, stage at diagnosis and degree of tumour differentiation. Early recurrence after primary treatment is a bad prognostic sign. Most patients who survive two years without recurrence are likely to be cured. Second primaries are common, occurring in perhaps one in eight patients, and associated with a poor prognosis. There are two possible explanations for the high frequency of second primaries:

- **Field change:** Carcinogens produce widespread epithelial changes which easily develop into malignancy
- **Clonal expansion and migration** of malignant cells

Common aetiological factors include:

- Smoking
- Alcohol

These two factors are synergistic and are the strongest factors in the causation of head and neck squamous cell carcinomas (HNSCC).
Tumours at particular sites also have specific risk factors e.g.:

- Betel nut chewing and vitamin deficiencies for oral cancer
- Nickel, hardwood dusts for airways tumours
- Epstein–Barr virus in nasopharyngeal carcinoma
- Iron deficiency: Patterson–Brown–Kelly syndrome (iron deficiency, koilonychia, glossitis, upper oesophageal web) associated with postcricoid carcinoma
- Familial: increased risk of head and neck squamous cell carcinoma if there are two or more first degree relatives with HNSCC

Histology

Most tumours are **squamous cell carcinomas**. This has a number of implications:

- often moderately chemosensitive but not curable with chemotherapy

- tend to develop hypercalcaemia. This is usually due to the secretion of parathyroid hormone related peptide (PTHrP), which causes mobilization of calcium from bone and reduction in the excretion of calcium by the kidneys

Less common tumours include adenocarcinomas, adenoid cystic carcinomas (salivary glands), anaplastic carcinomas, lymphomas, melanomas of the mucosa and other rare tumours.

Staging

Squamous cell carcinoma tends to progress from local disease, along lymph node levels in a stepwise manner to distant disease quite late. This allows radical treatment to be staged (see below). Treatment has now improved so substantially that the cause of death is changing: whereas forty years ago, only a small proportion died of disseminated disease, as local control has improved distant metastases are the cause of death in perhaps a third of patients, and are found in many others.[1] This has obvious implications for the likely problems to be encountered and the management of the terminal phase.

The patient with head and neck cancer

In the face of such overwhelming statistical possibilities, hypochondria has always seemed to me to be the only rational position to take on life.
John Diamond (died of carcinoma of the base of the tongue),
Because Cowards Get Cancer.

In cancer of the head and neck, both disease and treatment can cause disfigurement and major communication problems. Many of the vital functions of life such as breathing and eating are threatened, and the patient may run the risk of severe bleeding. Understandably, the psychological toll can be considerable.

Many, though far from all, patients with head and neck cancer will have a history of heavy alcohol and tobacco use, which may indicate poor coping strategies in difficult situations. It is important to obtain a psychiatric history, as past events may predict the reaction to new problems. Those with a history of heavy alcohol intake may also have poor family and social networks to fall back upon and sometimes very damaged close relationships. This must be kept in mind in assessment, rehabilitation and discharge planning, in order to provide adequate psychosocial support for the patient and their family.

- **Adjustment reactions:** can occur around the time of surgery or other treatment as well as when function alters rapidly in advanced disease. They can take the form of anxiety, depressive reactions or mixed states. Adjustment reactions are commoner and more marked if severe disfigurement or communication problems are anticipated. They often settle with time particularly in a supportive environment, but need active management if severe
- **Depression:** has been found in over half the patients with advanced disease. Diagnosis can be more difficult in cancer as the 'classical' physical signs (anorexia, disturbed sleep and fatigue) are also prevalent in cancer itself. Counselling and antidepressants may be needed

- **Suicidal ideation risk:** is said to be considerably higher than with other cancers. A professional psychiatric assessment should be sought if the risk is judged to be significant
- **Anxiety:** may be general or related to specific fears of the airway becoming blocked, or of an impending serious bleed. Underlying fears need to be addressed and consideration given to counselling, cognitive therapy, relaxation training and/or anxiolytic medication
- **Alcohol withdrawal:** can cause confusion and agitation and benzodiazepines may be necessary

Tumour treatment: implications for the palliative phase

While these tumours may metastasise (most commonly to the lungs), they also tend to recur locally. Given the site of these tumours, local relapse may cause major palliative problems. Primary therapy is directed at maximizing local control.

Surgical treatment

Where feasible, surgical resection of the tumour offers the best chance of long term local control and cure. Surgery often involves resection of large amounts of tissue; it may be cosmetically disfiguring and cause a number of functional problems including swallowing and speech difficulties. Postoperative support and a multidisciplinary approach with input from speech therapists, dieticians and physiotherapists will be needed. Surgical treatment operates on the principle that HNSCC spreads in an orderly manner through successive lymph node groups. En bloc dissection removing the tumour, lymph nodes and intervening lymphatics should therefore give the best chance of control. The extent of disease-free margin which needs to be excised varies from tissue to tissue: if a tumour involves bone (e.g. mandible), muscle (e.g. tongue) or submucosal soft tissue and lymphatics (e.g. hypopharynx), it requires wide excision even if the tumour itself is quite small. Furthermore, excision of structures invaded by tumour may be needed. Therefore major reconstruction is frequently required involving skin, muscle, and bone with the use of flaps, as well as prostheses. This can preserve appearance and function to an impressive extent for many patients.

Another important consequence is that salvage surgery, e.g. for recurrence after radiotherapy, usually has to be quite radical to give any chance of long term benefit to the patient. It is important to be radical when a substantial improvement in prognosis, function or quality of life is the goal but also to desist when the benefits are limited compared to the severe cost to the patient. This requires addressing issues such as quality of life and body image with the patient.

The treatment of neck nodes is a central issue in such burden/benefit equations.

- Cervical nodal metastases are found in 40 per cent of patients with HNSCC at diagnosis
- Radiotherapy can 'sterilize' small neck nodes or those from certain tumours (nasopharynx, thyroid) effectively, but surgery is needed in other cases

1 Taneja C., Allen H., Koness R. J., Radie-Keane K., Wanebo H. J. (2002) Changing patterns of failure of head and neck cancer. *Arch Otolaryngol Head Neck Surg*, **128**: 324–7.

- Radical neck dissection removes all the nodes on that side, sternomastoid muscle, internal jugular vein and the spinal accessory nerve, which supplies the trapezius and sternomastoid. This is effective but disabling, and more limited forms of neck dissection are now employed when appropriate, often associated with radiotherapy or chemotherapy

Radical radiotherapy often retains function better than surgery but causes other problems, such as mucositis and subsequently dry mouth (xerostomia). Tissue fibrosis makes later salvage surgery in the face of recurrence hazardous, and occasionally damage to other structures such as the spinal cord occurs.

Radiotherapy can be delivered by *external beam or brachytherapy* (radioactive implants, such as needles in the tongue). Various fractionation regimes are used. Fractionation into a larger number of small doses reduces adverse effects, but very prolonged radiation regimes can reduce effectiveness. *Hyperfractionation*, in which several small doses are given each day, is sometimes given in the hope of better disease control. In addition radiotherapy can be given preoperatively (neo-adjuvant), postoperatively (adjuvant), or as an accompaniment to chemotherapy.

Palliative radiotherapy is used for patients with inoperable tumours or those who are unfit for surgery and may also be used as an adjunct to surgery, particularly where resection has been incomplete.

Since the need to achieve local tumour control is so important, patients are frequently treated on 'radical' radiotherapy schedules even when the treatment is palliative in intent. Such treatments are associated with a high incidence of acute toxicity including oral mucositis, odynophagia, (pain on eating) loss of taste and dry mouth. This is particularly problematic in this population of heavy smokers and drinkers. Again, input from a wide range of professionals is essential to support patients through treatment.

Radiotherapy is also used for bone pain, dysphagia or stridor from paratracheal nodes, or bleeding or infection from fungating tumours.

Chemotherapy treatment

Chemotherapy is potentially curative in some tumours, such as lymphomas, but never in HNSCC. Nevertheless, adjuvant or neo-adjuvant chemotherapy has a place alongside surgery and/or radiotherapy. Platinum-based regimes may provide some palliation in fit patients with metastatic or locally advanced disease.

Specific head and neck cancers (with emphasis on advanced disease)

Oral cavity tumours site

- anterior two-thirds of tongue
- lips
- buccal mucosa
- alveola
- hard palate
- floor of mouth
- retromolar trigone

Oral cavity tumours are the most frequent head and neck cancers. They are usually well differentiated SCC, but tumours of minor salivary gland origin are also seen. Spread is predominantly local and to nodal groups in a stepwise manner. Larger tumours are more likely to have spread and have a poor prognosis. Midline tumours metastasize quickly to deeper cervical nodes and hence further afield. Anterior tongue carcinomas have an uncanny tendency to spread or recur despite adequate primary treatment.

Oral tumours can initially be treated with surgery, with or without radical neck dissection. Radiotherapy (external beam or brachytherapy) often gives equivalent results, with less functional impairment, but causes mucositis and xerostomia. Excellent dental care is essential with radiotherapy in order to avoid dental sepsis which can contribute to osteoradionecrosis. Tumour relapse or tumours which are advanced at presentation, require extensive surgery with major reconstruction. Late disease or treatment may cause dysarthria, dysphagia if the tongue is not mobile, and local ulceration. A third of patients with tongue tumours develop multiple primaries.

Carcinoma of the sinuses

Paranasal sinus malignancies (maxillary, ethmoid, frontal, sphenoid) are commonly well differentiated squamous cell tumours. They present late, with local swelling, pain and ocular, nasal or palatal or dental symptoms depending on the site of origin. Treatment is usually surgical with extensive reconstruction for cosmesis, followed by radiotherapy.

Salivary gland tumours

Malignancy is suspected if a parotid mass is associated with facial palsy, or if a salivary gland mass is rapidly growing, hard and infiltrative.

- **Adenoid cystic carcinoma** is the commonest salivary cancer. It is slow growing and ulcerative. It is the tumour most likely to spread along perineural sheaths, which can lead to nerve palsies and neuropathic pain. It also infiltrates marrow cavities and it may be difficult to demonstrate its true extent
- **Adenocarcinomas** often have a relatively good prognosis because of their differentiation
- **Squamous cell carcinomas** are more aggressive, cause pain, and metastasize early. They are more often metastatic from another cancer than primary
- **Undifferentiated carcinomas** progress rapidly, and may mimic sarcomas
- A small proportion of **pleomorphic adenomas** become malignant

Management is usually surgical, with radiotherapy for residual or recurrent disease, high grade tumours or lymphomas. The facial nerve may be involved by tumour or sacrificed at operation.

Malignant melanoma occurs most commonly on the hard palate but also occurs on the lower jaw, lips, tongue or buccal mucosa. It is infiltrative and metastasizes early to lymph nodes. It often ulcerates and bleeds.

Carcinoma of the larynx Carcinoma of the larynx, and its recurrence, may present with voice changes, dysphagia or stridor.

- Glottic (vocal cord) carcinoma is commonest. Nodal metastases occur late, because the cords have poor vascularity and lymphatic drainage, and the main determinant of prognosis is the T stage. Initial treatment consists of radiotherapy, which preserves function, or surgery which is equally successful but may cause voice changes, although the voice is often preserved with more conservative treatment. Combined radiosurgical or radiochemotherapeutic approaches are often needed in advanced disease

- Supraglottic carcinoma presents late, with vague dysphagia, referred ear pain, or cervical lymphadenopathy. Hoarseness may signify involvement of the vocal cords or adjacent structures. Progression is by local extension (to oropharynx, especially posterior third of tongue, hypopharynx, or glottis) or lymph node spread. Treatment is commonly radical radiotherapy. Surgery may have to be radical (total laryngectomy[2]), and to be used in certain settings such as airway obstruction. Radical neck dissection may be warranted. Voice restoration has to be considered after total laryngectomy (📖 see Chapter 10e)

- Subglottic carcinomas are rare but highly invasive. Pyriform fossa tumours behave like supraglottic tumours and have a poor prognosis. Postcricoid tumours may be associated with iron deficiency (Patterson–Brown–Kelly syndrome) and invade the hypopharynx circumferentially. Radiotherapy, radical surgery and chemotherapy have a rôle in management, depending on exact site and stage

Carcinomas of the pharynx are usually squamous cell, though lymphomas are fairly common, especially in the tonsils and nasopharynx

- Nasopharyngeal carcinomas cause nasal obstruction, epistaxis, and otitis media from eustachian tube obstruction. Lower cranial nerve palsies from base of skull extension, or third, fifth and sixth nerve palsies from cavernous sinus invasion, signify advanced disease. Growth into the posterior orbit also takes place. Some varieties of nasopharyngeal carcinoma have a tendency to haematogenous spread. Radiotherapy is the treatment of choice, giving as good results as *radical* neck dissection. Radiotherapy unless meticulously planned, very occasionally causes damage to the upper spinal cord. Xerostomia is common from salivary gland irradiation. Chemotherapy is sometimes very effective. Late recurrences (over two years) can be retreated

- Oropharyngeal carcinomas (posterior tongue, soft palate, fauces, tonsils, pharyngeal wall) frequently present late. They produce dysarthria, pain and risk of aspiration. Radical radiotherapy is usual, but extensive surgery with radical neck dissection followed by radiotherapy may be indicated in locally advanced disease

- Hypopharyngeal carcinomas are uncommon but present late and have a poor prognosis. Aggressive treatment has therefore to be used judiciously

2 Ward E. C., Bishop, B., Frisby, J., Stevens M. (2002) Swallowing outcomes following laryngectomy and pharyngolaryngectomy. *Arch Otolaryngol Head Neck Surg*, **128**: 181–6.

Symptoms in head and neck malignancy

Pain

Pain is widely prevalent in head and neck cancers, particularly in advanced disease. Diverse anatomical structures are compressed or invaded by tumour within in a small space. Thus pains are often mixed somatic (bone, muscle, skin) and neuropathic. 📖 See Chapter 6a.

Sources of pain in cancer of head and neck

- Local tumour infiltration e.g. ulceration, infection
- Vascular and lymphatic occlusion producing oedema/ lymphoedema
- Bone invasion or extension of soft tissue infection causing osteomyelitis
- Nerve involvement or pressure: adenoid cystic carcinoma in particular (but to a lesser extent most head and neck tumours) can show perineural invasion and extension
- Referred pain is very common e.g. earache from most structures in the face, neck and mouth
- Treatment related e.g. chemotherapy or radiotherapy-induced mucositis

Approach to pain assessment[3]

1 Take a detailed history of pain, with special emphasis on character, exacerbating factors and accompanying dysfunction. Functional disturbances are not only clues to diagnosis but also need treatment in their own right, since they are distressing and disruptive to the patient.
2 Examine head and neck for masses and deformities.
3 Check movement of involved joints.
4 Carry out cranial nerve assessment.
5 Occasionally radiology or other tests are helpful in elucidating the cause of pain.
📖 See Table 6h.1, pp. 346–7 for specific pain syndromes.

Further pain management options

Tumour mass reduction by surgery, radiotherapy or chemotherapy is usually the best way of reducing pain.

Radiotherapy is particularly useful for bone metastases e.g. base of skull.

Steroids e.g. dexamethasone 4–8mg p.o. mane may contribute to analgesia by reducing swelling inside restricted fascial spaces. They can also be a useful temporizing measure while effective doses of other agents for neuropathic pain are being titrated upwards.

Antibiotics can relieve pain by reducing pressure due to infection in tight fascial compartments, e.g. osteomyelitis.

Nerve blocks are often difficult due to the distorted anatomy following disease or treatment.

---

3 Vecht C. J., Hoff A. M., Kansen P. J., de Boer M. F., Bosch D. A. (1992) Types and causes of pain in cancer of the head and neck. *Cancer*, **70, 1**: 178–84.

The key in managing pain in patients with head and neck malignancy is careful assessment and differentiating as clearly as possible the nature of the pain/pains involved

Mouth problems in head and neck cancer (see Chapter 6b)

Head and neck cancer and its treatment are associated with severe oral problems. Contributory factors include:
- smoking and alcohol
- dry mouth: medication, treatment
- poor dental hygiene (made difficult by intraoral mucosal tenderness or friable tumour)
- infection and bleeding from fungating tumours
- trismus restricting mouth opening
- vitamin deficiencies associated with poor nutrition
- underlying osteomyelitis

Dry mouth (xerostomia) is extremely common and is due to:
- radiotherapy involving salivary glands
- antimuscarinic drugs, opioids
- blocked nose leading to open-mouth breathing
- dehydration, including diuretics

Xerostomia leads to many problems. Taste is diminished, appetite reduced, food becomes more difficult to swallow, and intraoral infections and dental caries become much more likely.
Management includes:[4]
- dental hygiene, see p. 238. May occasionally require specialist advice
- adequate hydration
- general measures e.g. sucking on fruit drops, pineapple chunks
- synthetic saliva e.g. saliva orthana (little evidence of effectiveness in these circumstances)
- simple sialogogues e.g. salivix tablets
- pilocarpine tablets[5] or eye drops instilled in the mouth (can induce sweating or gastrointestinal complaints)
- treating underlying causes when possible and reviewing medication

Drooling usually indicates either a problem with swallowing saliva or a mass in the mouth, such as an infected fungating tumour. It is also associated with poor lip closure, as in facial palsy.
Management:
- Antimuscarinic drugs e.g. transdermal or sublingual hyoscine, tricyclic antidepressants
- Occasionally the underlying problem may be treatable e.g. resuspension surgery with poor lip closure—rarely indicated in late stage

4 Seikaly H. (2003) Xerostomia prevention after head and neck cancer treatment. *Arch Otolaryngol Head Neck Surg*, **129**: 250–1.

Table 6h.1 Specific pain syndromes

Syndrome	Location/features	Causes	Notes
Shoulder syndrome	Pain in shoulder, difficulty with certain movements e.g. putting on jacket	Radical neck dissection (due to axillary nerve sacrifice/damage)	Patient can only abduct arm to 75° and flex arm to 45°
Trigeminal neuralgia-like syndrome	Lancinating, continuous/paroxysmal. Distribution of Va, Vb and/or Vc, not crossing midline, though very occasionally bilateral	Middle/posterior fossa tumours Base of skull metastases Meningeal metastases	Trigger areas on activities such as chewing, talking, breeze of air May be accompanied by neurological signs +/- diplopia, dysarthria, dysphagia, headache
Glossopharyngeal neuralgia	Severe unilateral paroxysmal pain in throat or beneath the angle of the jaw, may radiate to ear, often precipitated by swallowing	Meningeal metastases Disease around jugular foramen Local disease around the base of tongue or oropharynx	Occasionally associated with syncope or postural hypotension.
Jugular foramen syndrome	Pain occiput to vertex, ipsilateral shoulder or neck	Base of skull metastases Meningeal metastases	Horner's syndrome, lower cranial nerve signs +/- local tenderness Worse on head movement

Clivus syndrome	Vertex of head, worse on head flexion +/- VIn.–XIIn cranial nerve signs	Base of skull metastases Meningeal metastases	
Orbital syndrome	Retro-orbital/frontal headache	Orbital metastases Meningeal metastases Metastases around sella turcica, with sphenoid bone or cavernous sinus invasion	+/- diplopia, visual loss, proptosis, extraocular nerve palsies
Sphenoid sinus metastases	Bifrontal headache radiating to both temples, intermittent retro-orbital pain	Base of skull metastases: sphenoid sinus tumour Meningeal metastases	+/- nasal stuffiness, diplopia, VIn. Palsy
Occipital condyle invasion	Severe occipital pain exacerbated by movement	Occipital condyle invasion	+/- XIIn. Palsy

Sticky, viscous saliva is a much commoner problem than appreciated, and is more troubling than the actual volume of saliva.

- It is a frequent complication of radiotherapy, as serous salivary glands are more sensitive to its effects than the mucous glands
- Unfortunately antimuscarinics, in addition to reducing the volume of saliva, also render it more viscous
- Beta-blockers can make saliva less viscous

Antibiotics for intraoral infections and frequent meticulous oral hygiene appear to help. It is important to ensure adequate hydration

Mucositis usually follows radiotherapy or chemotherapy with certain agents e.g. 5-fluorouracil, methotrexate or cyclophosphamide. There are reports of reduction of mucositis by treating intraoral infections, suggesting that bacteria and fungi play a rôle in its genesis.[6] Treatment usually requires a combination of analgesics and topically applied local anaesthetic or anti-inflammatory agents. Benzydamine, an anti-inflammatory with local anaesthetic properties, is often used as a mouthwash and has been claimed to reduce the duration of mucositis. Sucralfate may also be useful, but a recent Cochrane review shows that neither of these two drugs nor chlorhexidine are significantly effective. On the other hand, allopurinol and vitamin E appear to be useful,[7] although the evidence is again weak.

Tracheostomy

A tracheostomy is a surgical opening in the anterior wall of the trachea for providing a patent airway.

Tracheal stoma—post laryngectomy

Patients may have a permanent tracheal stoma if they have had a laryngectomy (e.g. for carcinoma of the larynx). In this case the tracheal cartilages are brought to the surface of the skin and sutured to the neck as an end tracheostomy. The rigidity of the cartilage should keep the stoma open and a tracheostomy tube will not normally be needed. Since there is no connection between the trachea and pharynx, there is no risk of aspiration and the patient may eat safely (provided that any voice prosthesis, if used, is safely *in situ*—see later). Apart from removing the function of speech, laryngectomy also removes the function of the nose, which normally provides heat and humidity to the inhaled air, filters the air and increases breathing resistance. An artificial heat and moisture exchanger 'nose' may be applied over the stoma to redress these problems reducing mucus, coughing and psychosocial problems; air enters and exits through side openings of this device which can therefore easily be covered by clothing. The 'nose' may also have a valve that can be digitally occluded to improve maximum phonation time and dynamic voice range. A small number of patients with a stoma may need a tube or a button device to maintain patency of the stoma.

Tracheal stoma (without laryngectomy)

Patients may have a temporary tracheal stoma, either fashioned as an emergency or as a more elective procedure while waiting for a definitive surgical procedure. The patient will have a tube and in the palliative care setting, there may be no plans or possibilities of reversing the stoma and recreating a natural airway, usually because of persistent tumour in the upper airways. In this case, the trachea and upper airways are still intact, albeit probably partially obstructed. If the larynx is not adequately protected on swallowing, there is the potential for aspiration of pharyngeal contents into the lungs and a cuffed tube may be required. An outer tube remains *in situ* for a variable length of time according to the particular circumstances; a silver tube may remain *in situ* indefinitely. A non-metal tube will be used during a course of radiotherapy to the neck to avoid excessive radiation skin reactions and also during MRI scanning.

Types of tube

There are a variety of tracheostomy tubes all suited for different specific purposes. Cuffed tubes are usually used in theatre or for an emergency situation, the aim of the cuff being to prevent air escaping around the tube during mechanical ventilation and to reduce the risk of aspiration.

However, prolonged cuff inflation causes ischaemic damage to the tracheal wall. Prevention requires frequent pressure checks and periods of cuff deflation. Apart from some high aspiration-risk patients (in whom cuffs should be inflated for oral intake), all patients seen in general wards, palliative care settings or the home environment are almost certain to have *uncuffed* tubes.

Essential warnings about cuffed tracheal tubes

1 For resuscitation, the cuff must be inflated for bag ventilation to be effective. In most palliative care patients, of course, resuscitation may be inappropriate.
2 If the tracheostomy is occluded e.g. by secretions or a decannulation cap, and the balloon is inflated, the airway will be totally blocked and the patient will suffocate. Open the cap, deflate the balloon or remove the tracheostomy tube immediately.

Voice prosthesis

Patients with a laryngectomy may have a voice prosthesis. This is a one-way silicon valve that slots into a surgically created fistula connecting the trachea to the pharynx. Air is expelled from the lungs, up through the trachea, and then passes through the valve into the pharynx. When the patient wants to speak, the airflow causes the pharyngeal muscles to vibrate producing the voice. Since it is a one-way valve, pharyngeal contents should not be able to pass through the valve and cause aspiration.

5 Johnson J. T., Ferretti G. A., Nethery W. J., Valdez I. H., Fox P. C., Ng D., Muscoplat C. C., Gallagher S. C. (1993) Oral pilocarpine for post-irradiation xerostomia in patients with head and neck cancer. *New England Journal of Medicine*, **329**, **6**: 390–95.

6 Spijkervet F. K. L., van Saene H. K. F., van Saene J. J. M., Panders A. K., Vermey A., Mehta D. M. (1990) Mucositis prevention by selective elimination of oral flora in irradiated head and neck cancer patients. *Journal of Oral Pathology and Medicine*, **19**: 486–9.

7 Clarkson J. E., Worthington H. V., Eden O. B. (2004) Interventions for treating oral candidiasis for patients with cancer receiving treatment. *The Cochrane Database of Systematic Reviews*, **1**.

Location of tissue
vibration of voice

Tracheo-oesophageal
puncture and
Blom-Singer
voice prosthesis

Oesophagus

Trachea and
air from lung

Speech

Stoma closure with
thumb. (Low pressure
prosthesis pictured)

Adjustable machrostoma valve for
hands-free operation~
(Indwelling prosthesis pictured)

Figure 6h.1 Tracheo-oesophageal voice prosthesis

Care of voice prosthesis

The valve should be cleaned gently every day using a specialized brush and flush applicator to remove debris. Some patients are troubled by candida and may need frequent valve changes but others may be able to leave the valve in for 6 to 8 weeks. The valve will need to be changed if leaking occurs through the valve (which will be obvious if the patient coughs on eating or drinking) or if there is leakage around the valve or if the patient finds that voice cannot be generated. The valve is usually left *in situ* during a course of radiotherapy. Occasionally the prosthesis, which is normally held in place with a silicon retention collar, is dislodged accidentally on coughing or during cleaning. In this situation the patient should lie down and an introducer (which the patient should have) or, alternatively, a size 14 Foley catheter should be inserted into the fistula while a replacement prosthesis is being organized, this prevents aspiration through the fistula into the lungs and stops the fistula closing.

Guidance for trachesotomy care

- Good communication and patience. The patient knows his/her own tracheostomy better than anyone else!
- Find out the type of stoma i.e. Post laryngectomy or not
- Find out the type of tube e.g. cuffed/uncuffed, fenestrated/unfenestrated, disposable inner tube, speaking valve
- Check for risk of interference with tube function. Obese or fatigued patients who have difficulty extending the neck are at risk of occluding tubes and posture/position needs to be checked. Water must not enter the stoma and patients need to fix an adhesive covering before showering
- Most tubes now have a removeable inner tube which almost always prolongs the life of the outer tube, which will need changing at about 30 days (instead of 7–14 days with a single lumen tube). It also allows easy cleaning which reduces the risk of occlusion and infection. The inner tube should be removed, inspected for encrustation and cleaned regularly at least once a day, the timing depending on the needs of the individual. It should be cleaned with liquid detergent and hot running water and pipe brushes, cleaners or sponges should be avoided. If secretions are thick or crusted the inner tube should be cleaned with sodium bicarbonate first and then with hot running water
- Changing the outer tube (usually at about 30 days if used with inner cannula). Make sure that the replacement outer tube is the same size as the one to be replaced and that a smaller sized tube and tracheal dilator are available if necessary, since a stoma may close over. Some tubes have a lock to ensure that the inner tube cannot be displaced and a click should be expected as the inner tube is reinserted into the outer tube
- Suctioning—A suction catheter, that is no bigger than half the size of the tube, should not be inserted to more than one-third of its length, should not make the patient cough and should not be used for longer than a few seconds. Suction pressure should be no more than 100–120mm/Hg (13.5 and 20kPa). A sterile technique should be used and the catheter and gloves disposed after single use. If suctioning through a fenestrated tube, ensure there is a non-fenestrated inner cannula *in situ* to avoid sucking the tracheal mucosa into the fenestrations
- Avoiding infections—clean stoma site with normal saline using aseptic technique and ensure area is clean and dry before applying any dressings
- Humidification should be used with oxygen or air. Encourage patient to wear a bib sprayed hourly with water, particularly if they do not have a heat/humidifier exchanger. Regular normal saline nebulisers (via the tracheal stoma) may be needed to keep the mucosa healthy
- Secretions. Any change in the colour or odour of secretions may need antibiotic treatment. Forceps may be needed to remove thick encrusted plugs of mucus

Signs of problems with tracheostomy
- Stridor
- Bleeding
- Increasing thickness and volume of sputum
- Difficulty expectorating

If these develop, consult specialist ear, nose and throat teams and/or speech and language therapist.

Swallowing problems specific to patients with head and neck cancer[8]

Swallowing requires:
- good lip closure: prevents food leakage
- teeth: break food down
- mobile tongue: crushes bolus and pushes it back into pharynx
- saliva: lubrication
- an intact palate
- functioning cheek musculature to avoid food collecting in gingival sulcus
- intact oral and pharyngeal musculature and innervation (cranial nerves V, VII, IX, X, XI, XII)

Remember innervation:
- lingual nerve (V), supplies sensation
- chorda tympani (VII) supplies taste to anterior two-thirds of the tongue
- glossopharyngeal (IX) supplies sensation and taste to posterior third of the tongue
- hypoglossal (XII) supplies tongue musculature

A tongue lacking sensation produces more long-term swallowing difficulties than a tongue with restricted mobility. Obstruction by a mass or dysfunction (muscle dysfunction, nerve damage), pain, dry mouth or tooth loss all contribute to dysphagia.

Improving swallowing: Perhaps the commonest cause of difficulty swallowing is dry mouth—📖 see Chapter 6b)

Manoeuvres to help improve swallowing
- chilled food helps re-educate lost sensation e.g. after surgery
- encouraging the patient to chew or even just manipulate the bolus in the mouth for a few seconds facilitates initiation of the swallow reflex
- alternating temperature, taste and texture of food in a meal keeps awareness of the swallowing process high
- carbonated drinks increase sensation of the liquid bolus
- placement of food boluses in parts of the mouth where sensation is still intact
- viscous boluses e.g. thickened liquids and purées, permit poorly coordinated muscles to mount a more effective swallow than thin liquids
- head or body tilting in the appropriate direction can utilise gravity in the swallowing process or protect the airway

Is the patient at risk of aspiration?

Hints include:
- Wet or gurgling noises with breathing: fluid in the airways
- Altered voice during eating: food on vocal folds
- Cough associated with swallowing
- Fatigue during a meal: leads to prolonged meal times
- Lower cranial nerve palsies
- Aspiration pneumonia

Seek a speech and language therapy (SALT) assessment if appropriate, considering the patient's clinical state.

Reducing risk of aspiration

1 The patient should not eat unattended.
2 The patient should eat sitting up. Tilting the body or head may be useful, the direction depending on the exact disability.
3 Avoid distractions during meals.
4 Consider thickening fluids (e.g. Thick n'Easy) if thin fluids cause coughing, or other ways of increasing bolus viscosity.
5 Techniques that may reduce aspiration depend on the particular situation:
   - Turning head towards the paralysed side of the face or tongue encourages the passage of food down the competent side
   - Flexing neck while eating
   - Double swallowing
   - Supraglottic or super-supraglottic swallow: a SALT will teach these techniques

Gastrostomy

A gastrostomy is used for feeding when it is necessary to bypass the mouth. In head and neck cancer this happens with dysphagia, severe oral pain, or in some cases of chronic aspiration.

Nasogastric tubes

Nasogastric tubes can be used for feeding for up to four weeks, but beyond that, gastrostomies are preferable.

In the normal course of events, poor nutritional status parallels disease progression. With aggressive feeding through a gastrostomy, a patient may remain surprisingly well for a time only to be more aware of the gradual disintegration of their body through infected fungating wounds, total dysphagia with excessive dribbling, bleeding, pain and other symptoms. The pros and cons of ongoing management should be discussed regularly with patients.

8 Kendall K. (1997) Dysphagia in head and neck surgery patients. In R. Leonard, K. Kendall K (eds) *Dysphagia Assessment and Treatment Planning: A team approach*, pp. 19–27. San Diego, CA: Singular Publishing Group.

Communication problems

Head and neck cancer and its treatment impair communication in various ways:

- dysarthria e.g. tongue fixed by tumour
- laryngectomy
- recurrent laryngeal nerve palsies
- loss of facial expression: VII palsy, facial disfigurement
- kissing: tumour/body image problems
- reception of communication by others: hearing or visual impairment

Studies show that up to 92 per cent of patients with head and neck cancer have difficulties with speech. This has been found in surveys to be the single most important correlation with quality of life after treatment.

Production and articulation of speech

The vocal cords produce sound which is then modified by the action of tongue, lips and mouth to produce intelligible speech. For example good lip closure is needed to say 'p' or 'b' while a mobile tongue is necessary to produce 't' and 's'. Thus problems with any part of this apparatus can produce difficulties with intelligible speech.

Laryngectomy

This produces the most profound speech deficit, as the production of sound is removed. Various techniques have been developed to address this:[9]

- oesophageal speech is produced by swallowing air and then expelling it while mouthing the necessary sounds. Various techniques can be taught by a speech therapist. Only 25–50 per cent of patients master this technique, and it is useless in noisy environments or communicating from any distance
- Speaking valves e.g. Blom-Singer valve: an opening is made between the airway and oesophagus, and a valve is fitted which allows oesophageal air to be used to produce sound. Fluency rates of 70–90 per cent have been reported. However, the dynamics of sound production may change again if there is major local disease recurrence
- Electrolarynx: this produces clear intelligible words, although in an 'electronic' voice. It occupies one of the patient's hands to keep it against the neck while talking

Recurrent laryngeal nerve palsy

This causes hoarseness if unilateral which sometimes worsens as the day wears on.

- Bilateral nerve palsy reduces the voice to a whisper
- The recurrent laryngeal nerves are motor to the intrinsic muscles of the larynx and also supply sensory fibres to the mucosa below the level of the vocal folds. Therefore in bilateral palsy the sphincter effect of the vocal folds during swallowing is lost and aspiration can result. The aspiration will not be noticed by the patient due to the sensory loss, and the risk of aspiration pneumonia is high
- Bilateral abductor paralysis can also produce stridor which needs urgent attention

Techniques for treating vocal fold palsies
- Behavioural techniques and biofeedback may be taught by speech therapists
- Injection of Teflon, fat or collagen into a paralysed vocal fold
- More invasive techniques (thyroplasty, arytenoid adduction, reinnervation, vocal cord lateralisation) are very rarely indicated in patients with advanced disease
- Patients who aspirate from bilateral vocal fold paralysis are temporarily helped by vocal fold injection. More extensive surgery is unlikely to be indicated in this patient group with end-stage illness

Articulation difficulties result from:
- tongue problems: glossectomy, tumour
- facial palsy
- dry mouth
- poor lip closure
- poor control of jaw movement: e.g. V nerve palsy
- defect in palate (excision) or teeth
- other lower cranial nerve palsies: base of skull metastases

How to communicate with patients with articulation problems

(Remember to involve the speech therapist)
- Choose a quiet place where you can hear better
- Sit in a position where you can see the patient talk. Make sure there is enough light to see properly
- Sit close enough to hear
- Take time to get 'tuned in'
- Encourage use of gestures which give useful clues to the meaning
- If necessary, remind patient to keep sentences short and uncomplicated
- Encourage the patient to articulate each syllable clearly but not to overarticulate
- Learn lip reading
- Encourage the family to participate
- Be aware of range of procedures on offer

Remember Lack of fluency does not just result in loss of ability to speak. Patients are often embarrassed into reducing their communication so that the *content* of speech also becomes poorer and deals only with the concrete. These patients need time to express their deeper thoughts, and utilization of alternative means of communication. Also think about non-verbal expression: e.g. art therapy, which can often express feelings better than words.

Blalock D. (1997) Speech rehabilitation after treatment of laryngeal carcinoma. *Otolaryngologic Clinics of North America*, **30, 2**: 179–88.

Infection and fistulae

Local infection has devastating consequences in advanced tumours:

- septicaemia
- cancer wound extension
- pain—from inflammation, pressure build-up within fascial spaces, erosion into adjacent tissues, maceration e.g. of skin by exudates
- fistula formation
- vascular erosion: catastrophic bleeds
- cachexia in unchecked sepsis
- thick saliva—heavy intraoral exudate makes speech and breathing difficult
  - Osteomyelitis, particularly in the jaw, is common and produces discharging sinuses, pain, and tooth loss. Necrosis may be particularly extensive in irradiated bone
  - Base of skull infections spread via the *retropharyngeal space* to the anterior mediastinum, (the cervical vertebrae are protected by thick fascia). Such infections are, however, commonly caused by tuberculosis
  - Submental space infections (Ludwig's angina) cause pain, high fever, trismus and hypersalivation. Floor of the mouth swelling occasionally causes respiratory obstruction

Treatment

- Most infections are caused by anaerobic bacteria, and Gram positive cocci which are commensals in the mouth. Gram negative organisms are less frequent
- Options include metronidazole and a penicillin, or clindamycin (concentrates in bone but associated with pseudomembranous colitis), or a third generation cephalosporin
- Antibiotics have an indispensable rôle in analgesia and reduction of intraoral exudates enabling the patient to communicate and breathe easily, often for the first time in months
- The conditions which encourage the infection in the first place usually persist, and continuous prophylactic low dose antibiotics may be worth considering. There is little trial evidence for this, but clinical experience suggests that it is an effective ongoing symptomatic measure

Fistulae

Once formed, fistulae remain patent because:

- The wound is continuously discharging exudate that is usually infected, e.g. bone sequestrate in chronic osteomyelitis
- The chemical composition of the exudate prevents healing—e.g. saliva

In palliative care there is usually an untreatable deep necrotic tumour but treatable situations such as drainable abscesses and osteomyelitis should be considered. Exudate or saliva bathing the great vessels continuously (e.g. fistulae between oropharynx and skin), will increase the risk of catastrophic bleeding. This should be avoided by:

- Dressings
- Drying up saliva—see p. 345
- Continuous antibiotics

• Applying a silicone elastomer plug to fit a fistula associated with a large wound. Unfortunately, malignant fistulae enlarge, so this plug will need to be renewed regularly. Such plugs are only used in single, clean, open cavities. Plugging complex cavities impedes drainage, extending deep infection and encouraging new fistulae to form where they can drain freely

Specific pain problems in patients with head and neck cancer

• **Neuropathic pain** affecting the head and neck and radiating to the upper arm is not uncommon. This can be the result of direct compression of nerves by the tumour or a result of treatment. There may be associated hypersensitivity of the skin and oral mucosa, which may be so severe that the patient is unable to tolerate even a light breeze or chewing soft food. The pain syndromes are often complex and only partially respond to opioids. Adjuvant analgesia in the form of antidepressant and/or anticonvulsant medication is usually needed. Specialist advice is frequently needed to maintain symptom control, especially as compliance with medication may be a problem

• **Dysphagia** due to direct compression of a tumour mass or lymphadenopathy often means that feeding gastrostomies are needed to maintain nutrition and to allow the administration of medication, as the oral route may no longer be available. There may be ethical dilemmas, particularly with regard to the administration of feeds in the last days of life

• **Other problems** The tumour or the surgery performed often adversely affects a patient's *body image* in a site which is hard to hide from public view. Patients often become *socially isolated* as they feel disfigured and become reluctant to go out and socialize. *Depression* is a common feature. Relationship problems are not uncommon

• **Difficulties with articulation and speech production** are common. The quality of the voice may change significantly and make the patient self-conscious. All these problems need the regular input of specialist speech and language therapists. Communication aids may be needed after major surgery to enable a patient to express their needs and preferences

• **Fungating and malodorous tumours** can cause considerable distress. Radiotherapy may help in some cases, especially where there is bleeding. Topical antibiotics may help along with regular dressings sensitively applied to maintain dignity, covering the most disfiguring parts of the tumour. Tumours are often infected with anaerobic organisms for which appropriate antibiotics including metronidazole may be appropriate. The use of deodorizers in the patient's room may help to disguise the smell of the infected tissue

• **Major haemorrhage**. Patients with progressive tumours near the large blood vessels of the neck are at risk of a sudden massive bleed. This is rare, but difficult to manage and the early involvement of specialists should be considered

Emergencies

Catastrophic bleeds (partly based on British Association of Head and Neck Oncology Nurses guidelines)[10].

These are among the most feared complications of cancer of the head and neck, although they are rare.

Risk factors
- Previous neck irradiation
- Fungating tumour invading the artery
- Postoperative: flap necrosis
- Infection
- Salivary fistula
- Systemic factors, such as malnutrition, cachexia, elderly patients

Warning signs
- Minor bleeding from wound, tracheostomy or mouth
- 'Pulsations' from artery or tracheostomy or flapsite—false aneurysm formation
- Sternal or high epigastric pain several hours before rupture of carotid
- The patient may become restless and irritable

Management

1 If the patient is thought to be at risk, discuss a plan within the multidisciplinary team. Can the risk be reduced by e.g. embolization or ligation of the implicated artery?
2 What should the patient and family be told?

> #### To tell or not to tell about potential bleeding?
> Consider:
> - Bleeds are often feared but rarely occur
> - No preparation for a very severe bleed can make it any less frightening
> - Can anything be done to reduce the risk of bleeding e.g. embolization?
> - Are there special circumstances e.g. children in the house who would be especially traumatised by a catastrophic bleed?
> - Is the patient doing anything that might increase the risk e.g. neglecting an infection in a dangerous area?
> - Warning bleeds or other severe risk factors which would indicate that a major bleed is more likely?

If the patient or family ask specifically about what might be expected, this needs to be discussed, giving information in small steps and letting them decide how much they want to know. It is also useful to ask in a general way if they have any special fears about how the patient will die, as this may bring out unspoken fears. Otherwise one needs to be careful not to raise fears of unlikely complications which are terrifying and about which little can be done.

Checklist
- Stop anticoagulants, aspirin, NSAIDs (COX-2 inhibitors may be safe)—though this will make no difference to a major bleed. Correct any platelet abnormalities if warning bleeds occur

- Treat infection
- Ensure the family, and staff, know who to contact in an emergency
- Have emergency sedative drugs in the home: e.g. diamorphine, midazolam
- Ensure all professionals involved know the plan e.g. district nurses, GP etc.
- If in a hospice or hospital, nurse patient in a side room to avoid potential distress of other patients or relatives
- Discreetly have available blue/green towels, gloves, apron
- If there is a bleed, a senior member of staff must stay with the patient. Nothing is as reassuring as a calm human presence, nothing as frightening as panic. Call for help
- Be respectful of the family's wishes about whether or not they wish to stay with the patient. Support them
- Apply towels to bleeding site and absorb the bleeding if possible
- Apply gentle suctioning to mouth and trachea as necessary
- Give i/v or i/m midazolam e.g. 10mg, repeated in 10–15 minutes if necessary. Subcutaneous drugs are poorly absorbed in shock
- Occasional families might be taught to administer rectal diazepam or buccal midazolam. Few will be calm enough to do this, and the extra responsibility may be too much for them to cope with in most cases
- After the event, debrief family and staff, and point them in the direction of their normal supportive networks. Extensive counselling just after an event has actually been shown to be more likely to do harm than good
- Offer family and staff (including non-clinical involved staff, such as domestics who have witnessed the incident) a chance for a follow-up meeting later to deal with any questions they might have

Tracheostomy tube obstruction
Causes
- Infection
- Excessive mucus production
- Pressure sores
- Tube displacement
- Granulation tissue

Management
1 Call for help
2 Reposition patient to semi recumbent position
3 Ask patient to cough, use suction
4 Manipulate head to eliminate tube kinks
5 Give oxygen
6 Remove inner tube
7 Suction
8 Resuscitate if appropriate
9 If severe problems, sedate the patient

10 BAHNON website: *www.bahnon.org.uk*

Body image and sexuality

Slade[11] defined *body image* as the picture we have in our minds of the size, shape and form of our bodies, and our feelings concerning these characteristics and our body parts. This makes it clear that body image includes appearance but goes far beyond it; perceptual and subjective aspects of body image are deeply intertwined.

Indeed, some suffer from a deep dissatisfaction with their body, despite very minor or no disfigurement, whereas others with very major disfigurement have a very healthy self-image.

Perhaps surprisingly for some, there is little gender or age difference in the impact of appearance changes on body image. The degree to which people can be rehabilitated after facial disfigurement also does not depend on the degree of disfigurement, but correlates with perceived social support and with the degree of dysfunction.

Factors which have been associated with poor body image include:
- Poor self-esteem
- Social anxiety
- Self-consciousness
- Depressive features

Sexuality is a closely related field. One study found how, a year after head and neck surgery, marital and sexual relationships were still suffering and alcohol use (a marker of depression, particularly in men) was still high in a very significant number of patients. Almost half of patients at least a year after treatment in another small study had problems with libido, arousal, sexual activity; a significant minority still never or almost never kissed and held hands with their partner.

Questions about body image and sexuality feel difficult and embarrassing to raise, yet MUST be explored. Sometimes a broad question can be asked which the patient will often interpret as referring to their sexual relationship if it is preoccupying them:
- How has this affected your relationship with your wife/husband?
- What things that really matter to you do you miss?
- How did you feel about yourself after the operation?

Often a more direct approach, which tells the patient that it is all right to talk about issues of sex and intimacy, is needed:
- How did your husband/wife cope with the change in your appearance after the operation?
- What impact did it have on your sex life?
- How have you dealt with that as a couple?'

Normalizing embarrassing fears in this manner is one important step in dealing with them.

> Body image and sexuality depend more on perceived social support and the existence of supportive relationships than on the degree of disfigurement or disability. This again brings one back to one of the central, though often unsaid, tenets of palliative care: that ultimately what matters most to people is being cared for and respected and loved.

There is now good work showing how, after cancer treatment, social rehabilitation through a simple behavioural approach is effective. Medical staff play an important rôle by modelling attitudes and allowing patients to practice new behaviours in a safe environment. For example, patients can be trained to prepare a number of responses for when people inevitably comment to them about their appearance, or when they walk into a pub and everyone stares.

Changing Faces, a UK charity, runs courses to help patients manage this and has published very useful educational material.[12]

The situation in advanced cancer, where appearance is rapidly worsening rather than static as after surgery, and is accompanied by generalized bodily deterioration and by a shrinking social world, has not been explored properly yet.

Figure 6h.2 Price's body image triangle. Adapted from[13].

Price, one of the early writers about body image, presents a useful triangle of body reality, body presentation and body ideal which offers a programme for working on improving body image. Thus for example, prosthetic work or reconstructive surgery can improve appearance or 'body reality'; makeup and choice of clothes can improve 'body presentation'; and counselling and perhaps the presentation of rôle models can tackle 'body ideal'.

11 Slade P. D. (1994) What is body image? *Behaviour Research and Therapy*, **32**: 497–502.

12 Clarke A. (2000) *Psychosocial Rehabilitation After Head and Neck Cancer—A resource for health professionals*. London: Changing Faces. www.changingfaces.co.uk

13 Price B. (1990) A model for body-image care. *Journal of Advanced Nursing*, **15**: 585–93.

General medical problems in patients with head and neck cancer

When one recalls that the main risk factors for head and neck cancer are smoking and alcohol, it is not surprising that concurrent medical problems are common in these patients.

- Malignancies in other organs: these are common,[14] particularly lung, but also other smoking or alcohol-related tumours: bladder, kidney, pancreas, liver. This may both have physical consequences to the patient, for example due to metastatic disease from a distant malignancy, and have psychological morbidity. Patients are also more prone to other primary head and neck cancers
- Ischaemic heart disease: patients will be less tolerant of anaemia
- Alcohol-induced cardiomyopathies: may limit the use of some agents for neuropathic pain
- Cerebrovascular accident: if this is present in addition to neurological damage from the tumour, marked disability can result
- Chronic obstructive airways disease: airways problems from head and neck cancer can precipitate decompensation and respiratory failure
- Thromboembolic disease: may necessitate difficult decisions in continuing anticoagulation if there is a risk of bleeding. Sometimes conversion to heparin will allow more rapid control if bleeding occurs
- Alcoholic liver disease: may contribute to clotting problems or to altered handling of medication
- Nutritional deficiencies: from poor diet, dysphagia, alcohol, cachexia
- Psychiatric problems: depression, anxiety
- Substance abuse: watch out for alcohol withdrawal in particular
- **Syncope** is common among patients with cancer of the head and neck.[15] This may be carotid sinus syncope from metastatic compression or post-radiotherapy fibrosis. (Glossopharyngeal neuralgia can lead to sinus arrest, perhaps as intense glossopharyngeal nucleus stimulation overflows to the vagal nucleus leading to parasympathetic suppression of the cardiac pacemaker)

Many patients will have been on high doses of steroids for prolonged periods. In any crisis or period of physiological stress, steroids may need to be increased or restarted.

14 Crosher R., McIlroy R. (1998) The incidence of other primary tumours in patients with oral cancers in Scotland. *British Journal of Oral and Maxillofacial Surgery*, **36, 1**: 58–62.

15 MacDonald D. R., Strong E., Nielsen S., Posner J. B. (1983) Syncope from head and neck cancer *J Neuro-Oncology*, **1**: 257–67.

Further reading

Books

Close L. G., Larson D. L., Shah J. P. (1998) *Essentials of Head and Neck Oncology*. NY: Thieme.

Leonard R., Kendall K. (eds) (1997) *Dysphagia Assessment and Treatment Planning: A team approach*. San Diego, CA: Singular Publishing Group.

Watkinson J. C., Gaze M. N., Wilson J. A. (2000) *Stell and Maran's Head and Neck Surgery*, 4th edn. Oxford: Butterworth Heinemann.

Articles

Chua K. S. G., Reddy S. K., Lee M. C., Patt R. B. (1999) Pain and loss of function in head and neck cancer survivors. *Journal of Pain and Symptom Management*, **18, 3**: 193–202.

Forbes K. (1997) Palliative care in patients with cancer of the head and neck. *Clinical Otolaryngology and Allied Sciences*, **22, 2**: 117–22.

Endocrine and metabolic complications of advanced cancer

Understanding the association between endocrine and metabolic complications in advanced cancer is increasingly complex as knowledge of the processes involved at the genetic and biochemical level grows.

Malignancy produces endocrine effects in two ways:

1 Directly interferes with the function of endocrine glands by invasion or obstruction.
2 Remotely produces effects without direct local spread—paraneoplastic syndromes

Paraneoplastic syndromes are caused by:

- Tumour cells secreting hormones, cytokines and growth factors
- Normal cells secreting products in response to the presence of tumour cells (such as antibodies in the Lambert–Eaton syndrome)

Paraneoplastic syndromes

- Hypercalcaemia
- Cushing's syndrome
- Syndrome of inappropriate antidiuresis
- Hypoglycaemia (Non-islet cell)
- Carcinoid syndrome

Non-paraneoplastic

- Diabetes mellitus

Hypercalcaemia (see Chapter 15, *Emergencies in palliative care*)

Hypercalcaemia is the commonest life-threatening metabolic disorder associated with advanced cancer. In addition, as it is a condition which is usually amenable to treatment and untreated it is both distressing and fatal, hypercalcaemia must always be sought in patients who are deteriorating for no clear cause.

Epidemiology

- Ten per cent of patients with cancer develop hypercalcaemia
- Malignancy is responsible for 50 per cent of the patients with hypercalcaemia who are treated in hospital
- Up to 20 per cent of patients develop hypercalcaemia without bone metastases
- Most patients with hypercalcaemia of malignancy have disseminated disease—80 per cent will not survive beyond one year
- The prognosis is poor with a median survival of three to four months

Table 6i.1 Clinical features of hypercalcaemia of malignancy

General	Gastrointestinal	Neurological	Cardiological
Dehydration	Anorexia	Fatigue	Bradycardia
Polydipsia	Weight loss	Lethargy	Atrial arrhythmias
Pruritus	Nausea	Confusion	Ventricular arrythmias
	Vomiting	Myopathy	Prolonged P-R interval
	Constipation	Seizures	Reduced Q-T interval
	Ileus	Psychosis	Wide T waves

Treatment

Rehydration followed by the administration of calcium-lowering agents is the mainstay of treatment. Drugs promoting hypercalcaemia (thiazide diuretics, Vitamins A and D) should be withdrawn.

The corrected serum calcium should be calculated from the formula

$$\text{Corrected calcium} = \text{measured calcium} + [(40 - \text{serum albumin g/L}) \times 0.02]$$

Intravenous fluids

Dehydration due to polyuria and vomiting is a prominent feature of acute or symptomatic hypercalcaemia. While large fluid volumes will lower serum calcium, calcium levels will seldom return to normal by rehydration alone and care to avoid fluid overload must be taken.

Rehydrating with 2–3 l/day of fluid is now accepted practice, with daily serum electrolyte measurement to prevent hypokalaemia and hyponatraemia developing. There is little evidence that there is any benefit in using diuretics in conjunction with rehydration and they should be avoided.

Corticosteroids

While steroids have been shown to inhibit osteoclastic activity and calcium absorption from the gut in vitro, their use in vivo is limited. They are most effective in haematological malignancies when oral prednisolone 40–100mg/day is usually effective.

Bisphosphonates

These synthetic pyrophosphate analogues reduce bone resorption by inhibiting osteoclastic activity. They are highly effective at reducing hypercalcaemia, but take 48 h to be effective. Infusions of bisphosphonates following rehydration are the mainstay of hypercalcaemia treatment.

Oral bisphosphonates have been used for maintenance therapy, but low bioavailability and gastrointestinal side-effects have limited their widespread use. Oral Ibandronic acid 50mg orally daily is increasingly used. Tablets should be swallowed whole with plenty of water while sitting/standing, 30 minutes before breakfast or other medication. Many patients still receive monthly infusions as outpatients to maintain calcium levels within the normal range.

Twenty per cent of patients with hypercalcaemia of malignancy will be resistant to bisphosphonate infusion therapy.

- Disodium pamidronate 30–90mg/over 2–4 h
- Zoledronic acid 4mg over 15 minutes

- Clodronate 1.5 g over 4h
- Ibandronic acid 2–4 mg i/v 1–2 h

The newer more expensive zoledronic acid (4mg) has been found to achieve a normal corrected calcium in more patients, faster, and for longer (4–6 weeks).

Calcitonin

Calcitonin inhibits osteoclastic bone resorption and encourages calcium excretion. It is effective in around a third of patients and usually causes a fall in calcium within 4 h.

Doses of up to 8 IU/kg of salmon calcitonin can be used subcutaneously every 6 h. It is rarely used in palliative care.

Plicamycin (Formerly mithromycin)

This cytotoxic antibiotic blocks RNA synthesis and is toxic to osteoclasts. Given as an i/v infusion of 25mg/kg over 2 h it will produce normocalcaemia within three days in 80 per cent of patients. It is now rarely used due to its cumulative nephrotoxicity and hepatic toxicity.

Cushing's syndrome

- Ectopic secretion of corticotrophin (ACTH) by non-endocrine tumours is rare
- Associated pro-peptide secretion is more common producing a more complex mosaic of symptoms
- Up to 20 per cent of Cushing's syndrome is caused by ectopic ACTH, often from an occult tumour
- Fifty per cent of ectopic ACTH secretion is due to small cell lung carcinoma
- Fifteen per cent of ectopic ACTH secretion is due to carcinoid and neural crest tumours
- Long term survivors of malignancies with associated ectopic ACTH secretion will often continue to have elevated ACTH levels

Clinical features

Hypokalaemic metabolic alkalosis	Mental changes
Weak muscles	Glucose intolerance
Oedema	Weight loss
Raised blood pressure	

The more classical features of Cushing's syndrome e.g. truncal obesity moon facies and striae may suggest a benign tumour such as bronchial carcinoid or thymoma.

Investigations

- Increased free urinary cortisol
- Loss of diurnal variation of plasma cortisol
- Failure of cortisol suppression in low dose (2mg) dexamethasone test
- Failure of cortisol to suppress ACTH levels following high dose dexamethasone (2mg q.d.s. or 8mg nocte)

When the above investigations are still equivocal, more complex imaging techniques are available at specialist centres.

Treatment

The mainstay of treatment is inhibition of steroid synthesis.

Aminoglutethimide

At low doses (125mg b.d.), aminoglutethimide inhibits the enzyme aromatase which converts androgens to oestrogens, (hence its use in patients with post-menopausal breast cancer). At the higher doses (1.5–3.0g/day) which are needed in Cushing's syndrome, however, aminoglutethimide blocks the production of glucocorticoids, mineralocorticoids and androgens but produces unpleasant side-effects such as ataxia, sedation and rashes.

Metyrapone

250–750mg q.d.s. inhibits 11 β-hydroxylase, the final enzymatic step in steroid production, but again side-effects (nausea and vomiting) are common. In an effort to reduce drug toxicity, aminoglutethimide 250mg b.d. and metyrapone 250mg q.d.s. may be used in combination. The use of ketoconazole, bromocriptime and octreotide have also been advocated in case reports.

Treatment efficacy should be monitored by measuring 24h urinary cortisol excretion. As levels return to normal, hormone replacement therapy, as in Addison's disease, may be required, (e.g. hydrocortisone 20mg at 0800 and 10mg at 1800 h with fludrocortisone 0.05–0.15mg daily).

Syndrome of inappropriate antidiuresis (SIAD)

Hyponatraemia is common in patients with advanced malignancy due to many factors including cardiac and hepatic failure, hyperglycaemia, diuretics and sick cell syndrome. The presence of concentrated urine in conjunction with hypo-osmolar plasma, however, suggests abnormal free water excretion and the presence of the syndrome of inappropriate antidiuresis. (The SIAD acronym is more appropriate than SIADH, as there is no vasopressin hormone secretion in approximately 15 per cent of cases).

The vasopressin gene codes for peptide products including arginine vasopressin (AVP) and vasopressin-specific neurophysin II (NP II). In malignancy-related SIAD, tumours secrete ectopic AVP.

SIAD is most frequently associated with small-cell lung carcinoma or carcinoid tumours but has also been noted in pancreatic, oesophageal, prostatic and haematological cancers.

Causes of SIAD

- Ectopic AVP
- Infections
- Pulmonary, meningeal and cerebral
- Drugs

Morphine, phenothiazines, tricyclic antidepressants, NSAIDS, vincristine cyclophosphamide

Clinical features

Significant symptoms of hyponatraemia develop at plasma sodium levels below 125mmol/L with confusion progressing to stupor, coma and seizures. Nausea, vomiting and focal neurological signs may also develop.

The clinical features depend on both the levels of plasma sodium and the rate of decline. With gradual falls the brain cells can compensate against cerebral oedema by secreting potassium. Asymptomatic hyponatraemia suggests chronic SIAD whereas symptomatic hyponatraemia suggests acute SIAD.

Diagnosis

Essential criteria

- Plasma hypo-osmolality (plasma osmolality <275 mosmol/kg H_2O and plasma sodium <135 mmol/L)
- Concentrated urine (with plasma osmolality >100 mosmol/kg H_2O)
- Normal plasma/extracellular fluid volume
- High urinary sodium (urine sodium >20 mEq/l) on a normal salt and water intake
- Exclude (i) hypothyroidism, (ii) hypoadrenalism, and (iii) diuretics

Supportive criteria

Abnormal water load test (unable to excrete −> 90 per cent of a 20 mL/kg water load in 4h, and/or failure to dilute urine to osmolality −< 100 mosmol/kg H_2O).

Management

Management depends on the rate of onset of symptoms and neurological complications.

Acute symptomatic hyponatraemia has a mortality of 5–8 per cent and patients will need prompt correction with intravenous hypertonic saline with meticulous monitoring, as over rapid correction can lead to central pontine myelinosis with quadriparesis and bulbar palsy.

Chronic asymptomatic hyponatraemia is best treated with fluid restriction. In effect this means reducing dietary input or urinary output to less than 500mL/day, which may take several days to produce an effect. This may not be appropriate in the terminal care setting, when patients may prefer to eat and drink what they like without strict regimes.

Drug treatments involve the use of distal nephron inhibitors preventing water reabsorption (e.g. demeclocycline) and oral osmotic diuretics (e.g. urea).

Demeclocycline (desmethylchlortetracycline) inhibits vasopressin and causes nephrogenic diabetes insipidus: 900–1200 mg/day will reverse chronic SIAD over 3–4 days and should be followed by a maintenance dose of 600–900mg/day.

Side-effects include gastrointestinal disturbances, hypersensitivity reactions and reversible nephrotoxicity.

Urea is effective in controlling SIAD by both intravenous and oral routes. Oral urea, 30g dissolved in orange juice to mask the taste, is the daily dose. (Using urea obviates the need to fluid restrict the patient.)

Non-islet cell tumour hypoglycaemia

Hypoglycaemia in malignancy is often associated with beta cell tumours which secrete insulin. More rarely, non-islet cell tumours produce hypoglycaemia by increased tumour usage of glucose, secretion of insulin-like growth factors (IGFs) (formerly somatomedins) and disruption of the balance maintaining normal homeostasis.

Increased use of glucose by tumours has been clearly documented with daily consumption sometimes reaching levels of 200g/kg per day. Hepatic glucose production may also fall, and suppression of compensatory growth hormone and glucagons also contribute to the hypoglycaemic state.

In advanced malignancy the commonest cause of hypoglycaemia is oral hypoglycaemic medication.

Epidemiology
Insulin-secreting tumours are usually large (average 2.4kg), often retroperitoneal or intrathoracic with liver invasion. The tumours may be growing over a relatively longer time course than many other cancers (often several years).
- Approximately 60 per cent are mesenchymal tumours (mesothelioma, neurofibroma, leiomyosarcoma etc.)
  - Twenty per cent are hepatoma
  - Ten per cent adrenal carcinoma
  - Ten per cent are gastrointestinal tumours

Clinical features
Hypoglycaemic symptoms often do not appear until the terminal stage of the disease. Symptoms are associated with cerebral hypoglycaemia and the associated secondary response of catecholamine secretion. Neurological features include agitation, stupor, coma and seizures, usually following exercise or fasting and occur most often in the early morning or late afternoon. Other causes of hypoglycaemia should be excluded, such as overtreatment of diabetes.

Treatment
The reversal of symptomatic hypoglycaemia initially requires intravenous glucose infusion. Central lines may be needed for hyperosmolar glucose solutions. Up to 2000 g/day of glucose may occasionally be needed. Frequent feeding, including during the night, and steroids may be helpful.

Debulking surgery, arterial embolization of tumours or chemotherapy can all have a place in the palliation of tumor related hypoglycaemia.

Carcinoid syndrome
Carcinoid tumours are a diverse group of tumours of enterochromaffin cell origin. The incidence is 1.5 per 100,000. The carcinoid syndrome develops in up to 18 per cent of patients with such tumours and these patients almost invariably have hepatic metastases.

The commonest site of origin is the appendix (25 per cent) and rectum but they have also been reported in the pancreas, lungs, thymus and gonads. Tumours may be benign but 80 per cent greater than 2cm in diameter metastasize.

Clinical features
- Flushing and diarrhoea occur in at least 75 per cent of patients
- Cardiac manifestations involving the right side of the heart are late manifestations in a third of patients
- Wheeze/right ventricular heart failure (RVF) (tricuspid valve regurgitation +/− stenosis/pulmonary valve stenosis)
- Asthma and pellagra are less common

Clinical features are mediated by several active substances secreted by tumours including:
- Numerous vasoactive amines and hormones

- Serotonin (5-HT)   5-hydroxytryptophan (5-HTP)
- Prostaglandins
- Catecholamines
- Tachykinins (Substance P, neuropeptide K)
- Histamine

Alcohol or psychological stress may precipitate symptoms.

The features of carcinoid tumours vary by their sites of origin.

Table 6i.1 Comparison of carcinoid tumours by site of origin

	Foregut	**Midgut**	**Hindgut**
Site	Resp tract, pancreas, stomach, proximal duodenum	Jejunum, ileum, appendix, Meckle's diverticulum, ascending colon	Transverse and descending colon, rectum
Tumour products	Low 5-HTP, multihormones	High 5-HTP, multihormones	Rarely 5-HTP, multihormones
Blood	5-HTP, histamine, multihormones	5-HT, rarely ACTH, multihormones	
Urine	5-HTP, 5-HT, 5-HIAA, histamine	5-HT, 5-HIAA	Rarely 5-HT or ACTH
Carcinoid syndrome	Atypical	Frequently with metastases	Rarely occurs
Metastases to bone	Common	Rare	Common

5-HIAA, 5-hydroxyindole acetic acid

'Multihormones' include tachykinins, neurotensin, enkephalin, insulin, glucagons, glicentin, VIP, Somatostatin, pancreatic polypeptide subunit of human chorionic gonadotrophin.

Diagnosis is usually established by:

1 Measuring urinary excretion of 5-hydroxyindole acetic acid (metabolite of 5-HT)
2 Platelet 5-HT levels (unaffected by diet)

Tumour localization may be achieved with somatostatin scintography or PET scanning.

Palliative debulking surgery, hepatic artery embolization, and chemotherapy may be appropriate palliative treatment for selected patients, while symptomatic treatment of diarrhoea and wheezing using more traditional agents also have a place in the management of patients with advanced carcinoid tumours.

Ketanserin has been used in some centres, ameliorating flushing in 50 per cent but only 20 per cent relief of diarrhoea. Selective $5-HT_3$ receptor inhibitors may reduce diarrhoea.

Table 6i.2 Pharmacological management of carcinoid syndrome symptoms

Drug	Mechanism	May reduce diarrhoea	May reduce flushing	Comments
Octreotide	150–1500 mcg/day			CSCI +/–alpha interferon
Lanreotide	30mg every 7–14 days i/m			
Sandostatin LAR	20mg–30mg every 28 days Somatostatin analogues	yes	yes	First line therapy. 80% Reduced hormonal output and blocks action. Effects diminish with time. Doses need to be adjusted after three doses Very expensive
Verapamil 40–120mg t.d.s./q.d.s.	Calcium channel blocker	yes	(?)	Limited value
Cyproheptadine 4–10mg t.d.s.	5-HT₂ antagonism +/- Anti-histamine	yes (60%)	yes (47%)	Mean duration of response 8 months Limited value

Non-paraneoplastic complications

The incidence of hyperglycaemia in patients with cancer is higher than in the general population. Several theories to account for this have been postulated:

1 Increased gluconeogenesis
2 Increased conversion of lactate to glucose
3 Diminished glucose tolerance
4 Insulin resistance
5 Increased use of medications such as corticosteroids promoting hyperglycaemia

These changes may arise as a result of liver damage, altered glucose metabolism by tumour cells, and secretion of insulin antagonists.

Diabetes mellitus

Management of diabetes in palliative care

A limited prognosis for a patient makes *close* control of blood glucose (aimed at reducing long-term sequelae) unnecessary, thereby allowing a less invasive/interventional approach.

Changes in the patient's condition (e.g. cachexia), infection or treatment (e.g. corticosteroids) commonly alter the diabetic treatment needed—the management may have to change rapidly over time.

Aims of control

1 To prevent symptoms
   • Maintaining the blood glucose at <15mmol/L is usually sufficient to prevent symptoms of hyperglycaemia (polyuria, thirst, nausea and vomiting, feeling 'unwell', drowsiness). Hyperglycaemic patients are susceptible to infection
   • A dry mouth is commonly due to drugs (morphine or antimuscarinics) and is not a good indicator of dehydration
2 To prevent hypoglycaemia occurring
3 To minimize intervention i.e. frequency of blood sugar measurement and number of injections

Hyperglycaemia in advanced malignancy

In addition to pre-existing diabetes mellitus (including previously undiagnosed cases, which may present in the terminal stages), there are two particular causes of hyperglycaemia that may occur in patients with advanced malignancy:
• corticosteroid-induced diabetes
• insulin deficiency/resistance in pancreatic cancer

Hypoglycaemia

Common clinical changes that occur in patients with advanced malignancy, leading to reduced insulin or oral hypoglycaemic requirements in pre-existing diabetics are:
• cancer cachexia in advanced illness (reduced body mass)
• reduced food intake due to anorexia, dysphagia, 'squashed stomach' or nausea/vomiting etc.
• liver replacement by tumour causing low glycogen stores and limited gluconeogenesis

Corticosteroids

Corticosteroids are commonly used in advanced malignancy. They have a direct metabolic hyperglycaemic effect, but may also increase appetite, sometimes dramatically.

Hyperglycaemia is a dose-related effect in any patient (one in five patients on high doses will develop steroid-induced diabetes), but there is wide variability between patients in their response. The hyperglycaemia is usually asymptomatic and requires no therapy unless polyuria or poly-dipsia develop, in which case a short acting sulphonylurea (e.g. gliclazide) may be useful. The dose of steroids should be reduced to the minimum possible.

Treatment options for diabetes

Oral hypoglycaemic drugs

- Gliclazide is a short acting hypoglycaemic. It may be given once or twice daily at a starting dose of 40–80 mg mane
- Increase as required to a maximum total dose 160 mg b.d.
- Avoid metformin in patients with advanced cancer

Insulin

It is sensible to use only two or three insulins, such as:

- human insulin zinc suspension (mixed) (human monotard), insulin glargine long-acting half-life
- human isophane insulin (human insulatard or humulin I) medium-acting half-life
- human soluble insulin (human actrapid or humulin S) short-acting half-life

Use either:

- a single dose of human monotard daily (given at bedtime), or
- Isophane insulin: two-third daily dose mane, 1/3 rd dose nocte

If converting from mixed insulin regime (e.g. isophane + human soluble insulin) to single daily human monotard:

- calculate the total daily insulin requirement
- reduce the dose by approximately 20–30 per cent to account for the conversion
- adjust the dose as necessary if blood glucose has been high or low
- give this dose once daily as human monotard

For a patient who has been uncontrolled on oral hypoglycaemics, start with human monotard 10u daily.

> **Insulin glargine**, a human insulin analogue with a prolonged duration of action has been introduced and is given once daily in patients with type 1 diabetes.
> NICE guidelines (December 2002)
> Insulin glargine is not recommended for routine use with type 2 diabetes unless:
> - Patient requires assistance with injecting
> - Recurrent symptomatic hypoglycaemia
> - Need twice daily basal injections in addition to twice daily oral anti-diabetic drugs

Initiating treatment in new diagnosis hyperglycaemia
- Restrict diet *if overeating*: do not impose a strict diet on a patient with advanced illness. It is more important to try and achieve a regular caloric input from one day to the next
- Reduce dose of corticosteroids if appropriate
- Consider infection as a factor causing the hyperglycaemia
- Thin, cachectic patients are less likely to respond to oral hypoglycaemic drugs, and insulin should be considered early if not responding to simple measures e.g. gliclazide 80 mg o.d.
- If the patient is peripherally vasoconstricted, give insulin by i/m route, rather than SC

Sliding scale insulin regimen
Monitor blood glucose and give soluble insulin SC as indicated. Use 8-h if patient not eating, or before mealtimes. Adjust sliding scale doses according to response.

Fasting blood sugar mmol/L	Soluble insulin
10–14	4u
15–18	6u
19–22	8u
>22	10u

Drugs used in hyperglycaemia
Gliclazide
- Tabs. 80mg
- Dose: 80mg mane p.o.
- Blood levels increased by fluconazole and miconazole (hypoglycaemia)

Human insulin soluble
- Inj. 100u/mL (human actrapid or humulin S)

Human insulin glargine
- Inj. 100u/mL (Lantus)

Human insulin isophane
- Inj. 100u/mL (human insulatard or humulin I)

Human insulin zinc suspension (mixed)
- Inj. 100u/mL (human monotard)

Drugs used in hypoglycaemia
Glucagon may be ineffective in a starved patient, as it depends on adequate liver glycogen.

Glucagon
- Inj. 1mg
- Dose: 1mg i/m (<12yrs 0.5mg)
- Do not give by SC route, as the patient may be peripherally vasoconstricted

Glucose/dextrose
- Oral gel 10g (hypostop gel); Inj. 25 per cent 25mL 50 per cent 25mL
- Dose: 25mL of 50 per cent i/v or 10g p.o.

Blood sugar mmol/L	Action
11–17	Dietary advice.
	Reduce steroids if possible.
	Start gliclazide 40mg daily and increase as necessary every few days.
17–27	Start gliclazide 80mg mane if no, or mild, ketonuria.
	If moderate or severe ketonuria the patient will need insulin—start human monotard 10u nocte.
	If ketonuria and symptomatic, consider reducing blood glucose more rapidly using human soluble insulin 4–8u every 4h until glucose <17 mmol/L, or i/v regimen below.
>27	Consider if admission to acute medical unit is appropriate, especially if ketonuria present.
	Use i/v regimen as below if intensive treatment appropriate, or human soluble insulin 4–8u every 4h until glucose <17 mmol/L.

Table 6i.3 Managing diabetes when vomiting or not eating

Diabetes type	Action
Oral hypoglycaemics	Reduce dose by 50% if oral intake reduced, or discontinue if no oral intake.
Insulin dependent	Insulin is required to prevent ketosis even with no oral intake.
	Use i/v regimen below if intensive control is appropriate, or use sliding scale of Human Soluble Insulin 8-h.

Table 6i.4 Managing diabetes in the terminal days

Diabetes type	Action
Oral hypoglycaemics	Discontinue when unable to take oral intake.
Insulin dependent	Insulin is required to prevent ketosis, even with no oral intake.

For insulin dependent:

1 If patient unconscious/unaware, discontinue insulin and monitoring.
2 If the patient is still aware/conscious, several strategies may be appropriate, depending on the patients'/relatives' attitude to burden of treatment (and monitoring) and prognosis:
   • Use sliding scale soluble insulin 8-h
   • Give approximately half of the patient's recent insulin requirement as a single dose of human monotard as a single daily injection, with or without blood sugar monitoring

Further reading

Books

Back, I. (2001) *Palliative Medicine Handbook*. 3rd edn. Cardiff: BPM Books.

Doyle D., Hanks G., Cherny N., Calman K. (2004) *Oxford Textbook of Palliative Medicine*. 3rd edn. Oxford: Oxford University Press.

Watson M., Lucas C. (2003) *Adult Palliative Care Guidelines*. London: The South West London and the Surrey, West Sussex and Hampshire Cancer Networks.

Article

Poulson J. (1997) The management of diabetes in patients with advanced cancer. *Journal of Pain and Symptom Management*, 13, 6: 339–46.

Neurological problems in advanced cancer

📖 For spinal cord compression see Chapter 15 on Emergencies in palliative care.

Brachial plexopathy

Cause
Invasion or compression by tumour, or fibrosis secondary to radiotherapy.

Clinical features
Shoulder or arm pain (suggestive of tumour), numbness or allodynia in arm or hand, muscle weakness, atrophy, Horner's syndrome.

Investigations
CT scan or MRI scan of brachial plexus.

Management
Palliative radiotherapy or chemotherapy may reduce the pain if tumour is the cause, but there is rarely an improvement in function. Otherwise, appropriate analgesia, including an agent for neuropathic pain, will be necessary.

Lumbosacral plexopathy

Cause
Invasion or compression by tumour or radiation fibrosis (rare).

Clinical features
Lumbosacral pain radiating into the legs. Leg weakness is usually unilateral and sensory dysfunction is apparent.

Investigations
CT or MRI scan of pelvis.

Management
Palliative radiotherapy or chemotherapy, if tumour is the cause, reduces pain and can occasionally improve function.

Paraneoplastic neurological syndromes
- These are neurological disorders which occur in up to 7 per cent of patients with cancer
- The aetiology is unclear although the production of a specific antibody may be involved
- Syndromes can occur as a presenting feature, before the diagnosis of cancer is made
- The commonest implicated cancers include small cell lung cancer (30 per cent), breast and ovarian cancer and lymphoma
- Symptoms are usually subacute and there may be more than one syndrome in the same patient

Syndromes include:
- **Peripheral neuropathy** involving distal sensory and/or motor or autonomic nerves. Removal of tumour (which is usually SCLC, myeloma, Hodgkin's Disease, breast and gastrointestinal cancers) does not usually produce improvement in symptoms, which are usually progressive. Steroids may help
- **Cerebellar degeneration** may present rapidly, sometimes before the primary tumour becomes apparent. Response to treatment is disappointing
- **Lambert–Eaton myasthenic syndrome** is a disorder of neuromuscular transmission occuring in 3 per cent of patients with small cell lung cancer who account for 60–70 per cent of cases. It is seen occasionally with other cancers including thymoma, breast cancer and lymphoma. There is a presynaptic deficit in neuromuscular transmission caused by a reduction in the amount of acetylcholine released at the motor nerve terminal

  There is some evidence of an autoimmune aetiology, with the presence of autoantibodies to calcium channels at the neuromuscular junction. Common symptoms include proximal muscle weakness, particularly of the legs, and an associated waddling gait. Fatigue, diplopia, ptosis and dysarthria may also be a problem. Unlike classical myasthenia, weakness may be improved by repetitive activity and there is a poor response to edrophonium. It may improve with treatment of the underlying malignancy
- **Encephalomyelopathies** can affect the limbic system, brainstem and spinal cord
- **Other clinical presentations** include dementia, opsoclonus-myoclonus, limbic encephalitis (presenting rapidly with confusion, memory disturbance and agitation) and necrotizing myelopathy

Corticosteroid-induced proximal myopathy

- This can occur within a few weeks of starting dexamethasone 8–16 mg a day
- Patients experience difficulty in rising from a sitting position and in climbing stairs
- Disabling symptoms may not be readily volunteered and direct questioning may be needed. Management includes reducing the steroid dose to the minimum possible and considering a change to prednisolone, which may not cause as much muscle wasting (but is associated with more fluid retention)
- Weakness should improve in 3–4 weeks of steroid withdrawal

Drug-induced movement disorders

- Certain drugs may induce extrapyramidal symptoms and signs
- These include akathisia (motor restlessness in which the patient may frequently change position or pace up and down if able), dystonia and parkinsonism
- Implicated drugs are those which block dopamine receptors such as antipsychotics (particularly haloperidol and phenothiazines) and metoclopramide

- Antidepressants and ondansetron may also cause problems
- **All these drugs should be avoided as far as possible in patients with Parkinson's disease**

Convulsions and seizures

Common causes of seizures in palliative care include:
- Brain tumour (primary or secondary)
- Biochemical disturbance (e.g. severe hyponatraemia)
- Previous cerebrovascular accident
- Long-standing epilepsy

Isolated tonic-clonic seizures sometimes occur but rarely last more than a few minutes: treatment may not always be needed if they quickly settle and do not cause the patient distress.

Grand mal seizures should be treated promptly since it is very distressing and frightening for families to witness. Efficient management is therefore needed.

If a patient develops a grand mal seizure or status epilepticus, give:
1 Midazolam 5–10mg buccal/SC or slow i/v (dilute 10mg with water to 10mL) and repeat after 15 and 30 minutes if not settled. Midazolam is not licensed as an anticonvulsant, but is usually readily available in palliative care units. A number of alternative benzodiazepines can be used:
   - lorazepam 4mg slow i/v or SL
   - diazepam 10mg PR or diazemuls 2–10mg slow i/v
   - clonazepam 1mg slow i/v (into large vein)

If the patient has not responded to a repeated dose of benzodiazepine or seizures recur, consider:
   - phenobarbital 100mg SC, or 100mg in 100mL sodium chloride 0.9 per cent by slow i/v injection, over 30 mins
2 Repeat phenobarbital if necessary and set up syringe driver with phenobarbital 200–600mg SC over 24 h
3 Once seizures have been controlled, review anticonvulsant therapy.

General notes
- For patients with intracranial tumours, consider starting, or review dose, of corticosteroids
- Remember to advise the patient about restrictions on driving and to contact the DVLA
- Consider parenteral thiamine if alcohol abuse is suspected
- Consider and treat hypoglycaemia in at-risk patients
- Consider drug interactions that alter anticonvulsant levels (e.g. steroids)

Initiating anticonvulsant therapy
- It is usually appropriate to initiate anticonvulsant therapy after one seizure in patients with terminal illness
- Sodium valproate is an appropriate first line anticonvulsant for almost all types of convulsions or seizures, including focal and partial seizures, and those caused by intracranial tumours

- Aim to increase dose to lower end of quoted 'usual maintenance dose' unless side-effects occur, or the patient is frail and elderly. (Doses given below)
- Carbamazepine and phenytoin may be suitable alternatives

Patients unable to take oral medication

- Patients who are unable to take oral medication due to dysphagia, vomiting or in the terminal stages, may need anticonvulsants by another route
- The half-life of most anticonvulsants is quite long (>24h), therefore no parenteral anticonvulsant is usually needed if there is a low risk of seizures, **and** only a **single dose** is missed
- **The risk of seizures is higher if**:
  - patient has decreased or stopped steroids (intracranial tumours)
  - recent rise in headache or vomiting or other signs suggesting rising intracranial pressure (intracranial tumours)
  - myoclonus or other twitching is present
  - history of poor control of seizures or recent seizures
  - previously needing more than a single anticonvulsant to achieve control
- Because of the long half-life of anticonvulsants, parenteral treatment can be started at any time within 24h after the last oral dose

Choice of non-oral anticonvulsant

Choice may be determined partly by availability:

Table 6j.1 Choice of non-oral anticonvulsant

Phenobarbital CSCI or daily SC	Well-proven anticonvulsant for all types of seizures. Experience suggests it is effective in doses of 200mg/24h.
	Phenobarbital is incompatible with most other drugs in a syringe driver, therefore a second syringe driver may be necessary. Stat doses of 100mg SC or i/m can sting.
Midazolam CSCI	Midazolam is more useful as a sedative than as an anticonvulsant. Anticonvulsant efficacy of 'standard' doses is unknown, but probably requires 20–30mg/24h minimum. Unlicensed use.
	If low risk of seizures, and midazolam indicated for e.g. terminal agitation, then additional anticonvulsant probably unnecessary. If higher risk of seizures, use phenobarbital in addition.
Clonazepam CSCI	Main advantage is that clonazepam is compatible with many other drugs used in CSCI. Much less experience supporting its use in this way; doses recommended between 2–4mg/24h (4–8mg/24h if sedation acceptable or desired).
Carbamazepine or valproate suppositories	Occasionally suitable for patients well controlled on one of these drugs, who develop a temporary inability to take oral medication (e.g. vomiting and who would find rectal administration acceptable).

Phenobarbital as Anticonvulsant

- If a patient is dying, and sedation is acceptable, it is better to err on the generous side and give:
  - phenobarbital 200mg SC stat. as a loading dose
  - phenobarbital 200mg/24h by CSCI, or
  - if high risk of seizures—phenobarbital 400mg/24h by CSCI
- If needing to minimize sedation, use 100mg SC stat. as a loading dose followed by 100–200mg/24h by CSCI

Phenobarbital is compatible with diamorphine and hyoscine if given by CSCI

Management of seizures at home

Most seizures are self-limiting and require only supportive care. For more prolonged seizures occurring at home, a number of measures can be arranged in anticipation which can avoid inappropriate emergency admission to hospital.

- Diazepam rectal solution 10mg PR—administered by district nurse or carer
- Midazolam 5–10mg SC (or preferably i/m)—administered by district nurse
- Midazolam buccal 10mg/2mL can be administered by a carer if the rectal route for diazepam is unacceptable: it appears to be as effective and may be quicker-acting than rectal diazepam 10mg. Oral solution is available as a 'special' or the injectable preparation can be used

In an inpatient unit, midazolam 5–10mg SC (or preferably i/m) may be given first before treating status epilepticus as above.

Anticonvulsants

Carbamazepine and phenytoin levels are decreased (risk of fits) by corticosteroids. Carbamazepine, phenytoin and phenobarbital can reduce the efficacy of corticosteroids.

This two-way interaction is common when managing patients with cerebral tumours. Carbamazepine, phenytoin or phenobarbital plasma levels are also reduced by St John's Wort (risk of fits).

Sodium valproate
- Tabs.: 200mg, 500mg; syrup 200mg/5mL
- Dose: 200mg t.d.s. p.o.
- Increase 200mg/day at three day intervals. Usual maintenance 1–2g/24h. Max. 2.5g/24h in divided doses. Suppositories are available as special orders

Carbamazepine
- Tabs.: 100mg, 200mg, 400mg; liquid 100mg/5mL; Supps. 125mg, 250mg
- Dose: 100mg b.d. p.o.
- Increase from initial dose by increments of 200mg every week. Usual maintenance dose 0.8–1.2g/24h in two divided doses. Max. 1.6–2g/24h. Equivalent rectal dosage: 125mg PR $\cong$ 100mg p.o.
- Carbamazepine levels are increased (risk of toxicity) by clarithromycin, erythromycin, dextropropoxyphene (co-proxamol), fluoxetine and fluvoxamine

Phenytoin
- Caps.: 50mg, 100mg, 300mg; Susp. 30mg/5mL, 90mg/5mL
- Dose: 90mg b.d. p.o.
- Start 150–300mg daily. Usual maintenance dose: 300–400mg daily. Max. 600mg/24h. Single or two divided doses
- Phenytoin levels are increased (risk of toxicity) by clarithromycin, metronidazole, trimethoprim, fluconazole, miconazole, omeprazole, fluoxetine, fluvoxamine, aspirin, diltiazem, nifedipine and amiodarone
- Because phenytoin has a very long and variable half-life, it can take several days and even up to 3–4 weeks for changes in dosage to take complete effect: this should be borne in mind in determining the interval after dosage is altered before measuring the plasma phenytoin concentration again

Barbiturate
Phenobarbital (phenobarbitone)
- Inj: 60mg/1mL, 200mg/1mL; Tabs.: 15mg, 30mg, 60mg; elixir 15mg/5mL
- Elixir in various strengths can be made to order e.g. 10mg/mL
- Phenobarbital is a barbiturate with sedative and anticonvulsant effects. It is rarely used nowadays as a first line anticonvulsant, as it is too sedative. It can be given by CSCI, but usually needs to be given in a separate syringe driver. It can be given by daily SC or i/m injection, but the preparation is very viscous and stings on injection. Doses: see above

Benzodiazepines

Midazolam
- Inj: 10mg/2mL, 10mg/5mL
- Dose: 30mg/24h CSCI
- Oral solution available as special order, or use injection for buccal use
- Sedative effect markedly enhanced by itraconazole, ketoconazole and possibly fluconazole

Lorazepam
- Tabs.: 1mg, 2.5mg; Inj: 4mg/1mL
- Dilute inj. with equal volume of water or saline for i/m use

Diazepam
- Tabs.: 2mg, 5mg, 10mg; oral solution 2mg/5mL, 5mg/5mL
- Rectal tubes 5mg/2.5mL, 10mg/2.5mL; Supps. 10mg
- Inj: (emulsion) 10mg/2mL (diazemuls)—i/v use only
- Inj: (solution) 10mg/2mL—i/m use

Clonazepam
- Tabs.: 500mcg, 2mg; inj: 1mg/1mL
- Starting Dose: 1mg nocte
- Increase gradually to usual maintenance dose 4–8mg/24h. Oral solutions in various strengths are available from several sources

Further reading

Books

Back I. (2001) *Palliative Medicine Handbook.* 3rd edn. Cardiff: BPM Books.

Doyle D., Hanks G., Cherny N., Calman K. (2004) *Oxford Textbook of Palliative Medicine.* Oxford: Oxford University Press.

Watson M., Lucas C. (2003) *Adult Palliative Care Guidelines.* London: The South West London and the Surrey, West Sussex and Hampshire Cancer Networks.

Articles

Heafield M. (2000) Managing status epilepticus. *BMJ,* **320**: 953–4.

Newsom-Davis J. (1999) Paraneoplastic neurological disorders. *Journal of The Royal College of Physicians of London,* **33**: 225–7.

Sleep disorders

Sleep disorders are a frequent complication of medical illness, occurring in 50 per cent or more of those with advanced cancer, particularly where pain is a complicating factor. Night-time rest is an invaluable respite from the worries and pain of the day, allowing the patient to meet the next day with renewed energy. Despite this, it is not often taken seriously by healthcare professionals.

Human sleep is an essential, active, dynamic and complex physiological function in which stages are repeated in cyclical pattern throughout the night. There are two distinct states of sleep, non-rapid eye movement sleep (NREM) and rapid eye movement (REM). NREM sleep accounts for 75 per cent of the night, in a staged process from light to deep sleep, and is a period of relative physiological and cognitive quiescence. REM sleep, on the other hand, is characterized by muscle atonia, dreaming and autonomic variability.

The sleep–wake cycle is a component of the body's overall circadian rhythm, synchronized with other biological rhythms including temperature oscillation and cortisol and growth hormone secretion. The onset and maintenance of normal sleep patterns depend on the appropriate timing of sleep within the 24 hour circadian rhythm. Adequate physical comfort, an acceptable sleeping environment, an intact central nervous system function and relative absence of psycholological distress and psychophysiologic arousal is necessary for sleep.

The restorative functions of sleep are dependent on a well-organized and reasonably uninterrupted sleep structure. Sleep tends to be lighter with advancing age and in many medical conditions. The percentage of REM sleep, however, remains relatively constant in a healthy elderly population, but is decreased when cognitive impairment or certain other medical conditions are present.

Insomnia

Insomnia is a subjective complaint by the patient of poor sleep. This encompasses complaints of insufficient sleep, interrupted sleep, poor quality or non-restorative sleep or sleep which occurs at the wrong time in the day–night cycle. Physical, psychological and environmental factors contribute to poor sleep in medical conditions. Sleep deprivation may result in progressive fatigue, sleepiness, impairment of concentration, irritability and depression. Deep stages of NREM sleep may be critical in tissue restoration and in maintaining a healthy immune system.

Disorders of the sleep–wake cycle

A normal sleeping pattern is dependent on a well-established schedule of sleep and wakefulness. Patients who are terminally ill are prone to disturbances in the sleep–wake cycle because of frequent disruptions of night-time sleep, an absence of usual daytime schedule demands and relative inactivity during normal waking hours. A lack of sleep at night leads to late waking and daytime napping and late settling to sleep the following night (delayed sleep phase syndrome) or early morning waking and early bedtime (advanced sleep phase syndrome). Either way, a vicious disturbed cycle then emerges. For some a rhythm disappears altogether and is replaced by a pattern of multiple shorter sleep periods interspersed with wakefulness throughout the 24 h. It must not be forgotten that coming into hospital leads to highly fragmented sleep.

Excessive daytime sleepiness

It is very common for patients receiving palliative care to complain generally of tiredness and fatigue, but this must be distinguished from sleepiness. A degree of daytime sedation can be desirable in some cases, but excessive sleepiness can be disabling leading to inactivity and poor motivation. Patients may become less capable of participating in treatment and may find it difficult to retain information and to interact socially. They may also become unnecessarily depressed, irritable and withdrawn during the important last weeks or months of life.

Causes of disturbed sleep in the terminally ill which should be actively sought and treated where appropriate

- Uncontrolled pain—contributes to lack of sleep in up to 60 per cent of patients. Sleep deprivation lowers pain thresholds
- Medication—steroids, especially if taken late in the day; bronchodilators; enervating antidepressants e.g. fluoxetine; withdrawal from sedative hypnotics or analgesia; caffeine, nicotine and alcohol may also be contributory
- Depression—at least 90 per cent of depressed patients have abnormal sleep patterns. Depression is common and it is a significant cause of sleep pathology in the terminally ill
- Bladder or bowel discomfort and incontinence
- Anxiety and fears—anxiety may be directly related to the illness or treatment and is often associated with pain. Early delirium, withdrawal from drugs and breathlessness can frequently cause anxiety. During the daytime fears are masked by distractions
- Cognitive impairment disorder—delirium is not uncommon in the terminally ill and reversible causes should be actively sought. Sleep disturbance itself may lead to delirium. Patients with dementia sleep less deeply and have reduced REM and increased awakening after sleep onset
- Patients need constant reassurance and to be nursed in a lit room to minimize disorientation. Hypnotics may aggravate the situation. Drugs such as haloperidol 0.5–2.0mg or risperidone 0.5–1.0mg may be useful, particularly if given in the early evening, to pre-empt a restless period and give adequate time for the drug to take effect before settling for the night. NB Risperidone should not be used if there is a history of cerebrovascular disease
- Nausea and vomiting
- Respiratory distress
- Psychophysiological—conditional arousal response, poor sleep hygiene
- Sleep–wake schedule disorder—disruption of normal schedule, excessive napping during the day
- Restless legs syndrome—may be associated with potentially manageable causes such as sedative hypnotic withdrawal, anaemia, uraemia, peripheral neuropathy, iron deficiency, diabetes mellitus

Management

A full assessment must be carried out to define the individual's sleep characteristics and to address all possible reversible causes. In the absence of any obviously reversible causes, the aim is to achieve enough restorative sleep to ensure daytime alertness, concentration and energy. Attention must also be given to the carer, who may have fragmented nights for weeks and months yet still has to do the daytime chores and caring.

- **Sleep hygiene** Excessive arousal in bed is a frequent cause and effect of insomnia. Anxiety is exacerbated when lying isolated in bed, mind racing with all others asleep. Patients may need to undertake a relaxing activity to turn their minds away from the pressure to fall asleep, but may not be able to get out of bed to achieve this. They may lie awake, apparently asleep, fearful of moving and waking up their exhausted carers and bedtime may become a dreaded time. A chaotic, unpredictable pattern needs to be managed by reinforcing the rest–activity sleep–wake cycle. Physical, cognitively stimulating and social activity during the day may help to strengthen the difference between day and night

- **Non-pharmacological** Cognitive behavioural treatment is the mainstay of treatment for insomnia that is due wholly or in part to heightened cognitive or physiological arousal and poor sleep hygiene. Other techniques such as hypnosis and somatic imagery training, progressive muscle relaxation, psychotherapy and complementary therapy such as aromatherapy may help

- **Pharmacological** Benzodiazepines and other drugs that act on benzodiazepine receptors such as cyclopyrrolone (zopiclone) are the standard medications of choice in the treatment of transient or short term insomnia. Hypnotic medication is used frequently in palliative care and may greatly enhance quality of life. Choice of hypnotic depends on several factors including length of time of effectiveness, rate of absorption and metabolism and potential risks or side-effects. Daytime sedation with the shorter acting hypnotics is rarely a problem. Nocturnal confusion may be induced, particularly in individuals with baseline cognitive dysfunction.
  Most are absorbed quickly reaching peak concentrations within an hour or less. The non-benzodiazepine hypnotics have a very short half-life of about 1 hour. Temazepam, lorazepam and oxazepam have intermediate half-lives ranging from 8 to 15 h in healthy adults whereas diazepam is longer acting and is cleared more slowly.
  Chloral hydrate has modest short term efficacy but is more toxic than benzodiazepines. Sedating tricyclic antidepressants (e.g. amitriptyline) are often used but are associated with anticholinergic side-effects. Trazodone is a sedating heterocyclic with milder anticholinergic side-effects and a shorter half life than most tricyclics and can be administered over a longer period of time.
  Chlomethiazole is sometimes used.
  Sedative hypnotics in the elderly are associated with falls, cognitive impairment and worsening of nocturnal respiratory disturbance and should be used in low doses.

Haematological aspects

Anaemia

Anaemia is defined as a haemoglobin concentration in adults of less than 13.0g/dl in men and 11.5g/dl in women. It is a common problem, occurring in over 50 per cent of patients with solid tumours and in most patients with haematological malignancies such as multiple myeloma and lymphoma.

Symptoms caused by anaemia include:
- Fatigue
- Weakness
- Breathlessness on exertion
- Impaired concentration
- Chest pain
- Exacerbation of congestive cardiac failure
- Low mood
- Loss of libido
- Anorexia

There are no specific criteria for the functional assessment of anaemia. However, randomized controlled trials of the management of anaemia in malignancy have used validated tools in assessing its effect on quality of life (QOL) e.g.
- Cancer Linear Analogue Scale (CLAS)
- Functional Assessment of Cancer Therapy-Anaemia (FACT-An)

Causes of anaemia
- Reduced red cell production due to bone marrow infiltration
  - Multiple myeloma
  - Prostate cancer
  - Breast cancer
  - Leukaemia
- Chemotherapy-induced bone marrow suppression
- Anaemia of chronic disease related to malignancy
- Malnutrition/malabsorption e.g. post gastrectomy
  - B_{12} deficiency
  - Folate deficiency
  - Iron deficiency
- Blood loss:
  - Gastrointestinal
  - Haematuria
- Chronic renal failure
- Reduced red cell survival/haemolysis:
  - Autoimmune haemolysis—lymphoproliferative disorders
  - Physical haemolysis—micro-angiopathic haemolytic anaemia (MAHA) in some adenocarcinomas

- Anaemia of chronic disorder related to malignancy—a combination of effects
  - Suppressed erythropoietin production
  - Impaired transferrin production
  - Shortened red cell survival

Management of anaemia

Investigate cause of anaemia where appropriate

Diagnostic indicators
- Reduced marrow production/bone marrow failure
  - Full blood count—pancytopenia and reduced reticulocytes
  - Bone marrow examination—may show infiltration by non-haematological cells e.g. prostatic or breast carcinoma, or hypocellular marrow post-chemotherapy
- Bleeding
  - Clinical—haematuria, melaena
  - Acute—blood count and film: normochromic, normocytic anaemia, reticulocytosis and polychromasia
  - Chronic—iron deficiency anaemia
- Malabsorption/malnutrition
  - Low serum B_{12}
  - Reduced serum or red cell folate
  - Reduced ferritin
- Haemolysis
  - Blood film: polychromasia; autoimmune—spherocytes; MAHA—red cell fragments (schistocytes); reticulocytosis
  - Autoimmune—positive direct Coombs test
  - Bilirubin—raised

Table 6l.1 Differentiation between iron deficiency anaemia and anaemia of chronic disease

	Iron deficiency anaemia	Anaemia of chronic disease
Blood film	Hypochromic microcytic	Normochromic or hypochromic
Red cell distribution Width (RDW)	Increased	Microcytic +/− Normal
Total iron binding capacity (TIBC)	High	Normal/low
Plasma iron	Low	Low
Serum ferritin	Low	Normal/raised

N.B. The two causes can co-exist

Decrease bleeding risk
- Consider discontinuation of drugs that may increase risk of bleeding e.g.
  - aspirin
  - NSAIDs

- anticoagulants
- steroids
- Consider gastroprotection using:
  - proton pump inhibitors
  - H_2-receptor antagonists
  - prostaglandin analogues e.g. misoprostol
- Give vitamin K in liver disease-related coagulopathies as evidenced by prolonged prothrombin time (PT)
- Give tranexamic acid (antifibrinolytic agent) for mucosal bleeding. Tranexamic acid can be given topically and as a mouthwash. (Use with care in bleeding from the bladder or prostate as clot formation is enhanced and subsequent retention may become a problem.) Etamsylate may also be useful

Replace haematinic deficiencies

- Iron deficiency
  - Ferrous sulphate 200mg b.d. or t.d.s.
- Folate deficiency
  - Folic acid 5m.g. o.d.
- B_{12} deficiency
  - Hydroxycobalamin 1000mcg i/m every three months

Blood transfusion

Patients who are becoming terminally ill may receive blood transfusions inappropriately. The decision to transfuse should not be made on the basis of one haemoglobin result alone, but in the context of symptoms attributable to anaemia which are adversely affecting quality of life. It is important to document the clinical effect of the transfusion which will help in discussing the merits or otherwise of further transfusions. Blood transfusion helps about 75 per cent of patients in terms of wellbeing, strength and breathlessness.

- Since 1998, all red cells have been leuco-depleted, therefore an in-line blood filter is not now required. One unit of leuco-depleted packed red cells (approximately 300mL) results in a rise in haemoglobin of 1g/dl
- The aim should be to transfuse up to 11–12g/dl but this will vary according to the individual clinical situation
- Patients at risk of pulmonary oedema should have furosemide cover (20mg p.o. or i/v with alternate units)
- Patients should be told that the beneficial effects may not be apparent for a day or two post-transfusion

Indications for blood transfusion in patients with palliative care needs

- Haemoglobin of less than 10g/dl (patients may benefit from transfusion at higher levels)
- Prognosis greater than two weeks
- Reasonable performance status (i.e. not predominantly bedbound) (ECOG > 2)
- Presence of at least two of the following symptoms:
  - breathlessness on exertion
  - weakness
  - angina
  - postural hypotension
  - worsening cardiac failure
  - worsening fatigue

Blood transfusion reactions

Acute life-threatening transfusion reactions are very rare, however, new symptoms or signs that occur during a transfusion must be taken seriously as they may herald a serious reaction. As it may not be possible to identify the cause of a severe reaction immediately, the initial supportive management should generally cover all the possible causes. These include:

- Acute haemolytic transfusion reaction
- Infusion of a bacterially contaminated unit
- Severe allergic reaction or anaphylaxis
- Fluid overload
- Transfusion-related acute lung injury (TRALI)

Acute haemolytic transfusion reaction

Incompatible Group A or B transfused red cells react with the patient's own anti-A or B antibodies. This results in acute renal failure, and can cause disseminated intravascular coagulation (DIC) The reaction can occur after only a few mls of blood have been transfused

- **Symptoms:** acute onset pain at venepuncture site, loins, chest
- **Signs:** fever, hypotension, tachycardia, oozing from venepuncture sites
- A similar picture is seen with the transfusion of bacterially contaminated red cells
- **Action:** If a severe acute reaction is suspected:
  - Stop the transfusion, keep i/v line open with sodium chloride 0.9% infusion
  - Monitor temperature, heart rate, BP, respiratory rate, urine output
  - Recheck the patient's identification, the blood unit and documentation
  - Inform the blood bank
  - Further management will depend on the patient's developing clinical picture

Major allergic reactions

Rare but life-threatening complication usually occur in the early part of a transfusion. These complications are more common with plasma-containing blood components e.g. fresh-frozen plasma (FFP) or platelets

- **Symptoms:** chest pain, breathlessness, nausea and abdominal pain
- **Signs:** hypotension, bronchospasm, periorbital and laryngeal oedema, vomiting, urticaria
- **Action:**
  - Stop transfusion
  - High concentration O_2
  - Chlorphenamine 10–20mg i/v over 1–2 minutes
  - Hydrocortisone 100–200mg i/v
  - Adrenaline 0.5–1mg (0.5–1mL of 1 in 1000) i/m
  - Salbutamol 2.5–5mg by nebuliser
  - Maintain i/v access

Fluid overload

More common in patients with a history of heart or renal disease, but any patient with advanced malignancy is susceptible. In these patients, each red cell unit should be given over 3–4h and a maximum of two units given per day. Clinical signs to be aware of:

- **Symptoms:** Breathlessness with basal crepitations
- **Signs:** BP may be raised initially, tachycardia, raised jugular venous pressure (JVP) may be present
- **Action:**
  - Stop transfusion
  - High concentration O_2
  - Furosemide 40mg i/v

Transfusion-related acute lung injury (TRALI)

Usually caused by antibodies in donor's plasma that react strongly with the patient's leucocytes.

- **Symptoms:** Rapid onset of breathlessness and dry cough
- **Signs:** Chest X-ray shows bilateral infiltrates—'white-out'

- **Action:**
  - Stop transfusion
  - Give 100 per cent O_2
  - Seek expert advice and treat as Adult Respiratory Distress Syndrome (ARDS)

Febrile non-haemolytic transfusion reaction

Affects 1–2 per cent of patients
- A rise in temperature < 1.5°C from the baseline or an urticarial rash, +/– rigors
- Usually occurs towards the end of a transfusion or up to two hours after it is finished
- Treat with paracetamol
- Give chlorphenamine 10mg p.o. or i/v for rash
- Continue transfusion at a slower rate
- Observe for any deterioration

Iron overload is not often a concern in palliative care but if 50–75 units of red cells have been given, haemosiderosis may develop causing heart and liver dysfunction or failure of pancreatic endocrine function.

Contra-indications to blood transfusion

- Patient refusal
- No symptomatic benefit from previous transfusion
- Patient moribund with life expectancy of days

Erythropoietin

- This is a hormone made by the kidney. It stimulates the production of red blood cells and is licensed for anaemia of chronic renal failure and for patients undergoing chemotherapy
- It may also be effective in improving the chronic anaemia of cancer
- An injection of 150–300 Units/Kg SC three times a week for 4–6 weeks increases the Hb significantly in 50–60 per cent of patients with cancer. The patients most likely to benefit include those with a low erythropoietin concentration, adequate bone marrow reserve and an initial good response (i.e. an increase in Hb of >1g/dl within four weeks of starting treatment)
- The maximum benefit is achieved after about two months which may be a factor limiting its usefulness in palliative care patients where prognosis is short
- Patients should be given iron supplements during erythropoietin therapy to maximize the response

Complications

- Hypertension
- Thrombosis
- Iron deficiency, if not on iron supplements

Screening of donated blood products is inevitably becoming ever more stringent and blood transfusion may become justified only for the most needy. Erythropoietin may therefore become more commonly used. It is already used where appropriate for Jehovah's Witnesses.

Bleeding and haemorrhage

Bleeding occurs in about 20 per cent of patients with advanced cancer and may contribute to death in 5 per cent. Bleeding may be directly related to the cancer itself, e.g. local bleeding from fungating tumours, or indirectly related, e.g. peptic ulceration or nose bleeds secondary to treatment with NSAIDs or thrombocytopenia respectively.

A systemic deterioration in a patient's condition may be mirrored by a decline in the haematological profile.

Obvious bleeding

- Oral mucosa or nose
- Gums
- Nasopharynx
- Haemoptysis
- Haematemesis
- Skin/muscle

Hidden bleeding

- Gastrointestinal—melaena, anaemia, (raised urea may be noted)
- Pulmonary—worsening breathlessness, pleural effusion
- Urogenital—macroscopic or microscopic haematuria
- Cerebral—headache, visual disturbance, change in neurology
- Gynaecological—vaginal bleeding

General management of bleeding

Where possible and when appropriate, attempt to correct haemostatic factors that contribute to a bleeding tendency.

Haemostatic factors that contribute to bleeding

Platelets

Thrombocytopenia due to:
- Reduced marrow production
  - marrow infiltration
  - myelosuppression following chemotherapy
- Increased consumption/utilization
  - disseminated intravascular coagulation (DIC)
  - autoimmune
- Splenic pooling
  - hypersplenism

Abnormal function as seen in:
- Acute myeloid leukaemia
- Myelodysplasia
- Myeloproliferative disorders
- Paraproteinaemias e.g. multiple myeloma
- Treatment with NSAID, aspirin
- Renal failure

Coagulation factors

High level expression of tissue factor leading to:
- Extrinsic pathway activation
- Thrombin generation
- Consumption of clotting factors
- DIC

Metastatic liver disease results in:
- Reduced synthesis of vitamin K-dependent factors

Acute DIC is uncommon and presents as a mixture of thrombosis and bleeding. The skin may develop petechiae and purpura, and gangrene may occur in areas of end circulation such as the digits, nose and ear lobes. Bleeding may occur in areas of trauma such as at venepuncture sites or as haematuria in the presence of a catheter. Treatment includes platelet infusions, FFP and cryoprecipitate.

Chronic DIC is more common and may be asymptomatic (as measured by laboratory tests) but thrombotic symptoms of DVT, PE or migratory thrombophlebitis may occur. Treatment is usually heparin (low molecular weight).

Laboratory investigations
- **D-dimers**—more specific than fibrin degradation products (FDPs). Significant increase in D-dimers + prolonged PT, reduced fibrinogen, +/– thrombocytopenia necessary for diagnosis (D-dimers also increased in infection)
- **Prothronbin Time (PT)**—less sensitive, usually prolonged in acute DIC, but may be normal in chronic DIC
- **Activated Partial Thromboplastin Time (APTT)**—Less useful, as may be normal or shortened in chronic DIC
- **Platelets**—Reduced or falling count found in acute DIC
- **Blood film**—may show red cell fragments (schistocytes)

Thrombocytopenia
Spontaneous bleeding due to thrombocytopenia is rare if the platelet count is $> 20 \times 10^9/l$ but traumatic bleeding is problematic if the platelet count is less than $40 \times 10^9/l$. Sepsis will increase the bleeding tendency. If platelet function is abnormal, bleeding may occur at higher counts.
- A platelet transfusion may be considered if there is bleeding which is distressing. It will only raise the platelet count for a few days. This treatment should not be given routinely if there is no evidence of bleeding and the count is greater than $10 \times 10^9/l$. If the platelet count is less than $50 \times 10^9/l$ and the patient is bleeding, platelets should be given
- A pool of platelets is derived from four units of donated blood and is approximately 300mL
- Platelets must be kept at room temperature and transfused over 30min, using a sterile administration set or a platelet infusion set. Never use an in-line filter
- The donor should be ABO compatible with the patient

It is important to anticipate which patients are likely to require platelet transfusions and to decide appropriateness prior to a crisis. The whole team should be involved in decisions concerning ongoing regular prophylactic transfusions and their withdrawal. With platelet counts of $10–20 \times 10^9/l$ the risk of a major bleed is small, severe bleeding occurring mostly with counts less than $5 \times 10^9/l$

Tranexamic acid (inhibits fibrinolysis)can be used to control mucosal bleeding due to thrombocytopenia.
- 1g orally t.d.s. or slow i/v injection
- Mouthwash 1g every six hours for oral bleeding
- Topical tranexamic acid for superficial fungating tumours

On average it takes two days of therapy to slow down bleeding and four days for bleeding to stop.

Blood products

These are less commonly used in the palliative care setting and close liaison with the haematology department is essential when considering administration. The table below outlines some products and their indications.

Indications for blood products

Fresh frozen plasma (FFP)
- Disseminated intravascular coagulation
- Rapid correction of warfarin overdose
- Liver disease
- Coagulopathy due to massive blood loss

Cryoprecipitate
- In DIC when fibrinogen <1.0g/l
- For bleeding in cases of dysfibrinogenaemia

Bleeding directly related to cancer

Radiotherapy should be considered for local bleeding caused by cancer e.g. ulcerating skin tumours, lung cancer causing haemoptysis, gynaecological cancer causing vaginal bleeding and bladder/prostate cancer causing haematuria.

Specific situations
Nose bleeds
- Most nose bleeds are venous and when arising from the anterior septum can often be stopped by pressure.
- Silver nitrate caustic pencil can be applied to the bleeding point. The nose can be packed with calcium alginate rope (e.g. kaltostat) or with ribbon gauze soaked in adrenaline (epinephrine 1:1000 1mg in 1mL)
- If the bleeding is more posterior, and continues into the nasopharynx, a merocel tampon may need to be inserted for 36hours with antibiotic cover or the nose packed with gauze impregnated with bismuth iodoform paraffin paste (BIPP) for three days.
- The ENT department may need to be contacted for further management with a balloon catheter or cauterization under local anaesthetic.

Surface bleeding
The bleeding from tumour masses may respond well to radiotherapy. Other measures include the following:
Physical
- Gauze applied with pressure for 10 mins soaked in adrenaline (epinephrine) (1:1000) 1mg in 1mL or Tranexamic acid 500mg in 5mL
  - Silver nitrate sticks to bleeding points
  - Haemostatic dressings i.e. alginate e.g. kaltostat, sorbsan

Drugs
- Topical
  - Sucralfate paste 2g (two 1g tablets crushed in 5mL KY jelly)
  - Sucralfate suspension 2g in 10mL b.d. for mouth and rectum
  - Tranexamic acid 5g in 50mL warm water b.d. for rectal bleeding
  - 1 per cent alum solution for bladder
- Systemic
  - Antifibrinolytic e.g. tranexamic acid 1.5g stat and 0.5–1g b.d.–t.d.s. p.o. or slow i/v 0.5–1g t.d.s. **Do not use if DIC suspected.**
  - Haemostatic e.g. etamsylate 500mg q.d.s. (restores platelet adhesiveness).

Haemoptysis

Haemoptysis may be directly related to the underlying tumour or related to treatments or infection. A generalized clotting deficiency, seen in thrombocytopaenia, hepatic insufficiency or anticoagulation with warfarin, can also be contributory factors.

Treatments for **non-acute haemorrhage** include oncological, systemic and local measures. If radiotherapy is not appropriate, coagulation should be enhanced with oral tranexamic acid 1g t.d.s., but caution is necessary with haematuria since clots may form in the bladder, resulting in further problems The risks of encouraging hypercoagulation need to be considered carefully in patients with a history of a stroke or ischaemic heart disease.

Erosion of a major artery can cause **acute haemorrhage** which may be a rapidly terminal event. It may be possible to anticipate such an occurrence and appropriate medication and a red/green/blue towel to reduce the visual impact should be readily available. Relatives or others who witness such an event will need a great deal of support. If the haematemesis is not immediately fatal, the aim of treatment is sedation of a shocked, frightened patient.

It *may* be appropriate to have emergency medication in the home to sedate the acutely bleeding patient, but such a strategy can only be arrived at after discussion with the family, carers, and the patient's local GP, and needs to documented clearly.

Assessment

Consider the commonest causes:
- tumour bleeding
- clotting disorders
- infection
- pulmonary embolism

Treatment

- Treat any evidence or signs suggestive of infection
- Consider radiotherapy referral (not if multiple lung metastases) or brachytherapy, where the radiation sources are placed close to the tumour within the lungs
- Consider and treat other systemic causes of bleeding (🕮 see Chapter 15)
- blood tests for clotting screen and platelets
- Tranexamic acid 1g t.d.s. p.o.
  - stop if no effect after 1 week
  - continue for 1 week after bleeding has stopped, then discontinue
  - continue long term (500mg t.d.s.) only if bleeding recurs and responds to second course of treatment

Small bleeds can herald a larger massive haemorrhage; *consider* siting an i/v cannula to administer emergency drugs.
- One third of patients with lung cancer develop haemoptysis, although the incidence of acute fatal bleeds is only 3 per cent of which some occur without warning

- The patient is more likely to die from suffocation secondary to the bleed than from the bleed itself. Bleeding due to cancer is most commonly from a primary carcinoma of the bronchus and a massive haemoptysis is usually from a squamous cell lung tumour lying centrally or causing cavitation. Metastases from carcinoma of the breast, colorectum, kidney and melanoma may also cause haemoptysis
- Infection in the chest and pulmonary emboli are other causes of haemoptysis

Haematemesis

The incidence is 2 per cent in patients with cancer and may be associated with cancer and/or secondary to gastroduodenal irritants such as NSAIDs. The management includes stopping NSAIDs if possible or changing to celecoxib (reduced effect on platelets) and adding a proton pump inhibitor or H2 receptor antagonist a gastroprotective agent such as sucralfate may also be useful.

Major bleeds
- If patient's condition is not stable, with history of major haemorrhage or ongoing bleeding:
- Consider if appropriate to transfer to an acute medical/endoscopy unit
- Site an Iv i/v cannula to anticipate need for emergency drugs
- Treat anxiety or distress as needed:
- Midazolam 2–5mg initially by slow i/v titration (10mg diluted to 10mL with sodium chloride 0.9%)

If no i/v access, midazolam 5–10mg SC (give i/m if shocked or vasoconstricted).

Rectal bleeding

This may be associated with local tumour (radiotherapy may be the treatment of choice to stop the bleeding) and/or radiotherapy. Bloody diarrhoea may occur acutely with pelvic radiotherapy which causes acute inflammation of the rectosigmoid mucosa, but this should be self limiting. A predsol retention enema 20mg in 100mL o.d.–b.d. or prednisolone 5mg and sucralfate 3g in 15mL b.d. may help.

Bleeding from chronic ischaemic radiation proctitis may respond to tranexamic acid, etamsylate or sucralfate suspension given rectally.

Haematuria

This may occur with carcinoma of the bladder or prostate or as a result of chronic radiation cystitis. Urine infection will aggravate the situation. Tranexamic acid or etamsylate may be useful, although there is the risk of clot formation and urinary retention. Alum 50mL of 1 per cent can be useful if retained in the bladder via a catheter for 1 hour.

Massive terminal haemorrhage

Massive terminal haemorrhage occurs as a result of a major arterial haemorrhage and usually causes death in minutes. For patients who have undergone all possible treatment options, this inevitably terminal event should be treated palliatively, the main aim being comfort for the patient and support for the family.

It is usually associated with tumour erosion into the aorta or pulmonary artery (causing haematemesis or haemoptysis) or carotid or femoral artery (causing external bleeding). If a massive haemorrhage is unexpected, the only appropriate management may be to stay with the patient and attempt to comfort any distress. It may be appropriate to warn family members of the possibility.

Major haemorrhage may be preceded by smaller bleeds. Patients may have been receiving platelets and blood products, which have now been discontinued. If major haemorrhage is anticipated, it may be appropriate to warn family members of the possibility. Appropriate drugs, already drawn up in a syringe, should be kept available at the bedside to ensure fast administration. Blue or green towels (which mask the colour of blood) should be available to help control the spread of blood.

In the event of a massive bleed, the aim of treatment will be to rapidly sedate and relieve patient distress from what will, by definition, be the terminal event. Where possible drugs should be given i/v or else by deep i/m injection.

Drug options

Midazolam
Midazolam 10mg SC, i/v or bucally will sedate most patients. Heavy alcohol drinkers and patients on regular benzodiazepines may require larger doses.

Ketamine
The effect of ketamine is more predictable in palliative care patients than benzodiazepines and opioids, since the patient is unlikely to have been taking it regularly. Ketamine 150mg–250mg i/v will rapidly sedate a patient dying from a terminal haemorrhage. If the i/m route is necessary, a larger dose of 500mg will be required.

Opioids
These are less recommended for the management of terminal haemorrhage for the following reasons:
1 As a controlled drug, nurses may not be able to leave a dose by the bedside or to check doses quickly.
2 Diamorphine needs to be dissolved, leading to further delay.
3 Variable doses will be required depending on how opioid-naïve the patient is.

Summary
• Midazolam 10–20mg i/v, SC, i/m or buccal
• Ketamine 150–250mg i/v or 500mg i/m
• Diamorphine dose will vary.

Thromboembolism

It is over 130 years since Trousseau first noticed the association between cancer and thrombosis. Patients with cancer are at high risk of developing venous thromboembolism (VTE) and the risk increases as malignancy advances. It follows that palliative care patients are extremely thrombogenic.

Studies have suggested that the incidence of deep vein thrombosis (DVT) may be as high 52 per cent (with 33 per cent of those being bilateral) in palliative care.

Thrombogenic risk

Virchow's triad describes the predisposing factors for VTE as:

1 stasis,
2 endothelial perturbation,
3 hypercoaguability.

The table below suggests some of the reasons that patients with cancer are at such high risk.

Prothrombotic risk in cancer

- **Stasis**
  - Immobility due to weakness, lethargy
  - Compression of vessels by tumour e.g. pelvic disease
  - Extrinsic compression from oedematous legs
- **Endothelial perturbation**
  - Recent surgery
  - Central venous access
  - Direct tumour invasion of vessel
- **Hypercoagulable state**
  - Dehydration
  - Tissue factor/tumour procoagulant release
  - Increased platelet activation
  - DIC
  - Cytokine-related thrombotic changes
  - Prothombotic changes from certain chemotherapeutic agents

Deep vein thrombosis (DVT)

Signs and symptoms vary depending upon the severity of DVT. It should be suspected in patients with a swollen, tender, warm, erythematous leg, although it is unreliable to make a firm clinical diagnosis on the basis of these findings alone. Some are asymptomatic whilst extreme cases may lead to vascular insufficiency and gangrene. The risk of a pulmonary embolus from a distal DVT (i.e. below knee) is low, and only about 20 per cent of calf vein thromboses progress to a proximal thrombosis.

Differential diagnosis

- Cellulitis
- Lymphoedema
- Oedema due to hypoproteinaemia
- Ruptured Baker's cyst

Diagnosis

It is not always practical to confirm the presence of a DVT if the patient is in the terminal stages of illness or to treat all patients with VTE. If a patient is not going to be anticoagulated there is little point in investigating suspected thrombus. Anticoagulation carries risks as well as benefits and these should be weighed up on an individual basis first.

- Doppler ultrasound
  - Non-invasive. No ionizing radiation. Easily repeatable
  - Can be performed at the bedside if suitable equipment available.
  - Accuracy lower for non-occlusive iliac thrombus and calf vein assessment than ascending venography
- Venography
  - Invasive. Involves ionizing radiation. Contrast media is injected into a vein on the dorsum of the foot. Low risk of allergic reaction
  - No longer the first-line investigation. Useful when Doppler is inconclusive, for example in patients with large oedematous legs or with previous deep vein thrombosis
  - Gives excellent visualisation of all the leg veins
- Light reflection rheography
  - Non-invasive
  - Can be done at bedside
  - High sensitivity but poor specificity and therefore not used greatly in clinical practice
  - Cannot localize thrombus or distinguish between intrinsic/extrinsic compression
- D-dimers
  - Use in cancer patients is limited due to high false positive rate in malignancy
- Magnetic resonance angiography
  - Non-invasive
  - Good at imaging leg vessels
  - Use in palliative care patients is yet to be evaluated

Pulmonary embolus (PE)

Evidence from *post-mortem* studies suggests that pulmonary emboli are underdiagnosed clinically in the palliative care setting.

This may be due to several factors:
- Patient not well enough for investigation
- Other lung pathologies make radiological diagnosis problematic
- Concerns over anticoagulation in some patients
- Breathlessness assumed to be due to other causes

Most PEs occur as a complication of DVT in the legs or pelvis. The risk of PE from untreated DVT is estimated at 50 per cent and the mortality rate of untreated PE at 30–40 per cent. Most deaths from PE occur in the first hour.

Signs and symptoms will vary depending upon the extent of thrombus, general condition of the patient, other respiratory/cardiovascular co-morbidity and whether chronic pulmonary emboli or an acute event has occurred.

In some patients pulmonary emboli may go unnoticed, causing mild breathlessness, whilst in more severe cases, sudden cardiovascular collapse and death occur. Features suggestive of pulmonary emboli include:
- Breathlessness and cough
- Haemoptysis
- Palpitations
- Chest pain

Clinical signs may vary and are useful if present, but absence of signs should not exclude the diagnosis if there is a strong clinical suspicion. Likewise many of the signs could be accounted for by other co-morbidities. Signs may include:
- Tachycardia
- Tachypnoea
- Atrial fibrillation
- Raised JVP
- Hypotension
- Loud P2 heart sound
- Cyanosis
- Syncope

Investigations

It is important to decide whether an investigation is going to alter management and, if so, which test would be the most appropriate and best tolerated by the patient. A balance between the test most likely to confirm the diagnosis and that with the least disruption/burden to the patient may need to be considered. Several tests that may be done in the acute setting may be less appropriate near the end-of-life.

- Arterial blood gases. Painful and unlikely to give much useful information in the setting of co-existing lung disease

- ECG
  - Majority of ECGs are normal
  - Most common abnormality is sinus tachycardia
  - $S_1Q_3T_3$ phenomenon rare
  - Atrial fibrillation may be present
- D-dimers
  - High false positive results in cancer limit their usefulness
  - Chest X-ray
  - Useful in considering other causes of breathlessness besides PE

Objective testing for PE

All imaging techniques have their limitations and different degrees of burden on the patient

- **Spiral CT**
  - First-line investigation
  - Requires large volume of i/v contrast
  - Gives assessment of pulmonary veins
  - Other chest pathologies identified
  - Can be used to assess lower limb veins and Inferior Vena Cava (IVC) at the same time
- **Ventilation/Perfusion (V/Q) scan**
  - Usually well tolerated procedure
  - Use falling due to CT and pulmonary angiography
- **Pulmonary angiography**
  - Gold standard investigation
  - Invasive
  - Complication rate 0.5 per cent, mortality 0.1 per cent
  - Limited use in palliative care population
  - Rarely used now with advent of CT pulmonary angiography
- **Magnetic resonance angiography**
  - Under evaluation
  - Limited use in palliative population

Chronic venous thrombosis

Patients with hypercoagulability related to disseminated malignancy or with cancers obstructing veins may have chronic venous thrombosis requiring warfarin and/or low molecular weight heparin (LMWH). Migratory polyphlebitis affecting superficial veins, which is largely associated with disseminated bronchogenic and adenocarcinoma, may also cause venous and arterial clotting.

Treatment of VTE

Treatment goals should be to relieve symptoms and prevent further thrombotic events.

- **DVT**
  - Consider leg elevation
  - Analgesia for swelling and tenderness (NSAIDs may interfere with the INR)
  - Compression stockings if tolerated, ease the symptoms of venous hypertension
  - Consider anticoagulation
  - Venocaval filters may prevent PE if recurrent DVTs are a problem despite anticoagulation but are associated with painful engorgement of both lower limbs
- **PE**
  - Oxygen
  - Opioids +/− benzodiazepines for breathlessness and fear
  - Consider anticoagulation

Anticoagulation in a patient with advanced malignancy should be considered carefully prior to initiation. Palliative care patients are at a high risk of haemorrhage for several reasons:

- Presence of DIC
- Consumption of clotting factors
- Platelet dysfunction/thrombocytopenia
- Tumours may be vascular
- Liver metastases

Each patient should be considered on an individual basis taking into account the following:

- Prognosis
- Bleeding risk
- Ability to control symptoms and quality of life without anticoagulation
- Perceived burden of anticoagulation
- Patient's views

Local haematology department guidelines should be sought regarding anticoagulation. Traditionally in palliative care patients were initially treated with LMWH and, depending on the clinical circumstances, considered for commencing warfarin at the same time. Once the INR is stable at a therapeutic dose, the LMWH can be discontinued.

> **Important!**
> Never commence warfarin therapy without first checking the INR or platelet count.

Warfarin in patients with cancer

Despite being the mainstay of long term anticoagulation for VTE, extreme caution should be used when recommending warfarin. Several studies have demonstrated significant increases in rates of bleeding amongst cancer patients on warfarin (in the order of 20 per cent). More frequent monitoring of the INR (which should be maintained between 2 to 3) is often needed in patients with cancer (i.e. every 2–3 days) to reduce the risk of bleeding.

Problems with using warfarin in patients with advanced cancer:

- High risk of bleeding. Even higher if thrombocytopenia or liver metastases
- Unpredictable metabolism of warfarin
- Interaction with other drugs
- Difficulty maintaining stable International normalized ratio (INR)
- Burden of repeated INR checks to optimize safety
- Progression of thrombus despite therapeutic INR in a proportion of patients

Rapid reversal of warfarin
Give 12–50 mL/kg FFP, 1 unit 300mL—usually 3–4 units of fresh plasma and 10mg Vitamin K by slow i/v injection.

Low molecular weight heparin in patients with cancer
Although the mainstay of treatment of VTE in patients with cancer remains long term anticoagulation with warfarin, this is likely to change. There is now level 1a evidence comparing long term LMWH with warfarin in this patient group. LMWH has been shown to reduce the recurrence of VTE from 17 per cent to 9 per cent with no stastistical difference in bleeding when compared with warfarin.

LMWH may be of particular benefit in palliative care since there is no need to measure anticoagulation levels and the drug does not react with other medicines.

The progressive nature of advanced malignancy invariably heralds changing symptoms, which necessitate drug alterations. This is a particular area of risk in warfarinized patients, where drug interactions may increase the INR.

There have been concerns that the once daily injection of LMWH is too invasive, burdensome and detrimental to patients' quality of life, whilst others would argue that this is less of a burden than the alternate day INR checks that may be required to minimize the risk of warfarin-related haemorrhage.

A phenomenological study amongst palliative care patients receiving long term LMWH suggests it is an acceptable intervention and does not have an adverse impact on quality of life.

LMWH is more costly than warfarin, but this does not take into account costs of repeated blood monitoring and prolonged length of hospital stay whilst loading warfarin to therapeutic levels.

Potential benefits for LMWH
• Reliable pharmacokinetics
• Anticoagulant effect not altered by diet or concomitant drug use
• Fast onset of action
• Repeated blood test monitoring not required

At present there are no guidelines defining which patients should receive LMWH for long-term anticoagulation. Each patient should be considered individually, but the following patients should be considered for LMWH rather than warfarin:
• Continued thrombosis on therapeutic warfarin
• Liver metastases
• Symptoms that are difficult to control adequately with regular medication
• Regular INR checks considered too great a burden
• Poor venous access for blood testing

VTE and brain metastases
The management of VTE in patients with brain metastases is complicated and there is no consensus. Studies comparing the use of venacaval filters with anticoagulation, show that 40 per cent of patients with filters may have further thrombotic events and 7 per cent of those anticoagulated may develop neurological deterioration from intracerebral bleeding. The rôle of LMWH in these patients is yet to be clarified.

Length of anticoagulation
A patient should remain anticoagulated as long as the prothrombotic risk leading to VTE persists. In cancer, the prothrombotic risk increases as disease advances and so anticoagulation should, in theory, continue indefinitely. The decision should be made taking into account the patient's views, effect of treatment, logistics of treatment and complications. As disease progresses and the bleeding tendency increases, stopping anticoagulation may be the lesser of two evils.

Table 6l.2

Target INR	Indication
2.0–2.5	DVT prophylaxis
2.5	Treatment of DVT and PE (or recurrence in patients not on warfarin)
3.5	Recurrent DVT and PE in patients receiving warfarin
	Mechanical prosthetic heart valves

Developing a good relationship with haematology colleagues

- In order to provide the best possible care for patients with end-stage haematological disease, palliative care teams need to build close working relationships with colleagues in haematology
- Historically this relationship has been challenging, as there has been lack of understanding of respective rôles
- Many patients may benefit in terms of symptom control and prolongation of life from aggressive active haematological intervention (including invasive procedures and frequent infusion of blood products) even in the terminal stages. This may be difficult for palliative care teams, whose aim for dying patients is to control symptoms in the least burdensome manner
- The stereotypical prejudices inherent in both specialties are unhelpful
- It is crucial for the benefit of patients that there are good working relationships between haematology and palliative care specialists, so that patients and their families can have access and the support of both approaches, and are aware of all the issues and choices

There are reasons why palliative care involvement in haematological patients is challenging, as outlined below:

- There may be a misperception that palliative care teams only provide terminal care and therefore referrals should only be made when the patient is 'actively dying'
- Problems may have occurred previously with well intentioned but perhaps misguided palliative interventions, such as thrombocytopenic patients bleeding or myeloma patients developing renal failure having been started on NSAIDs
- Communication issues. The palliative care team may inadvertently question the patient's knowledge and understanding of their illness and attitude to continuation of treatment, which might overtly or covertly be seen to undermine the haematology treatment plan
- Fear that palliative care team will take over patients who have often been managed for many years by the haematology team
- It is important to fully appreciate that the haematology team may have looked after their patient through several near-death crises. Patients may have responded to previous treatments in extremis and, for instance, offering further chemotherapy may be totally appropriate
- During treatment and as disease progresses haematology patients can become very ill, very quickly. This may not be the terminal stage however as patients may respond to active support with antibiotics, fluids and blood products

In the haematology context it is often very difficult to identify when a patient is dying.

- Haematology colleagues need to be aware that palliative care specialists do not take over patients, or undermine their colleagues, or use medication to shorten the lives of patients
- Palliative care teams should work alongside haematology teams, amicably negotiating the treatment path with patients and families

Psychiatric symptoms in palliative medicine

Adjustment disorders

Adjustment disorders are defined as a maladaptive reaction to an identifiable psychosocial stressor which occurs within three months of the onset of the stressor and which does not persist for longer than six months. The symptoms are not specified, but the commonest presenting symptoms are depression and anxiety. Clinical presentations can include anger, bitterness and blaming others. A useful marker is that the patient with adjustment disorder feels bad about the situation, whereas patients with a depressive order feel bad about themselves.

Treatment

An adjustment disorder does not respond to antidepressants and generally improves as new levels of adaptation are reached. Certain interventions, such as problem-oriented psychotherapy, may be helpful. The symptoms may fluctuate in severity on a daily basis and patients can often be distracted from their distress. Beta blockers or a short course of benzodiazepines can be helpful.

Anxiety

It is normal to be anxious in certain circumstances, many of which pertain in the palliative setting. The spectrum of anxiety ranges from 'normal' through to persistent and severe anxiety. Anxiety becomes a problem when its duration and severity exceed normal expectations. It may be acute or chronic. Anxiety is common in the terminally ill for a variety of reasons, including the fear of uncontrolled symptoms and of being left alone to die.

Anxiety assessment

1 Is it severe?
2 Is it long-standing?
3 Is it alcohol withdrawal?
4 Is it situational?
5 Is it related to a specific fear?
6 Are the family anxious?[1]

Management involves assessing the patient for any reversible factors such as pain, or unfounded worries. Stimulant drugs or excessive alcohol intake or withdrawal may exacerbate the anxiety.

It is necessary to provide the time and opportunity for patients to express their worries and concerns and for these concerns to be addressed honestly and clearly. Relaxation techniques and various complementary therapies may help, as may the controlled safe atmosphere of a hospice with professional carers.

1 Kaye P. (1999) *Decision Making in Palliative Care*, pp. 34–5. Northampton: EPL Publications.

It is important for all members of the palliative care team to be aware of the 'infectious' nature of anxiety, which can distress individual members of the palliative care team and by default the whole team. These situations are often predictable, and extra effort should be made to support staff during potentially stressful situations and to avoid being driven to extreme management decisions.

Pharmacological treatment of anxiety

Benzodiazepines

These are very useful drugs but have received a bad press because of their addictive potential. They are traditionally divided between compounds which have more sedating effects and those which have more anxiolytic actions. However, there is considerable overlap on the anxiety/sedating spectrum.

They are useful to break the anxiety cycle, to restore sleep, and to reduce the suffering of the situation where a patient feels that he/she is 'losing control'. They are not a substitute for taking the time to allow a patient to ventilate fears.

- Diazepam: 1–5mg p.r.n. p.o.—diazepam has a long half-life and may therefore accumulate and be sedative. It should be possible to give it once a day at night
- Lorazepam: 1–2mg p.r.n, p.o.—lorazepam is short acting, rapidly anxiolytic and less sedating than diazepam
- Midazolam: 5–10mg p.r.n., SC or buccal—useful for emergency sedation

Drugs used for Anxiety

Diazepam is an appropriate first-line benzodiazepine.

Lorazepam is shorter acting, and (taken sublingually), has a faster onset of action, and is useful on a p.r.n. basis.

Midazolam can be used if a CSCI is required.

Propranolol is helpful, especially to control the somatic symptoms of anxiety e.g. tremor and palpitations.

The anxiolytic effect of buspirone develops over 1–3 weeks, and it probably has little place in palliative care.

SSRIs can be used for panic attacks if benzodiazepines are ineffective.

Diazepam

Tabs. 2mg, 5mg, 10mg; Oral solution 2mg/5mL, 5mg/5mL

Rectal tubes 5mg/2.5mL, 10mg/2.5mL; Supps. 10mg

Inj. (emulsion) 10mg/2mL (Diazemuls)—i/v use only

Inj. (solution) 10mg/2mL—i/m use

Blood levels increased by omeprazole (increased sedation).

Lorazepam

Tabs. 1mg, 2.5mg; Inj. 4mg/1 mL

Midazolam

Inj. 10mg/2mL, 10mg/5mL

Sedative effect markedly enhanced by itraconazole, ketoconazole and possibly fluconazole.

Propranolol

Tabs. 10mg, 40mg, 80mg, 160mg; Oral solution 40mg/5mL; Tabs. 80mg, 160mg

Antidepressants

Tricyclic antidepressants (TCAs) such as amitriptyline or dosulepin[2] may be useful as anxiolytics, often in 'sub-antidepressant' dosages. Selective serotonin re-uptake inhibitor (SSRI) antidepressants such as paroxetine and citalopram (must not be used <18y) are more expensive alternatives which have less reported side-effects and also have anxiolytic properties, though care must be taken to avoid enervating SSRIs such as fluoxetine, which can initially increase anxiety. Complementary therapies, e.g. aromatherapy, and massage and specific interventions, e.g. hypnosis, relaxation and imagery, may help increase the patient's sense of control.

Complex anxiety states with depression and psychosis may be more suitably treated with neuroleptics. The help of a psychiatric team may be needed.

2 Payne S. (1998) Depression in palliative care patients: a literature review. *International Journal of Palliative Nursing*, 4, **4**: 184–91.

Depression

Estimates of the prevalence of depression in patients vary greatly, but it is probable that at least 25 per cent may develop a significant mood disorder in advanced cancer. A review of 12 articles reported a range of depression rates from 3–69 per cent. Certain types of cancer, such as pancreatic cancer, are associated with an increased incidence of depression.[3] A spectrum ranging from sadness to adjustment disorder to depressive illness is recognized. There is concern that depression may be underdiagnosed. This may be due to a number of reasons including a diurnal variation in symptoms such that it may be missed, social 'cover-up', or presentation with physical symptoms. One of the main difficulties is distinguishing depression from appropriate sadness at the end-of-life.

In the physically *healthy* population, depression is diagnosed if patients have a persistent low mood and a least four of the following symptoms which are present most of the day for the preceding two weeks:

1 Diminished interest or pleasure in all or almost all activities
2 Psychomotor retardation or agitation
3 Feelings of worthlessness or excessive and inappropriate guilt
4 Diminished ability to concentrate and think
5 Recurrent thoughts of death and suicide
6 Fatigue and loss of energy
7 Significant weight loss or gain
8 Insomnia or hypersomnia

In patients with advanced cancer, symptoms 6–8 are almost universal, and it is doubtful whether physical symptoms should be included at all when diagnosing depression in the terminally ill.

Atypical presentations of depression

- irritability
- agitation and anxiety symptoms
- histrionic behaviour
- hypochondriasis
- psychotic features (delusions, paranoia) that are mood-congruent e.g. content of delusions consistent with depressive thoughts

Pharmacological treatment of depression

There is little information concerning the effectiveness of antidepressant medication in terminally ill patients. There is, however, a body of evidence showing that under treatment is common, with patients being prescribed antidepressants within the final six weeks of life, allowing little time for therapeutic benefit. Psychostimulants, which have a faster onset of action than classical antidepressants, are very rarely used in this terminal situation despite some evidence of benefit. Being younger and having breast cancer increase the chance of being prescribed antidepressants.[4]

Think list

- Corticosteroids—may help mild depression and low mood by improving sense of well-being, but can also induce psychosis or depression in others. Starting low dose dexamethasone e.g. 4mg daily

for a week followed by 2mg daily for a week can elevate a patient's mood whilst awaiting a response to antidepressants
- Psychostimulants (methylphenidate or dexamfetamine)
- ECT (electro-convulsive therapy)—response can be very rapid; very occasionally appropriate e.g. severe depression developing during chemotherapy
- Pathological crying may respond to citalopram

Tricyclic antidepressants (TCAs)

Tricyclic antidepressants may take several weeks to lift depression. Amitriptyline and dosulepin are relatively sedative in comparison with imipramine and lofepramine. They all have antimuscarinic properties to greater or lesser degrees and therefore may be associated with symptoms such as hypotension, dry mouth and difficulty in micturition. Doses should gradually be increased to avoid unnecessary side-effects.

Selective serotonin re-uptake inhibitors

- e.g. Citalopram 20mg o.d.
- Sertraline 50mg o.d.
- Fluoxetine 20mg o.d.

These drugs are less sedative than tricyclic antidepressants and have few antimuscarinic effects, low cardiotoxicity and may have a faster onset of action than the TCAs.

SSRIs may cause nausea, vomiting and headaches and extrapyramidal reactions can occur occasionally. Gastrointestinal side-effects are dose-related. There is little to choose between the SSRIs, but fluoxetine has a slower onset of action and may cause more agitation than other SSRIs: it is therefore not recommended as first line particularly in patients who are agitated.

- SSRIs may increase the risk of GI bleeding, especially in patients taking NSAIDs
- Serious reactions may develop with MAOIs and selegiline (serotonin syndrome)
- Increased serotonergic effects are seen with St John's Wort, which should be avoided
- Fluoxetine and fluvoxamine increase the blood levels of carbamazepine and phenytoin (risk of toxicity)

Use an SSRI unless other treatment is specifically indicated:
- Dose escalation is not usually needed, so more rapid control of symptoms may be possible
- The side-effects of SSRIs are generally better tolerated than TCAs in ill patients with cancer

A trial of at least three weeks, and preferably six or more, is needed to properly assess response to an antidepressant. Discontinuation symptoms (withdrawal) will not usually occur if stopped within six weeks of starting.

3 Doyle D. H., Hanks, G. W. C., Cherny N. (2004) *Oxford Textbook of Palliative Medicine*. 3rd edn. Oxford: Oxford University Press.

4 Lloyd-Williams M., Friedman T., Rudd N. (1999) A survey of antidepressant prescribing in the terminally ill. *Palliative Medicine*, **13**: 243–8.

Antidepressant discontinuation syndromes occur with both TCAs and SSRIs.

SSRI discontinuation symptoms include dizziness, light-headedness, insomnia, fatigue, anxiety/agitation, nausea, headache, and sensory disturbance. SSRIs should be withdrawn gradually when possible, using alternate day dosing if needed.

Symptoms of withdrawal are more common with paroxetine (short half-life), and least common with fluoxetine (half-life of weeks).

Paroxetine
- Tabs. 20mg; liquid 20mg/10mL
- Dose 20mg mane p.o.—increase by weekly increments of 10mg as necessary to max. 50mg o.d.

Citalopram
- Tabs. 10, 20, 40mg; oral drops 40mg/mL
- Dose: 20mg mane p.o.; max. 60mg o.d.

Sertraline
- Tabs. 50, 100mg
- Dose 50mg mane p.o.; max. 200mg o.d.

Other antidepressant drugs

Venlafaxine is a serotonin and noradrenaline re-uptake inhibitor (SNRI). It causes less side-effects than the SSRIs. The slow release capsules are preferable to use as they seem to be better tolerated. Mirtazepine is a noradrenergic and specific serotoninergic antidepressant (NaSSA) and is useful if there is marked anxiety/agitation. At lower doses the antihistaminic effect predominates producing sedation, which is reduced with higher doses when the noradrenergic transmission increases.

Venlafaxine
- Tabs. 37.5, 50, 75mg
- Dose: 37.5mg b.d. p.o. increased to 75mg b.d.
- Caps. m/r 75, 150mg
- Dose: 75mg o.d. p.o. increased to 150mg o.d.
- Dose should be increased gradually to the usual dose 150mg, and higher according to response; maximum 375mg daily (225mg if m/r)

Mirtazepine
- Tabs. (scored) 30mg
- Dose: 15mg nocte p.o. increased to 30mg nocte
- Dose should be increased gradually to usual dose 30mg, and higher according to response; maximum 45mg daily

Tricyclics and tetracyclics

The original tricyclics antidepressants (amitriptyline, imipramine etc.) are used in low doses as co-analgesics, but they are poorly tolerated due to side-effects in antidepressant doses and it is advisable to commence an SSRI and avoid TCAs for the treatment of depression in patients with advanced cancer. Dosulepin is a good first-line antidepressant, whilst lofepramine has a lower incidence of side-effects and is therefore useful in the elderly. Usual treatment dose of most TCAs is 150mg/day (perhaps less in elderly); lofepramine dose is 140–210mg/day.

Higher doses are associated with worse side-effects e.g. dry mouth, sedation, prostatism etc.

Tricyclic antidepressants used concomitantly with amiodarone increase the risk of ventricular arrhythmias and should be avoided.

Dosulepin
- Caps. 25mg; Tabs. 75mg
- Dose 50–75mg nocte p.o.

Lofepramine
- Tabs. 70mg
- Dose 70mg o.d.—b.d. p.o.

St John's Wort
A number of patients may be taking St John's Wort as an antidepressant. It is not a licensed medication, and has a number of significant drug interactions:
- Increases serotonergic effects with SSRIs; therefore avoid
- Reduces anticoagulant effect of warfarin
- Reduces plasma levels of carbamazepine, phenytoin, phenobarbital (risk of fits)
- Reduces plasma levels of digoxin

Screening for depression

There are no universally accepted criteria for diagnosing depression in the terminally ill. In patients with advanced cancer, many of the symptoms of depression, e.g. changes in appetite, energy levels and sleep pattern, are common and there is still considerable controversy as to whether these physical symptoms should be included. Depressed mood, irritability, loss of interest in anything, feelings of worthlessness and lack of hope for the future are more important in this population.

Rating scales to measure depression are increasingly used. Such tools are not diagnostic and can only serve to indicate whether a patient has particular psychiatric symptoms suggestive of a diagnosis of depression. The decision should then be taken whether to treat for depression or to refer the patient for further assessment. The majority of rating scales consist of a number of symptoms or feelings. Patients indicate their own response and the person administering the scale calculates the scores.

Several instruments have been developed which define a threshold score for the predictability of depression. However, a defined cut-off threshold suitable for patients with early cancer or those receiving treatment may not be valid for patients with advanced metastatic disease receiving palliative care. Recent work has suggested that a scale developed for use in the post-natal period (the Edinburgh Depression Scale) may be useful for screening in palliative care. It does not include somatic symptoms but does include symptoms such as sadness, feelings of helplessness and thoughts of self harm which may be particularly discriminatory in the palliative care population. Each item is scored from 0–3—the most negative response scoring highest. A cut-off threshold of 13 has a sensitivity and specificy of approximately 80 per cent.

The Edinburgh Depression Scale
Please UNDERLINE the answer which comes close to how you have felt IN THE PAST 7 DAYS, not just how you feel today

I have been able to laugh and see the funny side of things:
As much as I always could
Not quite so much now
Definitely not so much now
Not at all

I have looked forward with enjoyment to things:
As much as I ever did
Rather less than I used to
Definitely less than I used to
Hardly at all

I have blamed myself unnecessarily when things went wrong:
Yes, most of the time
Yes, some of the time
Not very often
No, never

I have been anxious or worried for no good reason:
No, not at all
Hardly ever
Yes, sometimes
Yes, very often

I get a sort of frightened feeling as if something awful is about to happen:
Very definitely and quite badly
Yes, but not too badly
A little, but it doesn't worry me
Not at all

Things have been getting on top of me:
Most of the time and I haven't been able to cope at all
Yes, sometimes I haven't been coping as well as usual
No, most of the time I have coped quite well
No, I have been coping as well as ever

I have been so unhappy that I have had difficulty sleeping:
Yes, most of the time
Yes, quite often
Not very often
No, not at all

I have felt sad or miserable:
Yes, most of the time
Yes, quite often
Not very often
No, not at all

I have been so unhappy, I have been crying:
Yes, most of the time
Yes, quite often
Only occasionally
No, never

The thought of harming myself has occurred to me:
Yes, quite often
Sometimes
Hardly ever
Never

Confusional states

Delirium: An etiologically, non-specific, global, cerebral dysfunction characterised by concurrent disturbance of level of consciousness, attention, thinking, perception, memory, psychomotor behaviour, emotion and sleep-wake cycle.

An acute confusional state (or delirium) is associated with mental clouding, leading to a disturbance of comprehension which is characterized by decreased attention, disorientation and cognitive impairment with poor short-term memory and concentration.

The prevalence of delirium may be as high as 85 per cent for hospitalized terminally ill patients and is particularly common in elderly patients moved from a familiar environment. It may be exacerbated by deafness and poor vision.

While delirium is normally understood as a reversible process, there may not be time for it to improve in terminally ill patients. Occasionally, irreversible processes such as multiple organ failure cause delirium.

The diagnosis may be obvious with a rapid onset of altered behaviour and incoherent rambling speech. The symptoms may fluctuate and there may be insight. Severe delirium can progress to psychotic features with hallucinations and delusions.

The differential diagnosis includes dementia, which is a more chronic condition, is not associated with mental clouding and is irreversible.

It may be appropriate, if done sensitively, to carry out a simplified mini-mental score test to help management and to monitor clinical progress.

Mini-mental score

A test devised for the serial testing of cognitive mental state on a neurogeriatric ward. A score of 20 or less was found in patients with dementia, delirium, schizophrenia or affective disorder.[5]

Instructions for administration	Max score

Orientation

What is the date (year) (season) (date) (day) (month)?   5

Ask for the date. Then ask specifically for parts omitted, e.g., 'Can you also tell me what season it is?' One point for each correct.

Where are we: (state) (county) (town) (hospital) (floor)   5

Ask in turn 'Can you tell me the name of this hospital? (town, county, etc.). One point for each correct.

Registration

Ask the patient if you may test his memory. Say the names of three   3
unrelated objects, clearly and slowly, about one second for each.
After you have said all three, ask him to repeat them. This first repetition determines his score (0–3; 1 point for each correct answer), but keep saying them until he can repeat all three, up to six trials. If he does not eventually learn all three, recall cannot be meaningfully tested. Count trials and record.

Attention and calculation

Serial 7's. Ask the patient to begin with 100 and count backwards by 7.   5
Stop after five subtractions (93, 86, 79, 72, 65). Score the total number of correct answers. 1 point for each correct. If the patient cannot or will not perform this task, ask him to spell the word 'world' backwards. Score the number of letters in correct order e.g. dlrow = 5, dlorw = 3.

Recall

Ask the patient if he can recall the three words you previously asked   3
him to remember.
Score 0–3. Give 1 point for each correct.

Language

Naming: Name a pencil, and watch.   2

Show the patient a wrist watch and ask him what it is. Repeat for pencil. Score 0–2.

Repetition: Ask the patient to repeat the sentence after you: 'No ifs,   1
ands or buts.' Allow only one trial. Score 0 or 1.

Three-stage command: 'Take a piece of paper in your right hand, fold it   3
in half, and put it on the floor'.Give the patient a piece of plain blank paper and repeat the command. Score 1 point for each part correctly executed.

Reading: Read and obey the following: 'CLOSE YOUR EYES'   1

On a blank piece of paper print the sentence 'Close your eyes', in letters large enough for the patient to see clearly. Ask him to read it and do what it says. Score 1 point only if he actually closes his eyes.

Writing: Give the patient a blank piece of paper and ask him to write   1
a sentence for you. Do not dictate a sentence, it is to be written spontaneously. It must contain a subject and verb and be sensible. Correct grammar and punctuation are not necessary.

Copying: On a clean piece of paper, draw intersecting pentagons,   1
each side about 1 in., and ask him to copy it exactly as it is. All 10 angles must be present and two must intersect to score 1 point. Tremor and rotation are ignored.

TOTAL SCORE

(Max. 30)

5 Folstein M. F., Folstein S. E., McHugh P. R. (1975) 'Mini-Mental State': a practical method for grading the cognitive state of patients for the clinician. *J Psychiatr Res*, **12**: 189–98.

Delirium and confusion

Treat reversible **cause** of confusion if possible.
Consider:
- hypercalcaemia
- hypoglycaemia
- hyponatraemia
- renal failure
- liver failure
- drug-related causes
  - opioids
  - corticosteroids AND withdrawal
  - alcohol withdrawal
  - benzodiazepine AND withdrawal
  - SSRI withdrawal
  - nicotine withdrawal
  - digoxin
  - lithium
- NB benzodiazepines and phenothiazines accumulate in liver failure and opioids in renal failure
- cerebral tumour, primary or secondary
- CVA or Transient Ischaemic Attack (TIA)
- anxiety/depression
- infection
- hypoxia
- disorientation of move to hospital (in pre-existing dementia)
- thiamine (vitamin B_1) deficiency
- non-convulsive status epilepticus

The cause is often multifactorial, and symptoms such as pain or those associated with constipation or urinary retention may aggravate confusion.

Prescribing for delirium and confusional states

- Drugs should only be prescribed if necessary
- Night sedation should be given only after an attempt to remove other causes of insomnia such as fear, noisy and unfamiliar surroundings, unrelieved pain, nocturia and stimulant medication such as steroids
- Reassurance and helping to orientate the patient and alleviate fear may be all that is required. The patient and family should be comforted by being told that the patient is not 'going mad', but that this is a temporary setback which is hopefully reversible. Daytime sedation should only be necessary if the patient is very distressed and not amenable to reassurance or is a danger to themselves or others
- Doses should be adjusted according to age and general condition, level of disturbance, and likely tolerance
- Antipsychotics are considered to be the drugs of choice for delirium, haloperidol being the most commonly used
- The risk of extrapyramidal side-effects (EPSE) is greatest in the elderly, and with the older antipsychotics such as haloperidol and chlorpromazine; newer drugs such as risperidone, olanzapine and promazine are better tolerated but may not be adequate if rapid control is needed of an acutely disturbed patient (Risperidone and olanzapine are associated with an increased risk of stroke in elderly patients with dementia.)

- Chlorpromazine and levomepromazine are more sedative than haloperidol
- Benzodiazepines carry a risk of paradoxical agitation (disinhibition with worsening of behavioural disturbance) especially in the elderly. Used in conjunction with haloperidol, lorazepam improves the control of the acutely disturbed patient, but used alone is less effective than antipsychotics in delirium
- Most antipsychotics decrease the convulsive threshold, and may increase the risk of convulsions in susceptible patients, but the actual risk is undetermined

Benzodiazepines in agitation and restlessness

Although antipsychotics are considered the treatment of choice for delirium, agitation and restlessness in the patient with advanced cancer may often be primarily an anxiety state, with secondary cognitive impairment or clouded consciousness. In this condition, benzodiazepines may be more effective than antipsychotics. A knowledge of the previous psychological state of the patient is vital in determining this.

Alcohol withdrawal

The best treatment for alcohol withdrawal in palliative care is usually alcohol if the patient is able to swallow. In practice, patients who have been deteriorating over months have usually gradually reduced their alcohol intake.

Clomethiazole ± benzodiazepines are the usual drug treatments. Alcohol withdrawal has also been treated with 10–20mL absolute alcohol made up to 50mL with saline/24h i/v using a syringe driver, but this type of management is rarely necessary in the palliative setting.

Wernicke's encephalopathy (thiamine/vitamin B_1 deficiency) may be more common than anticipated in the terminally ill. The diagnosis can be confirmed by red blood cell (RBC) transketolase estimation. The diagnosis should be considered in any patient with a history of alcohol misuse who develops unexplained:

- ophthalmoplegia
- nystagmus
- ataxia (not due to intoxication)
- acute confusion (not due to intoxication)
- memory disturbance
- seizures
- coma/unconsciousness

A presumptive diagnosis of Wernicke's encephalopathy should prompt treatment with high-dose parenteral B-complex vitamins.

Antipsychotics

Haloperidol

- Caps. 0.5mg; Tabs. 1.5mg, 5mg; liquid 2mg/mL; inj. 5mg/1mL
- (Indomethacin given with haloperidol can cause severe drowsiness.)

Levomepromazine (methotrimeprazine)

- Tabs. 6mg 25mg; susp. 25mg/5mL; inj. 25mg/1mL (nozinan)
- Dose 12.5mg nocte or b.d. p.o.; 12.5mg/24h CSCI
- 6mg Tabs. available on a named patient basis only

- Oral bioavailability of levomepromazine is approx. 40 per cent. Use half the daily oral dose by CSCI
- Avoid concurrent use with mono amine oxidase inhibitors (MAOIs)

Promazine

- Tabs. 25mg, 50mg; liquid 25mg/5mL, 50mg/5mL; inj. 50mg/1mL

Risperidone

- Tabs. 0.5mg, 1mg, 2mg, 3mg, 4mg, 6mg; liquid 1mg/1mL
- Avoid in patients with cerebrovascular disease

Olanzapine

- Tabs. 2.5mg, 5mg, 7.5mg, 10mg; dispersible 5mg, 10mg, 15mg
- Dispersible tablets can be placed on the tongue to dissolve/disperse
- Avoid in patients with cerebrovascular disease

Thioridazine and droperidol

Thioridazine has had its licence for treating agitation in the elderly removed because of the risk of cardiac arrhythmias, and should not be prescribed except under guidance from a psychiatrist.

Droperidol has been withdrawn for the same reason (prolonged QT intervals).

Benzodiazepines

Lorazepam

Lorazepam is shorter acting than diazepam, and is therefore safer in repeated doses; it can be given SC or sublingually for more rapid effect and in uncooperative patients.

- Tabs. 1mg, 2.5mg; inj. 4mg/1mL
- Dilute inj. with equal volume of water or saline for i/m use

Diazepam

- Tabs. 2mg, 5mg, 10mg; syrup 2mg/5mL; rectal soln. 5mg/2.5mL, 10mg/2.5mL
- Supps. 10mg
- Blood levels increased by omeprazole (increased sedation)

Midazolam

- Inj. 10mg/2mL, 10mg/5mL
- Dose: 20–30mg/24h *CSCI* (max. 100mg/24h)
- Sedative effect markedly enhanced by itraconazole, ketoconazole and possibly fluconazole

Vitamin B preparations

Pabrinex (vitamins B and C)

- Inj. Pair of ampoules containing 10mL
- Dose: 1 pair of ampoules daily for three days—for acute and severe vitamin B deficiency states
- Serious allergic reaction may rarely occur on i/v administration (probably <1 in 250,000, compared to incidence of 1–10 per cent allergy with penicillin). Inject slowly over 10 minutes

Table 6m.1 Treatment of delirium and confusion with antipsychotics when no reversible causes diagnosed

Presentation	Non-elderly	Elderly
Confusion ± drowsiness, or where sedation undesirable/unnecessary	Non-sedative antipsychotic Haloperidol 1.5–3mg nocte or b.d. SC/CSCI (Risperidone 0.5–1mg b.d.)	Non-sedative antipsychotic with lower risk of extrapyramidal side-effects (EPSE) Risperidone 0.5mg nocte or b.d. p.o Haloperidol 0.5–1mg nocte SC/CSCI.
Agitated confusion where sedative effects desired; mild—moderate agitation	Sedative antipsychotic Levomepromazine 25–50mg SC/CSCI/p.o. (Chlorpromazine 25–50mg b.d.–q.d.s. p.o.)	Sedative antipsychotic with lower risk of EPSE Promazine 25mg nocte or up to q.d.s. p.o. Levomepromazine 12.5–25mg/24h CSCI (Olanzapine 2.5mg nocte p.o.)
Acutely disturbed, violent or aggressive; at risk to themselves or others. Antipsychotic with proven safety record in repeated high doses for rapid titration; suitable for parenteral use*	Haloperidol 5mg SC/i/m ± lorazepam 1–2mg SC/i/m repeated after 20–30 minutes.	Haloperidol 2.5mg SC/i/m ± lorazepam 0.5–1 mg SC/i/m repeated after 30 minutes

* Risperidone and olanzapine must be avoided in patients with a history of cerebrovascular disease.

Equivalent doses of antipsychotic and benzodiazepine medication

Occasionally patients are taking antipsychotic drugs or benzodiazepines on a long term basis. The approximate equivalent doses are outlined below although, as ever, doses should be based on an overall assessment of the patient's individual needs. Switching antipsychotics or benzodiazepines, while not recommended, is sometimes required in the palliative care setting especially if the previous oral route is no longer available.

Table 6m.2 Benzodiazepine drug equivalence (an approximate guide)

Antipsychotic drug equivalence			
Antipsychotic drug	**Approximate equivalent daily dose**		
Chlorpromazine	100mg		
Haloperidol	2–3mg		
Levomepromazine	25–50mg		
Pimozide	2mg		
Risperidone	0.5–1mg		
Trifluoperazine	5mg		
	Equivalent dose anxiolytic/sedative	**Approximate duration of action**	**Approximate subcutaneous dose over 24 h**
Diazepam	5mg p.o. or PR	3 h to 4 days	N/A
Clonazepam	0.25mg p.o.	6–24 h	1mg
Midazolam	2.5mg SC	15mins to 4 h	10mg
Lorazepam	0.5mg p.o.	7–8 h	N/A
Temazepam	10mg p.o.	7–8 h	N/A

Psychostimulants

Potential uses for psychostimulants:
- Depression
- Opioid -induced sedation or cognitive impairment
- Fatigue
- Cognitive impairment due to brain tumours
- Hypoactive delirium
- Hiccups

Psychostimulants for depression

Psychostimulants have been shown to be effective in depression in medically ill patients including the terminally ill, although they do not seem to be effective in primary depression. They are rarely prescribed for depression in the UK. They are useful because of their rapid onset, and are generally well tolerated. The beneficial effects of these drugs are reported to occur within 36–48 h. Drug habituation is generally not a problem.

Methylphenidate appears to have been used more widely, but dexamfetamine is equally effective.

Doses of methylphenidate as low as 1.25mg daily have been used successfully in patients over 90 years old. Methylphenidate (average dose after titration 30mg daily) is as effective as imipramine 150mg o.d. in significantly reducing depressive and anxiety symptoms.

Psychostimulants have been used as adjuvants to reduce opioid-induced sedation and potentiate analgesia. It is not known whether this is due to a reduction in opioid-induced sedation, thus allowing dose escalation of the opioid, or to a direct potentiation of opioid analgesia.

Side-effects of psychostimulant drugs including agitation, dysphoria, insomnia, nightmares and hypomania have been reported.

Methylphenidate
- Tabs. 5, 10, 20mg
- Dose: 5mg b.d. p.o. (8.00am and 12 noon); increase every few days up to 30mg b.d. according to response

Dexamfetamine sulphate
- Tabs. 5mg
- Dose 5mg b.d. p.o. (8.00am and 12 noon); increase every few days up to 30mg b.d. according to response

Terminal restlessness/anguish (📖 see Chapter 13)

Spiritual distress (📖 see Chapter 9)

At the time of referral and transition to the palliative/terminal phase of an illness, many patients have an increased spiritual awareness. The concerns of these patients are often based on the existential questions:

- Who am I?
- What am I?
- Will I be remembered?
- How will I be remembered?

Patients experiencing emotional suffering often have 'Soul pain', but this may go unrecognized.

The integration of spiritual care into the palliative care team is therefore vital, to ensure that patients have the opportunity to disclose and discuss these concerns, which can cause great emotional distress. However, the spiritual needs are often not included in the assessment of quality of life of terminally ill patients, and may not be identified by health professionals.

Suicide

Depression is increased in patients with terminal cancer and the incidence of suicide and thoughts of self harm are increased in depressed patients. The incidence of suicide is therefore more common than previously believed.

Patients with cancer have twice the risk of committing suicide as the general population. Factors such as depression, advancing disease and hopelessness increase the risk of suicide. Other risk factors include actual suicidal thoughts, uncontrolled pain, exhaustion and fatigue, past suicidal attempts, substance abuse, recent bereavement, poor social support and family history of suicide. It is also thought that certain sites of cancer, i.e. oropharyngeal, lung, gastrointestinal, urogenital and breast, may increase the risk of suicide.

Patients with cancer tend to commit suicide by overdose of analgesia or sedative drugs. Many doctors believe that by inquiring about suicidal intent, they may precipitate a suicide. Contrary to this belief, talking and sharing his/her thoughts of self harm permits the patient to describe his/her feelings.

Suicidal ideation must not, however, be confused with patients who request death to be hastened—these patients may also be depressed, but may have other underlying fears e.g. of a painful or undignified death. 📖 see also the chapter on Euthanasia.

The initial assessment and evaluation of a patient with suicidal ideation should include the following:

1 Establish rapport and empathic approach
2 Assess the patient's understanding of illness and symptoms
3 Assess mental status
4 Assess other factors, e.g. poor pain control

5 Assess external support system
6 Establish prior psychiatric history
7 Obtain family history
8 Record past suicide attempts or threats
9 Assess suicide thinking and plans
10 Formulate treatment plan

Patients may require initial close supervision on a one to one basis. Careful attention should be paid to pain relief and relief of other distressing symptoms. It may be necessary to commence neuroleptic medication initially in addition to antidepressant medication. A psychiatric opinion should be obtained.

The patient's family and the palliative care team itself may require a lot of support.

Further reading

Books

Chochinov H. and Breitbart W. (eds) (2000) *Handbook of Psychiatry in Palliative Medicine*. Oxford: Oxford University Press.

Doyle D. H., Hanks G. W. C., Cherny N. (2004) *Oxford Textbook of Palliative Medicine*. 3rd edn. Oxford: Oxford University Press.

Kaye P. (1999) *Decision-making in Palliative Care*, pp. 34–5. Northampton: EPL Publications.

Kearney M. (2000) *A Place of Healing: Working with suffering in living and dying*. Oxford: Oxford University Press.

Lloyd-Williams M. (2003) *Psychosocial Issues in Palliative Care*. Oxford: Oxford University Press.

Articles

Ahronheim J., Morrison R., Baskin S., Morris J., Meier D. (1996) Treatment of the dying in the acute care hospital: Advanced dementia and metastatic cancer. *Archives of Internal Medicine*, **156**: 2094–100.

Breitbart W., Jacobsen P. B. (1996) Psychiatric symptom management in terminal care. *Clinics in Geriatric Medicine*, **12, 2**: 329–47.

Cox J., Holden J., Sagovsky R. (1987) Detection of postnatal depression: Development of the 10-item Edinburgh Postnatal Depression Scale. *British Journal of Psychiatry*, **150**: 782–6.

Folstein G. A., Folstein S. E., McHugh P. R. (1975) Mini Mental State. *Journal of Psychiatric Research*, 12: 189–98.

Kovach C., Weissman D., Griffie J., Matson S., Muchka S. (1999) Assessment and treatment of discomfort for people with late stage dementia. *Journal of Pain and Symptom Management*, **18**: 412–19.

Lloyd-Williams M., Friedman T., Rudd N. (1999) A survey of antidepressant prescribing in the terminally ill. *Palliative Medicine*, **13**: 243–8.

Lloyd-Williams M., Payne S. (2002) Can multidisciplinary guidelines improve the palliation of symptoms in the terminal phase of Dementia. *Int J of Palliative Nursing*, **8**: 370–5.

Index

Page numbers in *italics* indicate tables and figures.